Mental Disorders and Depression: A Clinical Guide to Diagnosis and Treatment

Mental Disorders and Depression: A Clinical Guide to Diagnosis and Treatment

Editor: Fernando Hogan

AMERICAN
MEDICAL PUBLISHERS
www.americanmedicalpublishers.com

AMERICAN
MEDICAL PUBLISHERS
www.americanmedicalpublishers.com

Cataloging-in-Publication Data

Mental disorders and depression : a clinical guide to diagnosis and treatment / edited by Fernando Hogan.
p. cm.
Includes bibliographical references and index.
ISBN 979-8-88740-260-4
1. Mental illness. 2. Depression, Mental. 3. Mental illness--Diagnosis. 4. Mental illness--Treatment.
5. Depression, Mental--Diagnosis. 6. Depression, Mental--Treatment. 7. Psychology, Pathological.
8. Psychiatry. I. Hogan, Fernando.
RC469 .M46 2023
616.890 75--dc23

American Medical Publishers,
41 Flatbush Avenue,
1st Floor, New York,
NY 11217, USA

ISBN 979-8-88740-260-4 (Hardback)

Contents

Preface

Mental disorders, also called mental illnesses, refer to conditions that affect the thinking, feeling, mood, and behavior of a person. Such disorders may affect a person occasionally or may be chronic. Such disorders can potentially impact a person's ability to perform their functions normally. There are various types of mental disorders such as anxiety disorders (panic disorder, obsessive-compulsive disorder, and phobias), depression, bipolar disorder, mood disorders, eating disorders, personality disorders, post-traumatic stress disorder (PTSD), and psychotic disorders. Depression is a serious mood disorder that that negatively affects how a person feels, thinks, and acts. There are multiple causes of mental disorders and depression such as genetics, family history, life experiences, stress, abusive past, traumatic brain injury (TBI), cancer, etc. Physical examination, laboratory tests, and psychological evaluation are used to diagnose mental disorders. The treatment of mental disorders and depression depends on the type of disorder and its severity. This book unravels the recent studies on mental disorders and depression. It will serve as a valuable source of reference for graduate and post graduate students.

All of the data presented henceforth, was collaborated in the wake of recent advancements in the field. The aim of this book is to present the diversified developments from across the globe in a comprehensible manner. The opinions expressed in each chapter belong solely to the contributing authors. Their interpretations of the topics are the integral part of this book, which I have carefully compiled for a better understanding of the readers.

At the end, I would like to thank all those who dedicated their time and efforts for the successful completion of this book. I also wish to convey my gratitude towards my friends and family who supported me at every step.

Editor

1

Rational Suicide in Late Life: A Systematic Review of the Literature

Carla Gramaglia [1,2,*], Raffaella Calati [3,4] and Patrizia Zeppegno [1,2]

1 Institute of Psychiatry, Università degli Studi del Piemonte Orientale, 28100 Novara, Italy; patrizia.zeppegno@med.uniupo.it
2 S.C. Psichiatria, Azienda Ospedaliero Universitaria Maggiore della Carità, 28100 Novara, Italy
3 Department of Psychology, University of Milano-Bicocca, 20126 Milan, Italy; raffaella.calati@gmail.com
4 Nîmes University Hospital, 30029 Nîmes, France
* Correspondence: carla.gramaglia@gmail.com;

Abstract: *Background and Objectives*: The complex concept of rational suicide, defined as a well-thought-out decision to die by an individual who is mentally competent, is even more controversial in the case of older adults. *Materials and Methods*: With the aim of better understanding the concept of rational suicide in older adults, we performed a systematic review of the literature, searching PubMed and Scopus databases and eventually including 23 published studies. *Results*: The main related topics emerging from the papers were: depression, self-determination, mental competence; physicians' and population's perspectives; approach to rational suicide; ageism; slippery slope. *Conclusions*: Despite contrasting positions and inconsistencies of the studies, the need to carefully investigate and address the expression of suicidal thoughts in older adults, as well as behaviours suggesting "silent" suicidal attitudes, clearly emerges, even in those situations where there is no diagnosable mental disorder. While premature conclusions about the "rationality" of patients' decision to die should be avoided, the possibility of rational suicide cannot be precluded.

Keywords: rational suicide; old age; late life; aging; ageism

---

1. Introduction

Suicide is a global phenomenon accounting for 800,000 deaths worldwide every year [1]. Considering the global aging trends in the world and that suicide rates increase with age, suicide in older adults cannot be neglected [2–4]. Older adults account for a disproportionately high number of suicide deaths because they are more successful at committing suicide compare to younger adults [5].

In older age there is a high risk of unrecognized and untreated psychiatric illnesses [6,7]. In particular, depression is the most common disorder and the most important risk factor associated with late life suicide [3,8–10]. However, most depressed older adults do not become suicidal. Furthermore, approximately 55% of late life suicides are associated with physical illness [3,4], and older people and those with chronic/terminal illness may not have psychiatric comorbidity. Physical illness is more likely to eventually lead to suicidal behaviour when it causes functional disabilities threatening the individual's independence, autonomy and dignity, quality of and pleasure with life, sense of meaning, usefulness and purpose in life, perceived personal value and self-esteem [11–13].

Aging may lead individuals to think back about their lives and to experience either feelings of integrity (if they feel their life has been meaningful) or despair (if they are unable to find meaning and achievement in their life) [14]. Moreover, notwithstanding what they have achieved in their life, older adults have to face changes, which are usually losses, in the context of several domains including health, employment, and relationships. Thus, the aging individual is compelled to go through grieving experiences and redefinitions of one's identity [13] which, if unsuccessful, lead to a damage of the individual's sense of self. The old age individual's skills in redefining their physical selves and integrating changes depends on their "historical" attribution of meaning to their body [13,15]. Amery defined aging as an incurable disease, where "the body becomes more and more mass and less and less energy. This mass ... is the new, enemy self", and "alien and authentically adverse self" which is opposed to the "self of the past"[16]: this sense of internal division between one's sick and healthy selves, with the first being perceived as "alien" by the latter, may lead the healthy self to wish the destruction of the sick one [13,15].

Furthermore, the current historical period is one marked by many new opportunities (including good hygienic conditions, availability of clean water, fresh food, quality public health, progress in medical knowledge and available treatments, starting from antibiotics) which have allowed a rapid increase of life expectancy and longevity, but also by the difficulties and ambiguities in facing what these opportunities have brought about. Life support technologies currently enable the prolongment of critically ill patients' life, often beyond a point where it can be experienced as meaningful and desirable [17]. Therefore, since living longer does not necessarily mean living a high-quality life, the need to balance benefits and harms of curative and, even more, palliative therapies, especially for painful, terminal illnesses, has opened new topics of legal, moral, and ethical concern.

In recent years, there has been much discussion (not only in the scientific community) about suicide and what has been named "rational suicide" in older adults. It is described as "rational" an action which is "sensible, appropriate, in keeping with one's fundamental interests, and perhaps even admirable"[18]. Rationality means being capable of deliberating, with no coercion, according to one's own values and purposes in life [19], and that motives and plans for a certain decision have been thoroughly explored, as well as alternative choices [20]. Therefore, rational suicide may be defined as a sane, well-thought-out and fairly stable decision by an individual who is mentally competent, and who is capable of reasoning and choosing the best alternative among the many available with no ambivalence (see Table 1 for the main definitions and criteria to define the construct of rational suicide).

Table 1. Definitions and criteria for rational suicide.

	Definition/Criteria of Rational Suicide
Siegel [21]	Realistic assessment of the situation on behalf of a person whose mental processes are not impaired by either psychological illness or severe emotional distress. The motivational basis for the decision could be understandable on behalf of uninvolved observers.
Cheung et al. [2]	Add further details about Siegel criterion (3): (1) The person understood the terminal nature of her/his condition. (2) The person consciously disengaged from treatment. (3) The person communicated the desire or made preparations to end her/his life. (4) A triggering event heightened a hopeless situation.
Werth & Cobia [22]	Presence of an unremitting hopeless condition (such as terminal illness, severe pain, both physical and psychological, deteriorating conditions, no longer acceptable quality of life, etc). The decision is a free choice. The decision results from a sound decision making process including the consultation with a mental health professional, and with objective and significant others; a non-impulsive assessment of alternatives, of the possible impact of the decision on significant others, and of the congruence of the decision with the individual's personal values.
Valente & Trainor [19]	Rational decisions reflect careful planning and consideration of adequate information (e.g., complete and accurate medical facts); preparations (e.g., wills, funeral arrangements); consideration of effect on others, treatment options and alternatives.
Motto [23]	A rational decision should be realistic (i.e., should be made after a realistic assessment of the individual's situation and after gaining full knowledge of options and consequences) and have minimal ambivalence (i.e., a decision should not be made on the basis of a transient desire and should not be inconsistent with the individual's longstanding and fundamental values).
Diekstra [24]	Enduring wish to die in a person with a condition of enduring unbearable physical and/or emotional pain, no hope for improvement. The person, who is not mentally disturbed, makes a free will decision which would not cause "unnecessary or preventable harm" to others.
Humphry [25]	"Considered decision" on behalf of a mature adult individual, after reasonable medical help has been sought and the treating physician has been informed. A will should be made and a note should be left. The suicide should not involve others criminally.
Weber [26]	Two meanings of right to die: - right to refuse life-sustaining treatment; - an "affirmative right to obtain death-a right to suicide".
Graber [27]	A reasonable appraisal of the situation reveals that one would be really better off dead.

The concept of rational suicide is controversial and difficult to define, so that some suicidologists and psychologists consider it as an oxymoron. The debate about this topic is even more complicated by emerging and complex to define concepts such as those of "good" or "gentle death", and of "silent suicide", defined as the intention to kill oneself by nonviolent means such as refusal of food and liquids or noncompliance with essential medical treatment. Such means of promoting one's death causes ambiguity in medical, clinical, personal, cultural, ethical, religious and historical interpretations [28]. Moreover, the concept of rational suicide is obviously linked to the debate about the hot topic of euthanasia, physician assisted death (PAD) and physician assisted suicide (PAS) (i.e., if suicide can be rational, then the right-to-die should be legal and regulated).

Given the ongoing debate about the possibility that a "rational suicide" exists, the concern represented by older adults' suicide and the world population aging trend, we performed a systematic review of the literature about rational suicide in late life, with the primary aim to offer an overview and better understanding of the concept of rational suicide in older adults through a description of the main related topics emerged from the literature.

2. Materials and Methods

We searched PubMed and Scopus databases from inception to April 16th and 19th 2019, respectively, with the following search keywords: rational AND suicid* AND (elderly OR older*). Two of the Authors (C.G., R.C.) reviewed and screened eligible articles according to the PRISMA (Preferred Reporting Items for Systematic Reviews and Meta-Analyses) flow diagram [29]. Any disagreement among reviewers was solved through discussion and with the supervision of the third Author (P.Z.). Studies were included if: (1) they focused on rational suicide defined according to one or more of the criteria mentioned in Table 1; (2) they focused on or included/mentioned older adults. To ensure the most complete reporting of the available literature about the topic, we decided to include all available study designs.

Studies were excluded if: (1) they were written in languages other than English; (2) their full-text was not available; (3) they were book chapters, commentaries and editorials/letters to the editor; (4) they were focused on euthanasia, PAD and PAS.

For each study, we extracted: year, design, sample features, used rating scales, reasons mentioned for rational suicide, rational suicide criteria and/or definition, main results, and conclusions.

3. Results

3.1. Main (Quantitative) Features of the Included Studies

The search retrieved 144 references; 24 full text articles were assessed for eligibility (see Figure 1 for the flow diagram); 1 full text article was not available for the assessment. We eventually included 23 published studies in the review.

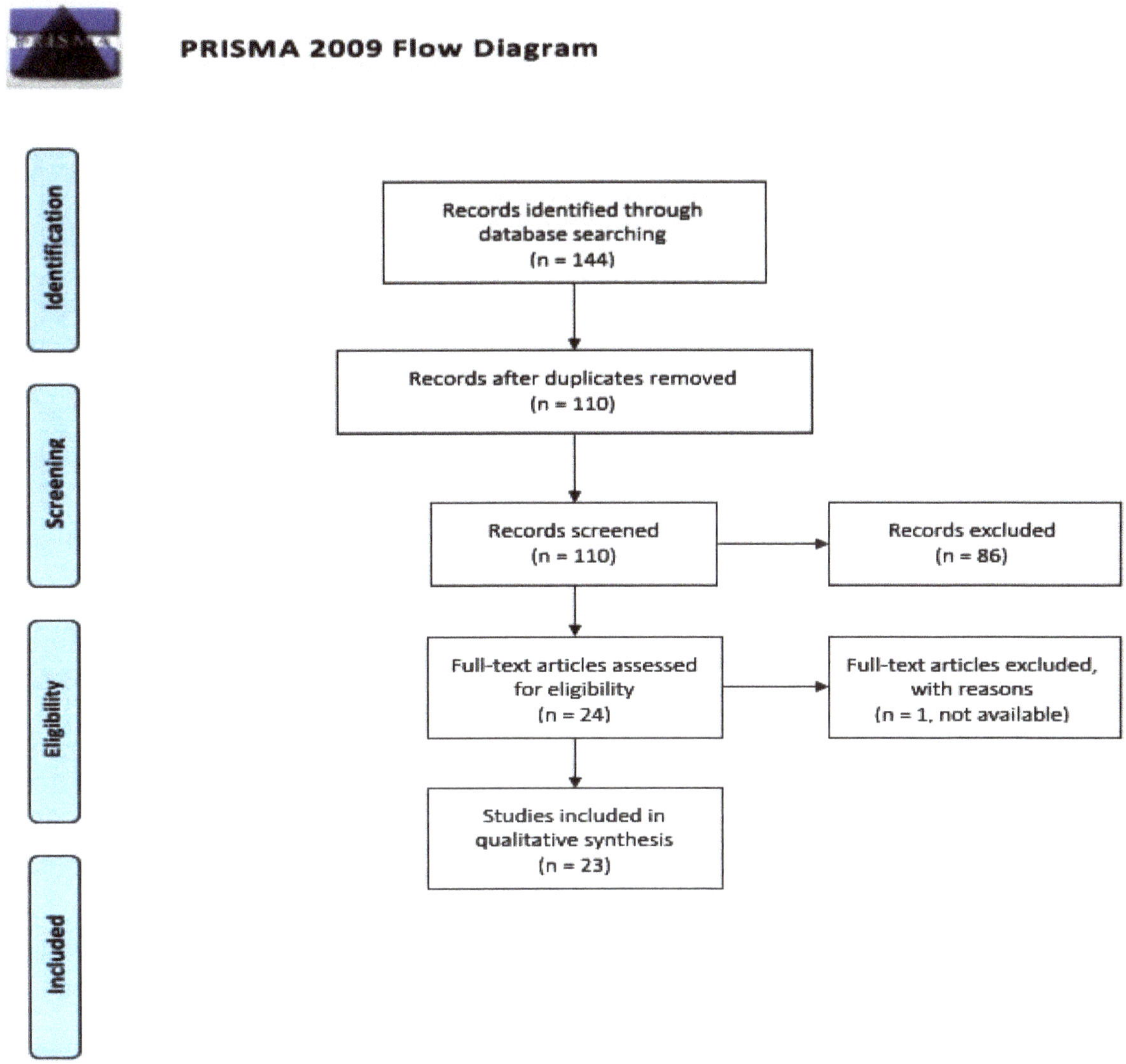

Figure 1. PRISMA 2009 Flow Diagram [29].

The data extracted for each of the studies are described in Table 2, where articles are presented in alphabetical order.

Table 2. Summary of the included articles in alphabetical order.

Empirical Studies Including Data						
Author, Year	**Perspective/Approach**	**Sample Features/Specialists**	**Rating Scales**	**Topics Covered/Reasons Mentioned for RS**	**RS Criteria and/or Definition**	**Main Results and Conclusions**
Cheung et al. 2017 [2]	Focus on the comparison between older people with and without terminal cancer who died by suicide, and analysis of motives for suicide. Hypothesis: in older people with terminal cancer, suicide can be considered a rational choice rather than the result of depression.	Source: Coroner records about suicides in ≥ 65-year-old 07/2007–12/2012, with available data about terminal cancer, N = 214, 74.3% males, 60.7% aged 65–79-year-old N = 23 (10.7%) terminal cancer.	n.a.	- Burden - Control (loss of) - Dependence - Dignity - Functional disability - Pain - Physical illness - Pleasure with life (loss of) - QoL - Sense of usefulness, purpose, value (loss of)	Siegel, 1986 [17] (3rd characteristic: a motivational basis that would be understandable to uninvolved observers) Werth & Cobia, 1995 [22]	- Older patients with terminal cancer who died by suicide were less likely than those without cancer to be depressed and to have had previous contact with mental health services. - 82.6% of terminal cancer cases had a motivational basis for suicide, understandable to uninvolved observers, due to physical (pain, functional disability) or psychological suffering. - Underdiagnosis of depression in patients with terminal cancer? - Choice to end one's life as a rational act to alleviate suffering?
Fortin et al. 2001 [30]	Focus on suicide prevention. Health care personnel (not mental health professionals) performing assessment.	N = 66 French-Caucasian older adults (age range between 69 and 96 y.o.) with no cognitive deficit, from 7 long-term facilities. N = 11 suicidal (N = 7 males). N = 55 non suicidal (N = 22 matched for age, gender, civil status).	PAQ GDS	- Control (loss of) - Decreased self-esteem - Helplessness - Hopelessness - Losses (physical, psychological, emotional, social, environmental) - Pain - QoL - Relationship problems - Satisfaction	Werth & Cobia (1995) [22], mentioned (but not used)	- No difference in self-determination between older adults with/without SI. - Differences on social subscale: SI have less consideration of own behaviour's impact on others and less satisfaction with relations with children and family relationships. - SI more depressed than non-SI. - Debate on RS warrants research on self-determination.

Table 2. *Cont.*

Empirical Studies Including Data						
Author, Year	**Perspective/Approach**	**Sample Features/Specialists**	**Rating Scales**	**Topics Covered/Reasons Mentioned for RS**	**RS Criteria and/or Definition**	**Main Results and Conclusions**
Gibbs et al. 2009 [31]	Focus on problem solving strategies, closely related to the topic of suicidality in old age.	N = 64 > 60-year-old MMSE >18 - N = 18 Depressed elderly with past SA. - N = 27 Depressed elderly never suicidal. - N = 19 Non-depressed elderly.	SPSI-R MMSE HAM-D BHS B-SIS SIS B-SLS CIRS-G	- Dependence - Loss - Physical illness	n.s.	- Depressed elderly SA perceived problem solving as dysfunctional and deficient compared to depressed non-attempters and non-depressed elderly: problems perceived more negatively and approached more impulsively and carelessly. This is in contrast with the common clinical view of late-life SA and those who die by suicide as being non-impulsive. - Both depressed groups compared to non-depressed elderly had lower rational and positive problem solving. - Depressed SA showed higher avoidant style than non-depressed elderly. - Lifetime diagnosis of SUD predicted lower total problem-solving score, higher negative problem orientation/impulsivity, and avoidance scores.
Uncapher and Arean 2000 [32]	To determine the influence of patients' age on primary care physician recognition of suicidal symptoms and the willingness to treat the suicidal patient.	N = 342 physicians (63% response rate), of whom N = 215 primary care physicians, asked to assess 2 vignettes of depressed suicidal patient, either geriatric, retired, age 78 y.o. (N = 100), or young, employed, 38 y.o. (N = 115).	21-item Suicidal Patient Treatment Scale	n.s.	n.s.	- Physicians recognized depression (99%) and suicidal risk (94%). - Physicians were less willing to treat the older patient, feeling that his SI was rational and normal. - Possible age bias?

Table 2. *Cont.*

Empirical Studies Including Data						
Author, Year	**Perspective/Approach**	**Sample Features/Specialists**	**Rating Scales**	**Topics Covered/Reasons Mentioned for RS**	**RS Criteria and/or Definition**	**Main Results and Conclusions**
Van Wijngaarden et al. 2016 [33]	Qualitative in-depth interview study aimed at a phenomenological characterization of the phenomenon "life is completed and no longer worth living".	N = 25, > 82 y.o., N = 11 males form the Netherlands, ideating on self-chosen death. Inclusion criteria: (1) considered their lives to be 'completed'; (2) suffered from the prospect of living on; (3) current wish to die; (4) 70 y.o. or older; (5) not terminally ill; (6) considered themselves to be mentally competent; (7) considered their death wish reasonable. N = 23 members of RTD organizations.	Interview HADS	- Burden - Control (loss of) - Dependence - Dignity (loss of) - Interpersonal theory of suicide: thwarted belongingness, perceived burdensomness - Loneliness - Meaning - Pain - QoL	n.s.	- Themes: detachment & attachment; rational & non-rational considerations; taking control & lingering uncertainty; resisting interference & longing for support; legitimacy & illegitimacy. - Rationality versus inner uncontrolled compulsion. - Ambiguities and ambivalence present after a putatively rational decision: need to develop careful policy and support for older people. - Results question the concept of rational suicide as an autonomous, free decision without pressure.
Winterrowd et al. 2017 [34]	To examine beliefs/opinions (most likely precipitants and protectors) and attitudes about older adults' suicide, in a cultural perspective.	N = 255 older adults (86% European American), 70.95 y.o. mean age, 38% males. N = 281 younger adults (81% European American), 19.04 y.o. mean age, 30% males.	Ad hoc attitudes Scale Personal Attribute Questionnaire-Short Form	n.s.	n.s.	- Precipitants: health problems, mostly in older adults; rational/courageous suicide, admissible (56.7%). - Most favourable attitude about older adult suicide: older adults, persons with more education, persons not identifying with a religion, persons with a history of suicidality. - Older adults suicide viewed as more admissible by males and with more sympathy by females. - Protectors: religiosity in older adults (21.1%); supportive relationships (37.9%) in younger adults. - Mental health care believed to play a preventative role by 6.7% respondents.

Table 2. *Cont.*

Case Studies Specifically Focused on Late Life Rational Suicide						
Author, Year	**Perspective/Approach**	**Sample Features/Specialists**	**Rating Scales**	**Topics Covered/Reasons Mentioned for RS**	**RS Criteria and/or Definition**	**Main Results and Conclusions**
Balasubramaniam 2018 [13]	Case presentation: 72 y.o. male, retired, widowed, with adenocarcinoma.	Geriatricians Psychogeriatricians	MCAS (used) DDRS and SATHD (mentioned)	Ageism Control (loss of) Dependence Frailty Gerontophobia Loss QoL Sense of identity/Sense of self (loss of)	n.s.	- Geriatricians increasingly encounter older adults expressing the desire to end their lives, who may have medical illnesses (not necessarily terminal ones), but no diagnosable mental illness. - Is the absence of a diagnostic category to describe a mental state in which suicide appears like the best option a flaw in nosology? - Is RS a rational entity that will be increasingly encountered as views about health, choice, and control continue to evolve?
Lerner 1995 [35]	Case Story of a Couple and Review of Humphry's Book Final Exit.	n.s.	n.a.	Autonomy (loss of) Terminal illness Terminal old age	n.s.	- Ageism and slippery slope. - Ambiguities surrounding elder suicide. - Need to approach elder suicide in the context of individual life experiences.
Simon 1989 [7]	Clinical/legal issues of silent S + 2 cases (clinical) + case law examples.	Clinicians	n.a.	Autonomy (loss of) Factors including psychological, social, ethical, cultural, economic and situational Losses Medical complaints	n.s.	- Silent S: by non-violent means as self-starvation or non-compliance with essential medical treatments. - Frequently unrecognized because of underdiagnosed depression and/or interjection of personal belief systems of healthcare providers and/or family members. - Cognitive and affective aspects of decision making. - Mental competency impaired (de jure or de facto) by depression: "Premature conclusions that the patient has made a 'rational' decision to die must be avoided"; anyway, "certainly every elderly patient who is depressed is not incompetent". - Treatment: ECT, antidepressants, psychotherapy.

Table 2. *Cont.*

				Case Studies Specifically Focused on Late Life Rational Suicide		
Author, Year	**Perspective/Approach**	**Sample Features/Specialists**	**Rating Scales**	**Topics Covered/Reasons Mentioned for RS**	**RS Criteria and/or Definition**	**Main Results and Conclusions**
Wand et al. 2016 [36]	2 cases discussed in the light of the importance of a narrative and bio-psycho-social approach to the management of the wish to die.	Psychiatrists Psychogeriatricians	MCAT	Autonomy (loss of) Burden Control (loss of) Coping strategies Dependence Disability External support Helplessness Hopelessness Loss of purpose/meaning/role in life QoL Scared of institutional care Tiredness of living	Battin 1984 [37] Conwell & Caine, 1991 [38]	- Open question about the possible differences between people expressing a wish to die and SA. Does a continuum exist, from wish to die, to SA, to S? - Rationality is probably dimensional rather than dichotomous (Conwell & Caine, 1991). - Requests for euthanasia may occur in older people in the absence of a significant mood disorder. - Ageism and medical paternalism. - Relevant topics: Narrative formulation: Crafting an advance care directive; Exploration of spiritual issues; empathic ongoing care/support; Support both for patients and families; Social interventions.
				Case Studies Not Specifically Focused on Late Life Rational Suicide (But Mentioning It in the Text)		
Author, Year	**Perspective/Approach**	**Sample Features/ Specialists**	**Rating Scales**	**Topics Covered/Reasons Mentioned for RS**	**RS Criteria and/or Definition**	**Main Results and Conclusions**
Fontana 2002 [39]	Historical and philosophical perspective + case description. RTD, PAS, euthanasia mentioned; Hemlock society mentioned.	Nurses	n.a.	Autonomy (loss of) Control (loss of) Dignity Loss of meaning/purpose in life Pain QoL Self-determination	Siegel, 1986 [17] Werth, 1995 [22]	- Good death as a right. - Problem of having no position and no guiding principle from AMA and ANA. - Implications for the meaning of care (in nursing).
Karlinsky et al. 1988 [40]	Psychological, ethical, legal issues + 2 cases, one advanced age, one terminal illness; euthanasia mentioned; Hemlock Society mentioned.	n.s.	n.a.	Competency Control (loss of) Dependence Disability, physical Mental state/psychiatric illness QoL	n.s.	- Contradictions between the principles of patients' autonomy and physicians' responsibility. - Living will.

Table 2. *Cont.*

				Case Studies Not Specifically Focused on Late Life Rational Suicide (But Mentioning It in the Text)		
Author, Year	**Perspective/Approach**	**Sample Features/ Specialists**	**Rating Scales**	**Topics Covered/Reasons Mentioned for RS**	**RS Criteria and/or Definition**	**Main Results and Conclusions**
Rich 2004 [28]	Historical, ethical + case description of chronic AIDS; PAS, euthanasia mentioned; Hemlock Society mentioned; VSED and terminal sedation mentioned.	Nurses	n.a.	Escape from life Terminal illness Disability, permanent Autonomy (loss of) Pain	Siegel, 1986 [17] Werth, 1999 [41] Werth & Cobia, 1995 [22]	- Ethics of care: "principles alone do not provide a comprehensive basis for the most important ethical decisions". - Slippery slope. - Autonomy versus beneficence principles. - Meaning of a caring relationship (exploration of feelings – including caregivers'; meaningful communication; thoughtful decision making). - Lack of guidelines from AMA and ANA.
				Opinion Studies Specifically Focused on Late Life Rational Suicide		
Author, Year	**Perspective/Approach**	**Sample Features/ Specialists**	**Rating Scales**	**Topics Covered/Reasons Mentioned for RS**	**RS Criteria and/or Definition**	**Main Results and Conclusions**
Conwell & Caine 1991 [38]	Critical position	Psychiatrists Psychogeriatricians Researchers Consultants	n.a.	Ageism Burden Physical illness QoL	n.s.	- Poor attention paid to the effects of psychiatric illness on rational decision making in the context of the debate on RS. - Personal biases possibly affecting the determination of a suicidal person's "rationality": about aging, old age, psychological effects of chronic disease. - Suicide in the absence of treatable affective illness is uncommon; critical depressive illness precludes rational decision making. - Differential diagnosis: depressed mood versus sadness developing as a natural response to serious illness. - Peculiar presentation of major depressive illness in old age, reduced use of mental health services on behalf of elderly.

Table 2. *Cont.*

Author, Year	Perspective/Approach	Sample Features/ Specialists	Rating Scales	Topics Covered/Reasons Mentioned for RS	RS Criteria and/or Definition	Main Results and Conclusions
				Opinion Studies Specifically Focused on Late Life Rational Suicide		
Gallagher-Thompson &Osgood 1997 [42]	Overview of epidemiology of late life S, demographics and risk factors, assessment, RS.	Healthcare professionals	BHS MSSI BDI GDS SCID	Autonomy (loss of) Control (loss of) Dignity (loss of) Disability Hopelessness Loss of meaning in life Losses Pain Poor self-esteem QoL Terminal illness	Diekstra, 1986 [24] Motto, 1972 [23] Battin, 1991 [43] Humphry, 1992 [25] Werth & Cobia, 1995 [22]	- Risk factors for old age S: > 60 y.o., Caucasian, divorced/widowed, no longer employed, poor health, depressed or not, alcohol, access to gun, reduced self-esteem, history of mental illness, history of S, poor relationships. - Arguments in favour: philosophy, autonomy, meaning in life. - Proposed interventions to reduce SI and increase QoL: medication, ECT, support groups.
Humphry 1992 [25]	Position of the leader of the National Hemlock Society, mentioning euthanasia and PAS + case narrative.	n.s.	n.a.	Choice (loss of) Control (loss of) "Living death"Pain/suffering, both physical and emotional Terminal illness	n.s.	- "Suicide and assisted suicide carried out in the face of terminal illness causing unbearable suffering should be ethically and legally acceptable". - Slippery slope.
Moore 1993 [44]	Historical perspective and discussion of supportive and opposing arguments; implications for nursing. "Old age in our society needs to be viewed once again as a valued status, rather than a cursed disease or a burden".	Nurses Psychologists	n.a.	Burden Control (loss of) Lack of satisfying role Meaning (loss of)	Weber, 1988b [26] Graber, 1981[27]	- Supportive: right to self-determination; evil of needless suffering; Battin's 17 considerations for assessment. - Opposing: ageism; slippery slope. - Having no alternative but suicide raises doubts about the rationality of older adults' decision. - Individual life histories, not aging, are critical for the understanding of suicide in later years.
Prado 2015 [45]	Philosophical and bioethical perspective; discussion of the author's position.	n.s.	n.a.	Conditions diminishing the individual as a person, irremediable Dependence Hopeless medical situations Irreversible deterioration Pain	n.s.	- "Life is not itself an unconditional good", and sheer organic survival is not an absolute value. - "Whatever the condition of our bodies, once our minds deteriorate beyond a certain point, we cease to exist as the person we are". - Proposed objections to S/SA: moral, religious, cultural, social, legal.

Table 2. *Cont.*

				Opinion Studies Specifically Focused on Late Life Rational Suicide		
Author, Year	**Perspective/Approach**	**Sample Features/ Specialists**	**Rating Scales**	**Topics Covered/Reasons Mentioned for RS**	**RS Criteria and/or Definition**	**Main Results and Conclusions**
Richards 2016 [46]	Empirical/theoretical overview to synthesize knowledge, including existential questions about the perception of complete life or tiredness of life.	n.s.	n.a.	Burden Control (loss of) Dependence Disability, functional Illness, chronic Loneliness Loss of meaning/purpose in life Losses Pain, suffering Personality and coping strategies Psychological issues (depression, cognitive decline) QoL Social isolation Tiredness of life	Werth, 1999 [41] Battin, 1991 [43] McCue & Balasubramaniam, 2017 [47]	- Not all SI or planning for S should be unquestioningly pathologized. - Decision making is not a purely cognitive process. - Not all motivating factors for old age RS are open to be remedied. - Importance of end of life care context in which older people find themselves.
Ruckenbauer et al. 2007 [48]	Critical revision of RS. Tension between medical care for patients and patients' autonomy.	Physicians	n.a.	Burden Conflict Illness Loss Pain Traditional family structures falling apart	n.s.	- Suicide as symptom of individually and/or socially conditioned lack of freedom, rather than of sovereign self-determination. - Underestimation of depression and suicidal potential in old age. - Cult of youthfulness versus old age, associated with weakness, deficiency, increased health costs.

Table 2. *Cont.*

				Opinion studies not Specifically Focused on Late Life Rational Suicide (but Mentioning it in the Text)		
Author, Year	**Perspective/Approach**	**Sample Features/Specialists**	**Rating Scales**	**Topics Covered/Reasons Mentioned for RS**	**RS Criteria and/or Definition**	**Main Results and Conclusions**
Battin 1991 [43]	S not interpreted as evidence of depression or mental illness; meaning and motivation.	Mental health professionals	n.a.	Terminal illness Disability, severe and permanent Advanced old age	Motto, 1972 (mentioned) [23]	- Presentation and discussion of 17 reasons which should be explored to understand whether S would be rational or not. - "[…] respectful and humane way" to approach "persons who, in a society now beginning to consider S as a rational and even responsible way of avoiding the degradations of terminal illness, severe permanent disability, or extreme old age, wish to explore this option with a trained and insightful professional".
Clark 1992 [49]	Overview of S and terminal illness, PAS, RTD and euthanasia mentioned; Hemlock Society mentioned. Critical position versus the "understandable reasons" for contemplating S.	Mental health professionals General internists Family physicians	n.a.	Dependence Deteriorating health Disability Helplessness Hopelessness Isolation Loneliness Outliving family members Pain Poverty Severe illness	n.s.	- The so called "understandable reasons" for S rarely stand alone, with no coexisting psychiatric illness, as causes of suicidal thinking. - Almost all persons who die by S evidence symptoms of major psychiatric illness. - Features of depressive illness often overlooked. - Possibility of RS not precluded, but there is likely a strong cultural bias to overlook the "forces and motives implicated in cases of S by older persons". - The question of mental competence to opt for S.

Table 2. *Cont.*

				Opinion studies not Specifically Focused on Late Life Rational Suicide (but Mentioning it in the Text)		
Author, Year	**Perspective/Approach**	**Sample Features/Specialists**	**Rating Scales**	**Topics Covered/Reasons Mentioned for RS**	**RS Criteria and/or Definition**	**Main Results and Conclusions**
Siegel 1982 [21]	Evolving societal values concerning death and S, RTD, RTS; Hemlock Society mentioned.	Clinicians	n.a.	QoL Pain Loss of meaning in life Lack of support Self-determination Control (loss of)	Hoche's "Balance sheet suicide"	- Living will. - Conflictual and ambivalent nature of SA. - Intervention appropriate if (1) the individual is not completely resolved in the decision to die (conflict, ambivalence); (2) the individual does not seem to be realistically appraising his/her problems or prospects for the future.

Legend: AMA: American Medical Association; ANA: American Nursing Association; BDI: Beck Depression Inventory; BHS: Beck Hopelessness Scale; B-SIS: Beck Scale for Suicidal Ideation; B-SLS: Beck Suicide Lethality Scale; CIRS-G: Cumulative Illness Rating Scale adapted for Geriatrics; DDRS: Desire for Death Rating Scale; GDS: Geriatric Depression Scale; HADS: Hospital Anxiety and Depression Scale; HAM-D: Hamilton Depression Rating Scale; MCAS: Montreal Cognitive Assessment Scale; MCAT: Montreal Cognitive Assessment Test; MMSE: Mini-Mental State Examination; MSSI: Modified Scale for Suicidal Ideation; n.a.: not applicable; n.s.: not specified; PAQ: Psychological Autonomy Questionnaire; PAS: Physician Assisted Suicide; QoL: Quality of Life; RS: Rational Suicide; RTD: Right to Die; RTS: Right to Suicide; S: suicide; SA: suicide attempt/suicide attempters; SATHD: Schedule of Attitudes Towards Hastened Death; SCID: Structured Clinical Interview for DSM; SI: suicidal ideation/individuals with suicidal ideation; SIS: Suicide Intent Scale; SPSI-R: Social Problem Solving Inventory-Revised – Short Version; SUD: Substance Use Disorder; VSED: voluntary stopping of eating and drinking; y.o.: years old.

Among the included articles, 6 were original papers [2,30–34], with different designs and aims: 1 was based on coroner records of suicides in older people with and without terminal cancer, and investigated motives for rational suicide [2]; 2 assessed suicidal and non-suicidal older adults, one with a specific focus on self-determination [30] and one on problem solving strategies [31]; 1 surveyed primary care physicians and the impact of patients' age on their ability in recognizing suicidal symptoms and willingness to treat patients [32]; 1 used qualitative in-depth interviews to assess older adults ideating on self-chosen death [33]; 1 examined older and younger adults' beliefs and attitudes about late life suicide [37].

Of these six articles, 2 referred to specific criteria or definitions for rational suicide [2,30], and only one out of these two actually used them [2]; in both cases Werth & Cobia's criteria were mentioned, and Cheung also mentioned Siegel's criteria; 1 did not mention rating scales [2].

Four out of the six studies explored and mentioned several reasons for rational suicide [2,30,31,33], with the concept of loss being explicitly or implicitly referred to in all these 4 studies. The following topics were mentioned: control, dependence, disability/illness, pain, quality of life (QoL) (3 studies); burden, dignity, loss of pleasure/meaning in life (2 studies) (see Table 2 for more details).

Eleven of the studies described in Table 2 did not include research data, but were specifically focused on old age rational suicide [7,13,25,35,36,38,42,44–46,48]: 5 included case(s) descriptions [7,13,25,35,36]; 7 specified the professionals involved in end of life and rational suicide issues.

Criteria for rational suicide and rating scales were mentioned respectively by 3 [13,36,42] and 4 [36,42,44,46] of these studies. Battin's and Werth/Werth & Cobia were the most frequently reported criteria for rational suicide. Regarding motives for rational suicide, the most frequently mentioned ones were: loss, including loss of meaning and purpose (9 studies); burden (5 studies); control (5 studies); pain (5 studies); QoL (5 studies); autonomy (4 studies); dependence (4 studies) (see Table 2 for more details).

The concepts of ageism and slippery slope effect were discussed by 2 [13,38] and 3 [25,35,44] studies, respectively.

Last, 6 papers were not specifically focused on late life rational suicide but mentioned it [21,28,39,40,43,49]; 3 included case(s) descriptions; all but one[40] specified the professionals involved in end of life issues. Four of these six studies [21,28,39,43] mentioned criteria for the definition of rational suicide: Motto's [23]; Siegel's [21] and Werth's [41]; Werth & Cobia's [22]; Hoche's "Balance sheet suicide"[21]. Among the reasons for rational suicide, loss (including loss of meaning) was implicitly or explicitly mentioned by all papers; other reasons included: pain (4 studies), disability (4 studies), control (3 studies), QoL (3 studies), dependence (2 studies), autonomy (1 study) (see Table 2 for more details).

All but one of these six papers [43] mentioned the Hemlock Society and either euthanasia, PAD, PAS, right to die; 2 [21,40] mentioned the Living Will.

3.2. Main Topics Covered in the Included Studies

The main topics emerged from the papers included in the review were: depression, self-determination, mental competence; physicians' and population's perspectives; approach to rational suicide; ageism; slippery slope.

Furthermore, Table 3 briefly summarizes arguments in favour versus arguments opposing rational suicide emerging from the included studies.

Table 3. Arguments in favour and opposing rational suicide.

Arguments in Favour of Rational Suicide	Arguments Opposing Rational Suicide
Moral right to self-determination [33]	Should death wishes, and ideation and action aimed at deliberately ending one's life ever be considered as "rational"?
Needless suffering [33]	Ageism: old age individuals as a burden; death as a solution for insoluble age-related suffering [12].
Exerting control over one's death: satisfaction and empowerment.	Slippery slope: from right to die to social obligation to die [9].
Suicidal ideation and behaviour may be the logical and understandable outcome of a balance sheet where death becomes preferable to life [33].	Is suicide *per se* an evidence of mental instability? [33] Having suicidal ideation is often the very reason why an individual is classified as having a mental illness.
Suicide can be a serious and legitimate answer to the individual's existential situation, which should not be dismissed as a depressive symptom [20]. A history of mood disorder (as well as of any other mental illness) does not mean that the individual's decision-making capacity is impaired and should be questioned forever [50,51].	Suicide itself is an emotional condition precluding the possibility of rationality: the suicidal individual is usually not capable to consider other option than suicide to a condition of perceived intolerable misery. One would rather live, if a better solution than suicide was at hand [22,52–55].

3.3. Depression, Self-Determination, and Mental Competence

Though in different ways and from different perspectives, almost all the included articles underscored ambiguities and possible biases regarding old age rational suicide. The point which is most discussed is the possible underestimation of depression in old age patients, either terminally ill or not, and its impact on patients' self-determination and mental competence. Actually, the current nosology includes suicidal ideation and attempts as symptoms of either major depressive episodes and of borderline personality disorder. Thus, the main emerging and unresolved question is whether suicidal ideation and attempt in late life should be always treated as symptoms of a psychiatric disorder or not.

The results about depression in suicidal older adults in the studies we assessed are mixed; while [2] found that among older patients who died by suicide, those with terminal cancer were less likely than those without to be depressed and to have had previous contact with mental health services [30] reported a greater likelihood of depression in elderly with suicidal ideation than in those with no such ideation. These two studies pointed to the question whether or not underdiagnosis of depression is an issue in older patients' suicide, and to the importance of assessing self-determination in the context of the rational suicide debate, respectively.

Consistent with the debate about decisions relying both on judgments and affective states [50], poorer problem-solving skills were found in depressed elderly suicide attempters, compared to depressed non-attempters and non-depressed elderly, in contrast with the commonplace belief that suicide attempt in late life would be non-impulsive [31]. Moreover, considering ambivalence, ambiguities and the contrast between rationality and inner uncontrolled compulsion in elderly ideating on self-chosen death, Van Wijngaarden et al. [33] indings seemed to question the concept of rational suicide as an autonomous, free decision without pressure.

Briefly, what emerges from the studies we assessed is that underdiagnosis of depression in old age and especially in terminal illness is a relevant problem [56–58] ecause it can be difficult to differentiate depressive disorders from old age-related cognitive impairment and from the normal emotional responses of a person coping with a terminal illness [59,60]. On the other hand, not all suicidal individuals are depressed and mental illness per se does not imply that the individual's self-determination and competency are compromised. So, even though a careful assessment of every single situation is mandatory, not every suicidal ideation and/or planning should be "unquestioningly" pathologized. Last, an approach focused on the concept of "understandability" of suicidal ideation and/or behaviour has been suggested as potentially more meaningful and useful than that of rationality, because an approach based on rationality might lead to overlooking the expressive and emotional meaning of the wish to die [52].

3.4. *Views of Rational Suicide: Physicians' and Population's Perspectives*

Two of the original studies assessed focused on views about rational suicide, on behalf of physicians [32] and of older and younger adults [34].

The first study found that primary care physicians' skills in recognizing depression and suicidal risk in late life were excellent, nonetheless physicians were less willing to treat older patients, likely due to an age bias leading them to consider suicide intent as rational and normal in that age group [32].

In the general population, a more favorable attitude towards late life suicide was found on behalf of older adults compared to younger adults. When asked about possible protective factors for late life suicide, interestingly, only a small percentage of respondents believed that mental health care could play a preventive role [34]. It is not clear whether this last result reflects mistrust in the possibility of suicidal individual to receive help, or rather the general population's actual belief that late life suicide is not a clinical issue. Mankind's history has witnessed changing views about death and suicide, which in clinical contexts have both turned out to be something which should be always prevented, fought and avoided; this is linked to the topic of the principles of autonomy versus beneficence, and of patients' autonomy and physicians' responsibility [28,40]. Conflicts inevitably surround the approach to rational suicide also from this standpoint, starting from the ethical principle guiding healthcare professionals, who should respect patients' autonomy as well as safeguarding their lives. On the other hand, the need of a reflection on the meaning and ethics of care in late life and end of life in the current society has been suggested [28,39].

3.5. *Approach to Rational Suicide*

A careful assessment of patients, a thorough and accurate investigation of the meaning of their attitudes towards end of life, and the development of appropriate supportive strategies to face the new emerging needs in the care of old age patients are described by most of the included papers.

It is clearly underscored that each situation and the actual meaning of the wish to die should be evaluated in the context of individual life experience and histories, which are critical elements for the understanding of rational suicide [2,35,44].

The position described by most of the articles reviewed is an "interlocutory" one, encouraging a thorough exploration of reasons for suicide in the context of a "respectful and humane" relationship between patient and "a trained and insightful professional" [43], based on the belief that most elderly persons "readily discuss their suicidal feelings and intentions and are glad to be able to share their thoughts with someone who cares enough to ask"[61]. Exploration of reasons and meaning of suicidal ideation and/or attempt is particularly important when it clearly emerges a conflictual and ambivalent nature of the decision to die, and when the individual is not realistically appraising her/his problems and prospects [21].

The approach to rational suicide should go beyond the mere assessment of the presence of a mood disorder, and address the whole range of issues possibly contributing to the individual's wish to die, in order to offer possible targets for interventions, and allow the implementation of approaches aimed at increasing QoL or decreasing pain, distress and suffering, which may eventually lead to a reduction of suicidal ideation [30,42,46,62,63].

3.6. *Ageism*

Albeit sometimes used inappropriately in the existing literature, the term "ageism" means a prejudice, stereotyped assumption, or discrimination made on the grounds of a person's age, possibly leading to unfair treatment of older ones. From a clinical standpoint, an ageist attitude may lead clinicians to consider older adults' suicides as rational choices (especially if the person has physical illnesses) and affect clinicians' ability to identify psychopathology [54]. For instance, depression may seem understandable in the context of an older person's health and living circumstances, but considering suicidal ideation and wishes to die as understandable just because of the person's old age is an ageist attitude which should be avoided. Nonetheless, some studies [32] have pointed out that while clinicians' skills in identifying suicidal behaviour in older adults seem to be preserved, what may be lacking is their willingness to treat patients in this age group, especially if the potential reversibility of their condition is underestimated. This attitude too may reflect ageism and therapeutic nihilism. On the other hand, the implementation of coercive life-prolonging measures with a poor consideration of the individual's autonomy is another potential form of ageism hidden behind medical paternalism [36].

Trying to find a balance between patients' autonomy and clinicians' responsibility, therapeutic nihilism and medical paternalism is necessary to face a phenomenon, which may be associated with increased longevity.

3.7. Slippery Slope

Several authors have expressed concern that recognizing the right to die would too easily shift to "a climate enforcing a social, obligatory duty to die", and novelists have well described this risk in science fiction stories such us Richard Matheson's The Test (1958).

Indeed, several of the selected papers mentioned the "slippery slope" argument, which is also debated in the end-of-life/euthanasia/PAS/PAD context and which refers to the possibility that acknowledging the right to die would eventually shift towards an obligation to die and/or lead older persons to feel guilty if they had no wish to end their life and decided not to commit suicide [21].

However, it has to be underscored that, in the context of the euthanasia debate, no consensus has yet been reached about the presence of the slippery slope effect [64,65].

4. Discussion

The aim of this review was to offer an overview and a better understanding of the concept of rational suicide in older adults.

Opinions are not consistent about whether older adults' wish to hasten death in the absence of a psychiatric disorder could be regarded as a rational choice. Suicide presenting in the absence of a clinically diagnosable depression (or of other conditions impairing mental function) and occurring in cases of adverse conditions such as physical illness and aging has been considered "rational" from the perspective of respect for individual autonomy, and the rational assessment of utility [52]. Suicide in these situations may be seen as a possibility to regain and exert control and autonomy in the face of a miserable existential condition marked by pain and suffering, before the progressive worsening of one's physical condition, thus finding an escape from a life which is no longer considered as such or worth living.

Even though Authors do not agree on the role of mental disorders in "rational suicide", usually those who adhere to the conventional psychiatric opinion think that mental disorders are preeminent with regard to suicidal ideation and that suicide is a manifestation of psychiatric illness, hence they do not consider suicide as a rational option [40,54]. The possibility to disentangle depression and suicidal ideation in old-age suicidal individuals would allow the identification of potential targets for ad hoc interventions, going beyond those specifically directed towards the treatment of depression. For instance, there might still be chances, even for terminally ill and/or disabled older adults, to find relief from their pain and suffering, which could eventually lead to a decrease in suicidal ideation and suicide risk [19]. Furthermore, the perspective considering suicide as a symptom of psychiatric illness overlooks the possibility that there may be circumstances in which suicide or the refusal of life-sustaining medical treatment may result from the rational decisions of autonomous individuals, and may lead to interventions aimed at preserving life which can sometimes be applied at the expense of individual autonomy[40].

Although life expectancy for those living in western societies is higher than ever before in human history, this has had the effect of making it difficult for medical professionals to find a balance between patients' autonomy and clinicians' responsibility, to admit when someone is dying and to know where to draw the line in terms of offering more treatment [66,67]. The improvement of late life palliative care and QoL should be possibly accompanied by changes in the medical organization and culture to better address the specific end of life related needs in old age.

Some valuable suggestions to face the problem of rational suicide emerge from the studies we assessed; for instance, Richman, quoted by Moore [44] underscored the primary importance, when meeting a suicidal individual, "to make contact rather than obsess over whether they have a right to live or die". The importance of an interlocutory and reflective attitude is described by Ruckenbauer and coworkers [48], who state that while suicidal individuals cannot be deprived of their autonomy, nonetheless they should not be fully and without protection be released into their autonomy. Moreover, they underscore that patients cannot be reduced to their medical or psychiatric illness, but at the same time, an overestimation of existential stock-taking should be avoided.

It should be underscored that a limitation of this work is that, since the available literature was very uneven and, despite the selection criteria, mainly based on opinions and theoretical papers, the reported quantitative synthesis is limited. Furthermore, we cannot exclude that the choice of not including editorials and book chapters in the current review might have limited the access to potentially relevant material. Further original research studies may help to better understand this complex topic.

5. Conclusions

In conclusion, despite contrasting positions and inconsistencies of the studies described in this review, what seems to emerge is that the expression of suicidal thoughts in older adults, as well as behaviours suggesting "silent" or indirect suicidal attitudes [68,69], should be carefully investigated and addressed, even in the absence of a diagnosable mental disorder. Clinicians should try to decode the possible communicative role of suicidal behaviour while avoiding premature conclusions about the "rationality" of patients' decision to die, and considering it by default as "reasoned behavioural expression of legitimate preference for an earlier death" [7,46,49,70]. Nonetheless, the possibility of rational suicide cannot be precluded.

Author Contributions: Each author made substantial contributions to the conception and design of the work; C.G. and R.C. searched the literature and read the papers, under the supervision of P.Z.; C.G. and R.C. drafted the paper and P.Z. revised it; AND each author has approved the submitted version; AND agrees to be personally accountable for the author's own contributions and for ensuring that questions related to the accuracy or integrity of any part of the work, even ones in which the author was not personally involved, are appropriately investigated, resolved, and documented in the literature.

References

1. WHO. Suicide in the Western Pacific. Available online: https://www.who.int/westernpacific/health-topics/suicide (accessed on 16 August 2019).
2. Cheung, G.; Douwes, G.; Sundram, F. Late-Life Suicide in Terminal Cancer: A Rational Act or Underdiagnosed Depression? *J. Pain Symptom Manag.* **2017**, *54*, 835–842. [CrossRef] [PubMed]
3. Conwell, Y.; Thompson, C. Suicidal behavior in elders. *Psychiatr. Clin. N. Am.* **2008**, *31*, 333–356. [CrossRef] [PubMed]
4. Zeppegno, P.; Manzetti, E.; Valsesia, R.; Siliquini, R.; Ammirata, G.; De Donatis, O.; Usai, C.; Torre, E. Differences in suicide behaviour in the elderly: A study in two provinces of Northern Italy. *Int. J. Geriatr. Psychiatry* **2005**, *20*, 769–775. [CrossRef]

5. Institute of Medicine (US) Committee on Pathophysiology and Prevention of Adolescent and Adult Suicide. *Reducing Suicide: A National Imperative*; Goldsmith, S.K., Pellmar, T.C., Kleinman, A.M., Bunney, W.E., Eds.; National Academies Press (US): Washington, DC, USA, 2002. Available online: http://www.ncbi.nlm.nih.gov/books/NBK220939/ (accessed on 16 August 2019).
6. Zeppegno, P.; Gramaglia, C.; di Marco, S.; Guerriero, C.; Consol, C.; Loreti, L.; Martelli, M.; Marangon, D.; Carli, V.; Sarchiapone, M. Intimate Partner Homicide Suicide: A Mini-Review of the Literature (2012–2018). *Curr. Psychiatry Rep.* **2019**, *21*, 13. [CrossRef] [PubMed]
7. Simon, R.I. Silent suicide in the elderly. *Bull. Am. Acad. Psychiatry Law* **1989**, *17*, 83–95.
8. Conwell, Y.; Duberstein, P.R.; Cox, C.; Herrmann, J.H.; Forbes, N.T.; Caine, E.D. Relationships of age and axis I diagnoses in victims of completed suicide: A psychological autopsy study. *Am. J. Psychiatry* **1996**, *153*, 1001–1008.
9. Turvey, C.L.; Conwell, Y.; Jones, M.P.; Phillips, C.; Simonsick, E.; Pearson, J.L.; Wallace, R. Risk factors for late-life suicide: A prospective, community-based study. *Am. J. Geriatr. Psychiatry* **2002**, *10*, 398–406. [CrossRef] [PubMed]
10. Sokero, T.P.; Melartin, T.K.; Rytsälä, H.J.; Leskelä, U.S.; Lestelä-Mielonen, P.S.; Isometsä, E.T. Suicidal ideation and attempts among psychiatric patients with major depressive disorder. *J. Clin. Psychiatry* **2003**, *64*, 1094–1100. [CrossRef] [PubMed]
11. Fässberg, M.M.; Cheung, G.; Canetto, S.S.; Erlangsen, A.; Lapierre, S.; Lindner, R.; Draper, B.; Gallo, J.J.; Wong, C.; Wu, J.; et al. A systematic review of physical illness, functional disability, and suicidal behaviour among older adults. *Aging Ment. Health* **2016**, *20*, 166–194. [CrossRef] [PubMed]
12. Rurup, M.L.; Pasman, H.R.W.; Goedhart, J.; Deeg, D.J.H.; Kerkhof, A.J.F.M.; Onwuteaka-Philipsen, B.D. Understanding why older people develop a wish to die: A qualitative interview study. *Crisis* **2011**, *32*, 204–216. [CrossRef]
13. Balasubramaniam, M. Rational Suicide in Elderly Adults: A Clinician's Perspective. *J. Am. Geriatr. Soc.* **2018**, *66*, 998–1001. [CrossRef] [PubMed]
14. Erikson, E.H. *Childhood and Society*; WW Norton & Company: New York, NY, USA, 1993.
15. Muskin, P.R. The request to die: Role for a psychodynamic perspective on physician-assisted suicide. *JAMA* **1998**, *279*, 323–328. [CrossRef] [PubMed]
16. Arie, T. On Aging. In *Revolt and Resignation*; Jean Amery; Indiana University Press: Bloomington, IN, USA, 1994; p. 132.
17. Siegel, K. Psychosocial aspects of rational suicide. *Am. J. Psychother.* **1986**, *40*, 405–418. [CrossRef]
18. Mayo, D.J. The concept of rational suicide. *J. Med. Philos.* **1986**, *11*, 143–155. [CrossRef] [PubMed]
19. Valente, S.M.; Trainor, D. Rational suicide among patients who are terminally ill. *AORN J.* **1998**, *68*, 252–258, 260–264. [CrossRef]
20. Moody, H.R. *Ethics in an Aging Society*; Johns Hopkins University Press Books: Baltimore, MD, USA, 1992; Volume 1, Available online: https://jhupbooks.press.jhu.edu/title/ethics-aging-society (accessed on 17 August 2019).
21. Siegel, K. Rational suicide: Considerations for the clinician. *Psychiatr. Q.* **1982**, *54*, 77–84. [CrossRef]
22. Werth, J.L.; Cobia, D.C. Empirically based criteria for rational suicide: A survey of psychotherapists. *Suicide Life Threat. Behav.* **1995**, *25*, 231–240. [PubMed]
23. Motto, J.A. The Right to Suicide: A Psychiatrist's View. *Suicide Life Threat. Behav.* **1972**, *2*, 183–188.
24. Diekstra, R.F.W. The significance of Nico Speiler's suicide: How and when should suicide be prevented? *Suicide Life Threat. Behav.* **1986**, *16*, 13–15. [CrossRef]
25. Humphry, D. Rational suicide among the elderly. *Suicide Life Threat. Behav.* **1992**, *22*, 125–129.
26. A Cliff, Not a Slope: A Response to Margaret P. Battin. Centre for Suicide Prevention. Available online: https://www.suicideinfo.ca/resource/siecno-19890235/ (accessed on 17 August 2019).
27. Graber, G.C. The rationality of suicide. In *Suicide and Euthanasia: The Rights of Personhood*, 1st ed.; Wallace, S.E., Eser, A., Eds.; University of Tennessee Press: Knoxville, TN, USA, 1981; pp. 51–65.
28. Rich, K.L.; Butts, J.B. Rational suicide: Uncertain moral ground. *J. Adv. Nurs.* **2004**, *46*, 270–278. [CrossRef] [PubMed]
29. Moher, D. Preferred Reporting Items for Systematic Reviews and Meta-Analyses: The PRISMA Statement. *Ann. Intern. Med.* **2009**, *151*, 264. [CrossRef] [PubMed]

30. Fortin, A.; Lapierre, S.; Baillargeon, J.; Labelle, R.; Dubé, M.; Pronovost, J. Suicidal ideation and self-determination in institutionalized elderly. *Crisis* **2001**, *22*, 15–19. [CrossRef] [PubMed]
31. Gibbs, L.M.; Dombrovski, A.Y.; Morse, J.; Siegle, G.J.; Houck, P.R.; Szanto, K. When the solution is part of the problem: Problem solving in elderly suicide attempters. *Int. J. Geriatr. Psychiatry* **2009**, *24*, 1396–1404. [CrossRef]
32. Uncapher, H.; Areán, P.A. Physicians are less willing to treat suicidal ideation in older patients. *J. Am. Geriatr. Soc.* **2000**, *48*, 188–192. [CrossRef]
33. Van Wijngaarden, E.; Leget, C.; Goossensen, A. Caught between intending and doing: Older people ideating on a self-chosen death. *BMJ Open* **2016**, *6*, e009895. [CrossRef]
34. Winterrowd, E.; Canetto, S.S.; Benoit, K. Permissive beliefs and attitudes about older adult suicide: A suicide enabling script? *Aging Ment. Health* **2017**, *21*, 173–181. [CrossRef]
35. Lerner, B.H. Knowing when to say goodbye: Final Exit and suicide in the elderly. *Suicide Life Threat. Behav.* **1995**, *25*, 508–512.
36. Wand, A.P.F.; Peisah, C.; Draper, B.; Jones, C.; Brodaty, H. Rational Suicide, Euthanasia, and the Very Old: Two Case Reports. *Case Rep. Psychiatry* **2016**, *2016*, 4242064. [CrossRef]
37. Battin, M.B. The Concept of Rational Suicide. 1984. Available online: https://scholar.google.com/scholar_lookup?title=The+concept+of+rational+suicide&author=M.+P.+Battin&publication_year=1984 (accessed on 16 August 2019).
38. Conwell, Y.; Caine, E.D. Rational suicide and the right to die. Reality and myth. *N. Engl. J. Med.* **1991**, *325*, 1100–1103. [CrossRef]
39. Fontana, J.S. Rational suicide in the terminally ill. *J. Nurs. Scholarsh.* **2002**, *34*, 147–151. [CrossRef] [PubMed]
40. Karlinsky, H.; Taerk, G.; Schwartz, K.; Ennis, J.; Rodin, G. Suicide attempts and resuscitation dilemmas. *Gen. Hosp. Psychiatry* **1988**, *10*, 423–430. [CrossRef]
41. Werth, J.L. *Contemporary Perspectives on Rational Suicide [Internet]*; Brunner/Mazel: Philadelphia, PA, USA, 1999. Available online: https://trove.nla.gov.au/work/8768140 (accessed on 16 April 2019).
42. Gallagher-Thompson, D.; Osgood, N.J. Suicide in later life. *Behav. Ther.* **1997**, *28*, 23–41. [CrossRef]
43. Battin, M.P. Rational suicide: How can we respond to a request for help? *Crisis* **1991**, *12*, 73–80.
44. Moore, S.L. Rational suicide among older adults: A cause for concern? *Arch. Psychiatr. Nurs.* **1993**, *7*, 106–110. [CrossRef]
45. Prado, C.G. Ageism and elective death. *Ethics Med. Public Health* **2015**, *1*, 442–449. [CrossRef]
46. Richards, N. Old age rational suicide. *Sociol. Compass* **2017**, *11*, e12456. [CrossRef]
47. McCue, R.; Balasubramaniam, M. *Rational Suicide in the Elderly—Clinical, Ethical, and Sociocultural Aspects*; Springer Ebooks: New York, NY, USA, 2017; Available online: https://www.springer.com/gp/book/9783319326702 (accessed on 16 August 2019).
48. Ruckenbauer, G.; Yazdani, F.; Ravaglia, G. Suicide in old age: Illness or autonomous decision of the will? *Arch. Gerontol. Geriatr.* **2007**, *44* (Suppl. 1), 355–358. [CrossRef]
49. Clark, D.C. "Rational" suicide and people with terminal conditions or disabilities. *Issues Law Med.* **1992**, *8*, 147–166. [PubMed]
50. Den Hartogh, G. Two Kinds of Suicide. *Bioethics* **2016**, *30*, 672–680. [CrossRef]
51. Torre, E.; Zeppegno, P.; Usai, C.; Rudoni, M.; Ammirata, G.; De Donatis, O.; Manzetti, E.; Marangon, D.; Migliaretti, G. Suicide in Verbano-Cusio-Ossola province: Decade 1990–2000. *Epidemiol. Psichiatr. Soc.* **2002**, *11*, 277–283. [CrossRef] [PubMed]
52. Clarke, D.M. Autonomy, rationality and the wish to die. *J. Med. Ethics* **1999**, *25*, 457–462. [CrossRef] [PubMed]
53. Maris, R. Rational Suicide: An Impoverished Self-Transformation. *Suicide Life Threat. Behav.* **1982**, *12*, 4–16. [CrossRef]
54. Richman, J. The Case against Rational Suicide. *Suicide Life Threat. Behav.* **1988**, *18*, 285–289. [CrossRef] [PubMed]
55. Shneidman, E.S. Psychotherapy with suicidal patients. *Suicide Life Threat. Behav.* **1981**, *11*, 341–348.
56. Stiefel, F.; Die Trill, M.; Berney, A.; Olarte, J.M.; Razavi, A. Depression in palliative care: A pragmatic report from the Expert Working Group of the European Association for Palliative Care. *Support. Care Cancer* **2001**, *9*, 477–488. [CrossRef] [PubMed]
57. Passik, S.D.; Dugan, W.; McDonald, M.V.; Rosenfeld, B.; Theobald, D.E.; Edgerton, S. Oncologists' recognition of depression in their patients with cancer. *J. Clin. Oncol.* **1998**, *16*, 1594–1600. [CrossRef] [PubMed]

58. McDonald, M.V.; Passik, S.D.; Dugan, W.; Rosenfeld, B.; Theobald, D.E.; Edgerton, S. Nurses' recognition of depression in their patients with cancer. *Oncol. Nurs. Forum* **1999**, *26*, 593–599. [PubMed]
59. Block, S.D. Assessing and managing depression in the terminally ill patient. ACP-ASIM End-of-Life Care Consensus Panel. American College of Physicians—American Society of Internal Medicine. *Ann. Intern. Med.* **2000**, *132*, 209–218. [CrossRef]
60. Periyakoil, V.S.; Kraemer, H.C.; Noda, A.; Moos, R.; Hallenbeck, J.; Webster, M.; Yesavage, J.A. The development and initial validation of the terminally illgreif of depression scale (TIGDS). *Int. J. Methods Psychiatr. Res.* **2005**, *14*, 202–212. [CrossRef] [PubMed]
61. Osgood, N.J. *Suicide in the Elderly. A Practitioner's Guide to Diagnosis and Mental Health Intervention*; Aspen Systems Corporation: Rockville, MD, USA, 1985.
62. Kerkhof, A.; de Leo, D. Suicide in the elderly: A frightful awareness. *Crisis* **1991**, *12*, 81–87. [PubMed]
63. Schneewind, E.H. Of ageism, suicide, and limiting life. *J. Gerontol. Soc. Work* **1994**, *23*, 135–150. [CrossRef]
64. Reggler, J. The slippery slope argument and medical assistance in dying. *CMAJ* **2017**, *189*, E471. [CrossRef] [PubMed]
65. Potter, J. The psychological slippery slope from physician-assisted death to active euthanasia: A paragon of fallacious reasoning. *Med. Health Care Philos.* **2019**, *22*, 239–244. [CrossRef]
66. Kaufman, S.R. *Ordinary Medicine: Extraordinary Treatments, Longer Lives, and Where to Draw the Line (Critical Global Health: Evidence, Efficacy, Ethnography)*; Duke University Press: Durham, NC, USA, 2015.
67. Gawande, A. *Being Mortal Illness, Medicine and What Matters in the End*; Profile Books Ltd.: London, UK, 2014.
68. Farberow, N.L. (Ed.) *The Many Faces of Suicide: Indirect Self-Destructive Behavior*; McGraw-Hill: New York, NY, USA, 1980.
69. Shneidman, E.S. *Deaths of Man*; Quadrangle: New York, NY, USA, 1973.
70. Conwell, Y.; Pearson, J.; De Renzo, E. Indirect self-destruptive behavior among elderly patients in nursing homes: A research agenda. *Am. J. Geriatr. Psychiatry* **1996**, *4*, 152–163. [CrossRef] [PubMed]

2

Keeping in Touch with Mental Health: The Orienting Reflex and Behavioral Outcomes from Calatonia

Anita Ribeiro Blanchard [1,*] and William Edgar Comfort [2]

[1] Faculty of Psychology, University of Barcelona, 08035 Barcelona, Spain
[2] Social and Cognitive Science Laboratory, Centre for Health and Biological Sciences, Mackenzie Presbyterian University, São Paulo 01241, Brazil; 9032936@mackenzie.br
* Correspondence: aribeiri8@alumnes.ub.edu

Abstract: Physical and psychological therapy based on touch has been gradually integrated into broader mental health settings in the past two decades, evolving from a variety of psychodynamic, neurobiological and trauma-based approaches, as well as Eastern and spiritual philosophies and other integrative and converging systems. Nevertheless, with the exception of a limited number of well-known massage therapy techniques, only a few structured protocols of touch therapy have been standardized and researched to date. This article describes a well-defined protocol of touch therapy in the context of psychotherapy—the Calatonia technique—which engages the orienting reflex. The orienting reflex hypothesis is explored here as one of the elements of this technique that helps to decrease states of hypervigilance and chronic startle reactivity (startle and defensive reflexes) and restore positive motivational and appetitive states.

Keywords: orienting reflex; motivational system; touch therapy; integrative psychotherapy; somatic psychology

1. Introduction

The limitations of verbal psychotherapy have become more evident in the past thirty years [1], giving rise to a large number of somatic and body-based modalities aimed to address treatment-resistant disorders [2–4]. Recently, there has been an interest in developing somatically informed research methods to support a wide range of these integrative practices [5,6]. Accordingly, this article discusses the significance of integrating a structured touch therapy (Calatonia) into psychotherapy to facilitate an orienting reflex (OR) [7]. The OR leads the individual to direct their motivational system towards appetitive and exploratory states, which can, in turn, positively influence affective and cognitive states.

Motivation—a concept derived from the biological sciences—has not been explored for its potential strength in mental health treatments, although motivation as a cognitive concept was well developed by Miller [8]. Affective responses comprising an organism's underlying motivational state have been broadly categorized in terms of defensive and appetitive systems, evolving either separately or in conjunction to engage with environmental stimuli indicative of threat or opportunities for survival, respectively [9]. In this perspective, emotional experiences occur within a range of appetitive-pleasant or defensive-unpleasant valence and have levels of arousal that indicate the degree of activation in response to that emotional valence [10]. These two basic dimensions of affective responses support mobilization for action, attention and social communication, according to the motivational system that is engaged (defensive or appetitive), its intensity of activation and its emotional context [9–13].

While several findings have identified distinct brain networks for approach/avoidance behavior and pleasant or aversive affect in healthy subjects [14,15], mental health continues to be studied primarily from a symptomatological perspective, with little research into long-term behavioral outcomes linked to the patient's motivational state.

As an illustration, depressive disorders—from their biological symptoms to their emotional and cognitive expression—can be understood as dysfunctions of the motivational system, in which (appetitive) motivation is reduced. Anxiety disorders may also be viewed from a motivational system perspective, in which there is either strong behavioral inhibition or impulsivity, based on aversive, defensive or avoidant motivation [16]. In such cases, touch therapies may prove useful to redirect the individual's motivational state toward more approach-oriented behavior, in conjunction with conventional psychotherapy and/or pharmacological treatment.

It is in this context that we introduce the therapeutic potential of Calatonia, a long-standing technique of touch therapy which aims to re-orient the individual toward a more open behavioral approach through activation of the appetitive motivational system and concomitant inhibition of startle and defensive states. This integrative approach has been used to treat disorders unresponsive to verbal psychotherapy alone, such as PTSD and other forms of trauma.

The primary mechanism through which Calatonia is thought to exert changes in the individual's motivational states is by eliciting an orienting reflex (OR) within the context of psychotherapy [17]. The OR is activated through touch experienced as a novel, sustained and non-threatening stimulus. Calatonia (described in Section 3) is a therapeutic technique based on a structured sequence of touches applied bilaterally to distinct regions of the body [18–20]. Since its inception, Calatonia has purported to induce a state of deep relaxation and increased unconscious processing with a net result of altering the patient's motivational and affective states [19–21].

However, Calatonia has yet to be submitted to rigorous scientific testing for the direct therapeutic benefits accrued from its application. One potential avenue for such research is the Research Domain Criteria (RDoC) framework for evaluating novel treatments for mental health put forth by the National Institute of Mental Health (NIMH) [22]. Within the RDoC framework, an upward level of analysis constitutes mapping functional measures of neural activity to variation in clinical symptoms on a distinct spectrum of mental health such as anxiety [22]. In line with this approach, a study utilizing near-infrared spectroscopy (fNIRS) to investigate alterations in neural markers of anxiety following Calatonia is currently under preparation.

2. History of the Technique

During WWII, the Hungarian physician Pethö Sándor (1916–1992) structured a sequence of ten light touches while treating the psychological and physical suffering of refugees and other displaced persons at Red Cross refugee camps. This sequence of touches emerged from the combined biomedical knowledge and feedback from patients about the points of tactile contact that appeared to balance their sympathetic and parasympathetic responses and foster autonomic regulation [18–20].

After being treated with this technique—then named Calatonia—patients spontaneously shared their feelings, thoughts, worries, memories and traumatic experiences with a scale of trust and openness that had not happened before the treatment—a clear validation of its usefulness in psychotherapy [19,20]. Following a few applications of Calatonia, patients showed decreased symptoms of traumatic stress (shell shock), anxiety, depression, pain and other ailments that afflicted most war survivors at the time. Patients' improvements manifested in terms of increased morale, acceptance, well-being, hope, will to live, overall motivation and resilience [21], defined as the ability to adequately adapt and respond to homeostatic disturbances [23]. These touches seemed to promote global changes, which led Sándor [19,20] to describe Calatonia as a technique for psychophysical regulation and reorganization.

After the end of the war, Sándor worked for two years in the psychiatric wards of German hospitals, using Calatonia to successfully treat depression, suicide ideation, post-traumatic stress disorder, anxiety, catatonic states and other mental disorders [18,21,24,25]. Later, in São Paulo, Brazil [26], he expanded the repertoire of techniques to include many other "light touch" sequences, grouped under the name subtle touch (ST) [27–30]. Another ST technique, Fractional Decompression, works by gradually releasing pressure from a touch applied to hairy skin on the back, arms or legs [27]. Fractional decompression is thought to primarily target the affective-affiliative touch system associated with hairy non-glabrous skin [31]. Calatonia continues to be the most widely used ST technique. At times, subtle touch and Calatonia are used interchangeably to denote the whole gamut of techniques developed by Sándor and subsequently expanded by other clinical psychologists [32]. Sándor's subtle touch method has produced numerous qualitative studies published over the past four decades (reviewed in [32]), as well as quantitative research in the past fifteen years [32–34].

Sándor had previously hypothesized [19,20] that the experience of physiological regulation, mood stabilization, inflow of adaptive cognition and neuromuscular relaxation induced by Calatonia were linked to the associative activation of somatosensory representations in the frontotemporal cortex, the engagement of peripheral proprioceptive nerve fibers, particularly in the skin and cortical mediation by the ascending reticular activating system. Furthermore, he associated its effects with psycho-affective elements mobilized by the configuration of dyadic regulation through the touch therapy protocol.

Given the barriers to many forms of social and affiliative touch in social interactions, particularly in the context of psychotherapy, it can be useful to compare the touch sequence employed in Calatonia with other common forms of "pleasant" touch found in everyday encounters. In particular, a recently discovered category of slow-response unmyelinated nerve fiber, C-tactile afferents, have been implicated in many forms of innocuous touch [35], as well as touch in social contexts [31]. C-tactile afferent projections terminate in the ventral medial nucleus of the thalamus and posterior insular cortex [36,37], associated with the contextual and affective components of touch [38]. While the primary areas of contact in Calatonia are to the glabrous skin areas of the feet or hands (see below), the sequence employed also includes contact to hairy skin containing C-tactile afferent connections. Several other ST techniques similarly activate CT connections by contact with the arms, calves, back and head. As such, Calatonia may act on both a common affiliative system for social touch as well as on more discriminative neural pathways in glabrous areas of the hands and feet. However, the perceptual characteristics of touch in these regions are specifically modulated in Calatonia to induce large-scale novelty-related activation in addition to more familiar responses to CT touch primarily in thalamic and insular regions.

3. The Calatonia Technique

Touch therapies differ in their goals. Some focus on achieving body awareness, structural readjustment, functional improvement, emotional-affective regulation, release of pent up energy, healing of trauma, among other issues [2]. Calatonia has an open-ended goal, in contrast to more narrowly defined ST techniques: one geared toward spontaneous adaptive adjustments in one's idiosyncratic psychophysical needs and imbalances, prompted by the sequence of touches. As an example, for some, stress will manifest as insomnia or excessive worrying; for others, it will manifest as addiction, overeating or overreacting emotionally in relationships. Each maladaptive style will lead to different responses to Calatonia's applications, despite being caused by the same underlying problem—stress.

A description of this technique (Figures 1–5) may be useful to integrate the elements that will be discussed in this article. Calatonia is performed in silence (unless the patient feels discomfort or the need to speak) after the patient has been briefed on the steps of the protocol [19,20]. The patient removes his or her shoes and socks and lies on a massage table in a supine position, with his or her eyes closed, fully dressed (Figure 1). Preferably, the therapist applies the technique on the lower limbs, or, alternatively, on the hands and forearms. Excluding the tenth point (the head), the first nine points of tactile contact are bilateral (the same tactile stimulus is simultaneously held on each side of the body). The seven first touches (Figure 2) are extremely light (as if the therapist were holding a "soap bubble") and sustained in place for one to three minutes (preferably three minutes on the few initial applications). The eighth, ninth and tenth tactile contacts (respectively Figures 3–5) are supported and held in place for one to three minutes on the heels, calves and head (in that order). At the end, patients are coached back to awareness of the environment and themselves and instructed to sit up and walk back to their seat, at which point they are invited to share their observations or impressions, if any, which may have manifested during or after the application of the technique.

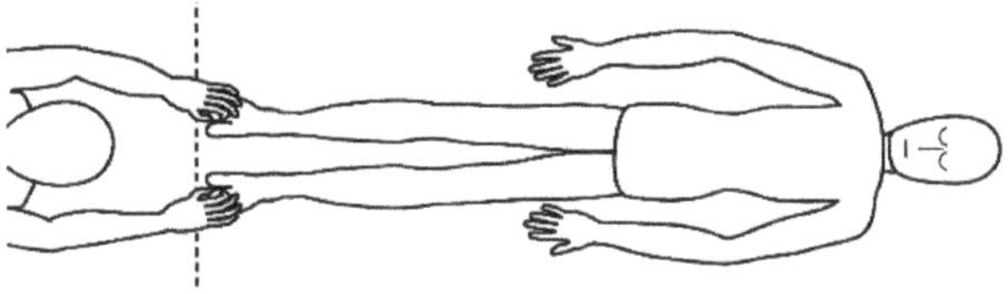

Figure 1. Resting state (task-free) supine position.

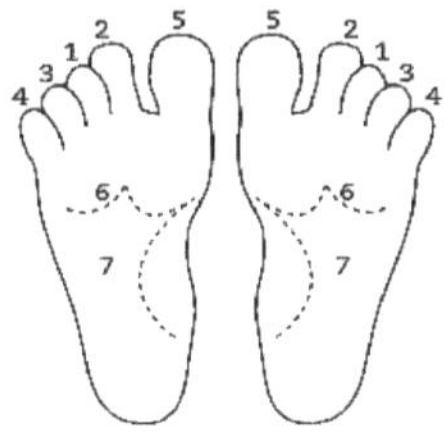

Figure 2. Sequential order of bilateral points of tactile contact.

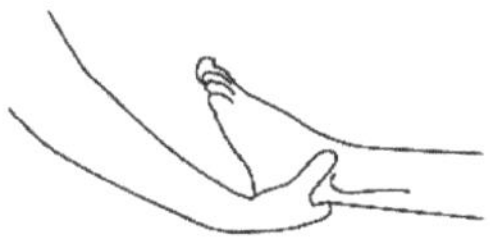

Figure 3. Ankle support, eighth bilateral touch.

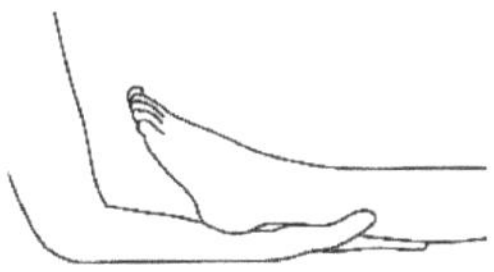

Figure 4. Calf support, ninth bilateral touch.

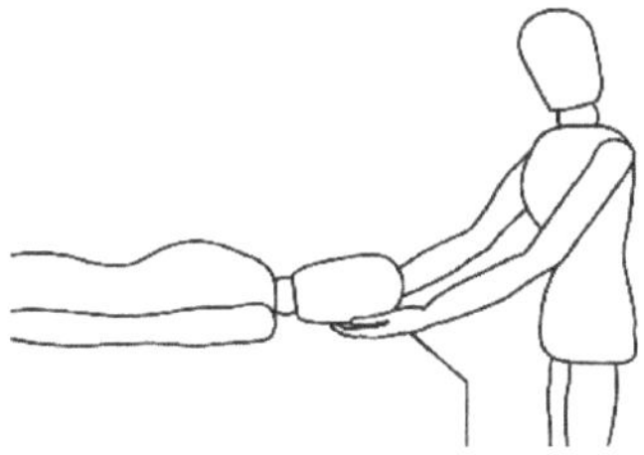

Figure 5. Head support, tenth and last touch.

4. Touch to the Feet or Hands

While it appears unusual to propose tactile contact with the patient's feet or hands in psychotherapy, there is strong empirical support for doing so. Contact is made to these specific sites, as nowhere else on the body is there found a similar configuration of neurobiological and physiological variables, including the distinctive dermo-mechanical features and receptors found on the glabrous skin of the feet and hands [35–44]. This combination of features frequently results in the activation of an orienting response by eliciting a pattern of neural activation associated with novelty, of either a neutral or pleasant nature, through both conscious and unconscious perceptual pathways.

The glabrous (non-hairy) skin of the hands and feet is indirectly connected to several perceptual subsystems involved in the detection of vibration, temperature changes and differences in texture and pressure, as well as somatosensory and proprioceptive responses [43,44]. The areas targeted in Calatonia contain the most numerous populations of skin receptors, collectively known as the discriminative–spatial system [41–46], distinct from receptors of the affective–affiliative system found primarily in non-glabrous skin. Glabrous skin is a dedicated site of very precise tactile perception geared toward the exploration of and adaptation to novel stimuli, as well as the evaluation and appraisal of a spectrum of touch pleasantness and roughness mediated by the somatosensory cortex [47–49].

For example, to read and attribute meaning to the raised dots of the Braille system requires language, touch and spatial coding to be transformed into semantic, lexical and haptic processing. This in turn engages highly associative areas of the brain to produce concrete and abstract thinking, symbols and ultimately communication [50].

Hands are also especially involved in the formation of procedural memory, which makes them potential "roads" for the emotional retrieval of such implicit memories—in particular, early childhood memories linked to independence, mastery, self-care, reaching out and so forth. These memories may be accompanied by emotional and relational contexts of frustration, impatience, among many other emotions and behavioral patterns [51,52]. Similarly, the locomotor system is in many ways involved in early childhood developmental milestones (standing, walking, running, bike riding, etc.).

The feet bear the total gravitational force imposed on the body and function as an integrated system with the cerebellum and vestibular system to control posture, coordination, equilibrium and the generation of locomotor rhythm; the proprioceptive control of posture is chiefly initiated in the feet [53]. Drew, Prentice and Schepens [54] state that these essential mechanisms of control of postural muscle tone and locomotion "are located in the brainstem and spinal cord, in which a range of locomotor behaviors are achieved by the projections from the forebrain structures (cerebral cortex, basal ganglia and limbic-hypothalamic systems) and cerebellum to the brainstem-spinal cord". As such, despite the role of these mechanisms in voluntary movement and locomotion, a significant portion of the adjustment of balance is made involuntarily, based on information that does not require conscious attention to be processed. When the feet are in an unloaded position (i.e., lying down), there is no background discharge activity in any of the cutaneous receptors unless there is intentionally applied stimulation [49,53–55]. This may be indicative of how Calatonia on the feet facilitates the reorganization of the individual's global posture and muscle tension.

5. Novel Stimuli in Psychotherapy

There are several common elements to Sándor's many ST techniques, yet two elements can be immediately perceived as fundamental: (a) their non-invasiveness, by respecting an individual's boundaries and even their resistance to therapy, while gently supporting the individual towards gaining resilience toward the integration of crucial personal issues; (b) their novelty, through the application of atypical sensory stimuli—not merely an oddball protocol for the sake of novelty itself, but a meaningful stimulus that engages global responses and multidimensional aspects of a person's life.

The combination of these two aspects, non-invasiveness and novelty, is hypothesized as generating an orienting reflex or an orienting response [7], also known as the 'what is it response?' or the exploratory response. The OR is an involuntary response of an organism to a stimulus that is 'out of the ordinary' but not alarming or menacing. ORs are an adaptive feature of cognition present since infancy [56] that play a major role in many aspects of motivation, emotion and attention [57–62].

Sándor purposefully developed different methods for creating ORs by using an unusually light and static form of touch or other forms of stimulation in his techniques. These included passive movements that were mechanically impossible for the patient to perform voluntarily (e.g., rotating the patient's finger sideways); atypical but non-threatening sounds directed towards specific parts of the body, small vibrations applied to bone projections and protuberances, such as the spinous processes [27] and many others. His approach was geared toward the enhancement of neural plasticity and the generation of 'dedicated neural circuitries' for experiencing well-being, leading to increased self-confidence and a sense of safety within one's own body [17,18].

6. The Orienting Reflex in Calatonia

An orienting reflex is triggered when a sensory stimulus is perceived as novel, innocuous or pleasant [58,63]. This may be seen in opposition to defensive reflexes initiated when a sensory stimulus is perceived as painful, aversive and potentially dangerous—or startle reflexes activated in response to abrupt, unexpected or overly intense stimuli. All of these responses, whether defensive/startle or orienting, will activate the executive network for regulation or action if necessary [64,65].

In animals, the OR is a survival reflex that does not burden the organism with a full-blown alert response but entices them to explore the environment. Pavlov [66] saw the OR as the biological basis for the highest form of curiosity, imagination, science and knowledge of the world around us. At the basic end of this spectrum, the OR encourages human curiosity, which drives child development and "involves an indissoluble mixture of cognition and motivation" [67]—a key prerequisite for learning and the formation of top-down predictions in perceptual processing. To achieve this level of exploration, the OR tunes the organism toward a specific stimulus by enhancing perceptual awareness [68–70]. In contrast, the defensive and startle reflexes limit the impact of the stimulus on the organism by functionally raising perceptual thresholds [68–70].

The OR halts all non-essential brain activity to allow the individual to orientate their primary senses towards the source of stimulation, focusing on possible means of interaction with the stimulus through the activation of the autonomic nervous system (ANS) [68,69]. It produces an unintentional shift of attention that interrupts the ordinary flow of awareness and leads us to attend to the novelty of a stimulus for the appraisal of its meaning and/or significance. This phase of the reflex has been classified by researchers as an "information-gathering", "analyzing", "modelling" or simply "sensory" phase [7]. One of the key physiological markers of an OR is the initial deceleration in the heartbeat, which is a sign of enhanced perceptual processing and is mediated by the parasympathetic branch of the ANS [71,72]. This initial slowdown allows the organism to more easily detect the potential significance of stimulus features to estimate 'uncertainty'. An OR is triggered if uncertainty is detected concerning the biological value or perceptual features of the stimulus [73].

As mentioned above, Calatonia triggers an OR due to its non-invasive nature (experienced as either of a neutral or pleasant affect), extended duration of passive tactile stimuli and the novelty of its touch. Sustained attention to a body location results in the enhanced processing of the tactile stimuli presented at that location compared to other unattended locations [74]. A light touch is often a strange sensory perception, particularly on the feet, accustomed to supporting the individual's body weight and rough contact with stimuli on the ground. The palms of the hands and the soles of the feet are instruments of self-agency [75–77] and rarely the object of passive interaction. Receiving a passive gentle touch in these areas may easily throw the organism into a state of perceptive, emotional and cognitive surprise yet still feel innocuous within a safe context. The neutral affect associated with the surprise response works to reset attentional processes [78]—with attention defined in cognitive terms as the ability to selectively attend to some stimuli while ignoring others [79].

Individuals have different forms of appraisal and emotional responses to touch based on their personal history and cultural biases [80]. However, it is highly likely that most people will experience an OR in response to an unexpectedly static, sustained and light touch that conveys neither personal meaning nor affection. Such a response is dependent on the therapist adopting an appropriately responsive but neutral affective state during the application of Calatonia.

7. Brain Areas Associated with the Orienting Reflex

Sándor's hypothesis concerning reticular formation mediation in the large-scale neural response activated during Calatonia has been borne out by subsequent research based on brain imaging (fMRI-PET, EEG, NIRS). Here, we articulate an updated argument in the light of this evidence for the therapeutic benefit of engaging the orienting reflex through novel stimulation and the cognitive re-evaluation this may engender.

The functional circuitry of the reticular formation (RF), known as the reticular activating system (RAS), has long been recognized as a central component within a multitude of subcortical and cortical neural circuitry [81]. The RAS has been implicated in cognitive functions such as the orienting reflex to novel stimuli [7], attention, sleep, homeostatic regulation, as well as the transmission and modulation of pain, alongside other brain structures [82–85]. Essentially, the RF plays a major role in the modulation of attention to the extremely light sensory stimuli of Calatonia, which takes the organism by surprise and induces an orienting reflex, with extensive engagement of the RF and related networks in this process.

The OR triggers an extensive search for possible associations to previous contexts and meanings within the individual's history, beginning with short-term memories and moving on to those that may be embedded in implicit memory. With the aim of associating the new stimulus to previous memory representations, the brain quickly 'explores' the memory via the hippocampus and sensory association areas in the central-parietal cortex. In this process, a set of neocortical limbic interactions occur to resolve the significance of the stimulus [73,86,87].

Uddin and colleagues [88] note that the insula is commonly involved in detection of novel stimuli across sensory modalities. The insula, dorsal anterior cingulate (dACC) and other subcortical structures form part of the 'salience network' (SN), which is activated in response to out-of-the-ordinary or "oddball" stimuli. The function of the SN is to identify "the most homeostatically relevant among multiple competing internal and external stimuli" [88]. Most importantly, for the higher-order cognitive processes produced with Calatonia [17] where more complex stimuli require greater cognitive processing, the dorsal anterior insula will be recruited. Insular activation primarily functions "to integrate external sensory information with internal emotional and bodily state signals to coordinate brain network dynamics and to initiate switches between the default mode network (DMN) and central executive network (CEN)" [88].

If no associations are formed between the tactile stimuli in Calatonia and previous experiences recorded as memories, then the significance of the event will be assessed primarily by the amygdala. The amygdala plays an important role in encoding, storing and retrieving emotionally charged events and controlling the hormonal cascade triggered by defensive responses [89]. Amygdalar structures are activated by both emotionally salient and novel stimuli. This activation may occur regardless of whether the stimuli are emotionally valent and/or pleasant or unpleasant. In addition, the salience of the emotion is central to determining whether either a fight-or-flight or other motivational or appetitive response is triggered [90–94].

8. The Appraisal of New Stimuli

A stimulus or event is significant if it is helpful in satisfying a need, reaching a goal, or sustaining an internal value. The opposite holds true for negative significance, whereupon the stimulus is unhelpful for achieving any of the aforementioned goals. In ANS terminology, significance can be equated to homeostasis, whereby a stimulus or event positively influences homeostatic mechanisms, leading to that stimulus being attributed a high level of significance [92,95,96].

Scherer [97] asserts that the appraisal of significance is defined by one's needs, goals, values and general wellbeing, which leads to a cascade of motivation-related changes. In particular, emotionally-laden appraisals of pleasantness and well-being (or the opposite valence) lead to somatovisceral changes via the ANS and changes in motor facial expression, as well as voice and bodily tensions, conveyed through the somatic nervous system [97–99]. Over the course of Calatonia, adjustments in body tension are frequently reported in the form of twitching, sudden jerks, spontaneous jolts felt in the diaphragm, lung expansion (a respiratory reflex) and fluttering eyelids, while at the end of Calatonia, the facial muscles are often notably relaxed [17–20,32].

In the presence of a pleasant OR, several somatic responses may occur, such as a deceleration in heart rate, salivation, pupillary responses, pharyngeal expansion and a relaxation of the tract walls ('wide voice') [97]. These many somatic reactions are conducive to a trophotropic response (a relaxation response for resting and replenishing energy) and increased stability. This may in turn lead to a decrease in respiration rate, a slight decrease in heart rate, sphincter relaxation, a decrease in general muscle tone, relaxation in facial muscle tone and overall relaxation of the vocal apparatus ('relaxed voice'), comfort and resting posture. If this relaxation response leads to changes in one's motivational state and plans for action, an ergotropic shift (the activation response and usage of energy) may occur as a result of experiencing well-being [97]—in this way, one feels motivated to become proactive. This fact may explain why Calatonia is a method of psychophysiological regulation and not exclusively a relaxation technique because, ultimately, it takes the organism where it needs to go. Whether positively activated (ergotropic) or relaxed (trophotropic), Calatonia fosters the organism's optimal state [17–20].

9. ORs in Clinical Practice

The emotional significance of a stimulus, defined by its level of pleasantness and importance, can frequently affect OR intensity when focusing one's attention on a stimulus [7,100,101]. One example of the use of OR in clinical practice is a simple technique designed by Sándor: a sequence of three slow and sustained 'insufflation (blowing) on and above the seventh cervical vertebra (C4–C7)'. The therapist applies the technique while the patient remains in a sitting or standing position. This somatosensory contact at C4–C7 affects the entirety of the brachial plexus, which innervates the arm muscles, thus affecting a large area of the brain, as well as cervical vagus branching [102], causing an immediate and involuntary shift in attention with a pleasant affective tone. This is an effective way of peacefully redirecting disruptive behavior in children in less than a couple of minutes and one that has been applied on many previous occasions to institutionalized children in foster care when they felt themselves unable to engage in emotional regulation [17]. For these children, the novelty of tactile stimulation diverted their attention from an overwhelming state of emotional reaction, offering them a state of adaptive relief directly proportional to this initial state.

The process of neocortical-limbic connectivity and integration linked to an OR is not a standard occurrence in children and adults with histories of abuse and/or PTSD [103–105]. These patients frequently show symptoms of excessive limbic system activity (particularly an abnormally overactive amygdala) with less activity in the neocortex, which causes them to react impulsively to the minor triggers of daily life [106]. However, in several cases of PTSD, the opposite pattern of activation is observed, with over-activation of the prefrontal systems and over-inhibition of the amygdala and insula, leading these patients to experience flat affective states and anhedonia.

When the amygdala is chronically activated in response to trauma, stress and/or overwhelming fear, the individual's emotional response to sensory inputs becomes compromised and often requires re-setting [68,69,83]. The effects of exposure to traumatic events on brain structure and function are extensive and very specific brain regions have been implicated in trauma and PTSD [107–111]. Significant research has been dedicated towards investigating a variety of psychological treatments to address specific types of such neural dysregulation [3,112–117].

In the treatment of trauma, by prompting a neutral/pleasant OR, Calatonia shifts the patient's experience away from defensive states, leading to the re-setting of vigilant states and attentional processes and facilitating the reinstatement of neocortical–limbic interactions.

By enhancing the perception of a stimulus, Calatonia also activates motivational (or appetitive) systems that support survival, adaptation and tending to one's needs and, consequently, attentional processes based on 'interest', 'curiosity' and 'well-being'. This seemingly simple process conceals a complex reorganization of the individual on physical, emotional and cognitive levels—a process of great psychotherapeutic utility [28–30,32–34,112].

In terms of its general application in psychotherapy, the OR has been hypothesized as one of the key drivers for successful clinical outcomes following eye movement desensitization and reprocessing (EMDR) [117]. This technique aims to gradually expose the patient to the stimuli underlying PTSD and other trauma disorders, similar to other forms of cognitive-behavioral therapy. Hypothetically, EMDR pairs the recall of a traumatic event with a supposedly emotionally-neutral motor stimulus—eye movements. EMDR appears to show similar improvements in post-therapy outcomes to other cognitive-behavioral therapies particularly for the treatment of PTSD, however the functional mechanisms underlying its action remain unclear [117–120].

To many patients who suffer from PTSD, the idea of re-experiencing the trauma as proposed in EMDR is unbearable. Unlike EMDR, Calatonia does not target a specific event or memory. Consequently, there is no resetting of new homeostatic values based on previous traumatic experiences, thus amplifying the effects of Calatonia beyond specific trauma memories. Instead, there is a decrease in startle and defensive reflexes and a reinforcing of the "benign present", allowing the individual to be spontaneously released into a 'stream of consciousness' state corresponding to the emergence of the default mode network (DMN) of broad frontoparietal activation in the brain [17]. In this context, high-priority psychological issues may emerge spontaneously and rescript themselves in light of this new experience, producing the myriad of idiosyncratic reports that demonstrate the nonlinearity of psychological processes, followed by a sense of well-being [30].

10. Habituation: Does Repeated Calatonia Cease to Generate an OR?

What happens when Calatonia is repeated on a weekly basis? Does it lose its novel impact and stop triggering an OR response?

First, a description of the technique and the consent given by the patient are always requirements to minimize the possibility of a startle or defensive response by making the technique 'cognitively safe' and, evidently, this technique is offered only once a good therapeutic relationship is formed. However, a description of this technique does not prevent an OR from occurring as the OR is a result of the direct tactile stimulus and frequently resistant to top-down modulation.

In time, the sequence of touches becomes predictable and thus provides a sense of safety to the patient. Most importantly, what happens within one's mind, body and emotions during each Calatonia session may become an element of significance for an OR. The route taken towards eliciting an OR may be the same, but the journey is always different. This approach places emphasis on the significance of the event and its capacity to continue to generate a significant OR response. It is very common for patients who receive regular Calatonia to say, "today was different, I didn't feel the same way I felt last week", "today the touch seemed much lighter", "the left side of my body seemed to be heavier", or similar such observations. These comparisons can be accounted for by Friston's free energy principle [121], in which the brain is constantly trying to predict events to minimize errors. In this hypothesis, bottom-up processes are thought to compare previous events (memories) to current perceptual inputs to estimate the error in deviation between the internal model and novel input, thus recognizing minimal differences in deviation. Any changes in the representation or original "neural model" of an event that triggered an OR will retrigger the OR by establishing a comparison to what was previously experienced [122,123].

11. A Clinical Vignette

The reorganization of the (appetitive) motivational system prompted by Calatonia can be seen in action in a clinical case presenting a dysfunction of the primary motivational behavior for survival, eating. For three consecutive sessions, a fifteen-year-old female patient suffering from anorexia nervosa reported that she "knew exactly what she was going to eat for dinner". She proceeded to describe to the therapist the meal that came to her mind during the session of Calatonia.

She spontaneously sent pictures of her meals to the therapist shortly following these sessions. These included pictures of her breakfast on the mornings following therapy, revealing nutritious and complete meals. It can be hypothesized that the neurobiological mechanisms set in motion by ORs bypassed her voluntary resistance to homeostatic self-regulation and allostatic behaviors [17], restoring a biological imperative, via "neural circuits in the mammalian brain that prompt specific somatic and autonomic responses associated with motivated behavior" [9].

As the sessions of Calatonia progressed, the sadness and depression she felt surrounding her self-destructive behavior emerged—and her menstrual periods returned, along with these emotions.

In her ninth session, she reported a dream in which she "had been kidnapped by a skinny and weak man, from whom she escaped to a shopping mall together with a beautiful girl of the same age who was also his hostage".

The attentional and motivational processes set in motion during Calatonia seemed to have redirected her perception of her physical needs, revealing the pain she inflicted on herself. In the dream, the self-destructive dynamics that required her awareness were depicted by the skinny and weak man (anorexic thought patterns) and the beautiful girl (her idealized version of herself). She also began to go out more often instead of staying at home watching videos of other anorexic girls. This process suggests what Schomaker and Meeter [124] describe as an "attentional response to novelty, possibly mediated by the amygdala, an arousal-like response to deviance, which could be mediated by the noradrenergic system and a slower upregulation of exploration, motivation and learning, mediated by the dopaminergic system", as well as a possible reorganization of thalamic functional connectivity [125,126].

12. Conclusions

Calatonia and other ST techniques appear to function through the re-calibration of a subset of attentional processes. These include a reduction in the startle response to anxiety- and fear-inducing stimuli and may help to orient the patient towards novel unknown stimuli in a context of adaptation. The redirection of alerting and defensive responses towards motivational and appetitive states through innocuous, pleasant and unusual touch sequences allows the patient to implicitly process past states of trauma. A necessary prerequisite for this technique to be considered a safe psychotherapeutic approach is for the psychotherapist to have adequate training and observe strict adherence to the established protocol of touch and engagement with the patient.

Many studies discuss whether the novelty or significance of an event is the actual trigger of an OR and the consensus is that both novelty and significance are involved in the generation of an orienting response. However, significance was found to be a key factor in sustaining engagement in an OR [7,127], only a relevant/significant novel stimulus will continue to trigger an OR.

In summary, novelty-driven stimulation can support reward processes, drive exploration and other adaptive cognitive processes and enhance perception and sharpen its responses. Most importantly, an OR has a lasting and strong impact on memory and on the attentional system mediated by the amygdala, resulting from neural plasticity and deep changes to the motivational system [124].

13. Final Considerations

Beyond the impact of orienting reflexes, there are several other neurobiological, neuro-cognitive and neuro affective-emotional elements that influence the results and responses to the complex stimuli proposed in Calatonia, as listed in a previous publication [30] and briefly mentioned below.

Among these elements, dyadic regulation proposes a fine-tuned, non-verbal, inter-brain synchronization, whereby inter-brain synchronization between two individuals is defined as a natural occurrence that impacts interpersonal communication [128–132].

The importance of establishing a conscious pace of communication in therapeutic relationships cannot be emphasized enough [133–135] as several physiological systems follow a preset tempo or rhythm (heartbeat, respiration, thalamo-cortical oscillations) and "rhythms are a prominent signature of brain activity" [136]. The modulation of cortical oscillation via paced somatosensory stimuli may also facilitate integration of the individual's basic notion of selfhood. From early infancy to adulthood, selfhood is built through physical contact and proximal interaction with others via skin-to-skin interactions—before one develops the ability to share mental states in distal face-to-face interactions [137–140].

Other hypotheses about the possible elements involved in the complex mental stimuli and contexts observed in Calatonia include:

The use of (task-free) resting-state functional connectivity to facilitate access to spontaneous and pertinent (to psychotherapy) self-reflective cognitive processes [141,142];

(a) The modulation of global brain connectivity and patterns of synchronization (identified as an aspect of brain self-regulation) through the rhythmic segregation and integration of neural populations acting in concert to code for complex stimuli [143–149];
(b) The engagement of cross-hemispheric communication via the corpus callosum, which facilitates integrative higher-order neural network processes and is implicated in the ability to verbally identify, interpret and communicate emotions [150–154].
(c) The simultaneous engagement of low threshold (sensitive to light touch) skin receptors from the affective-affiliative system in the mammalian nervous system, primarily composed of C-tactile fibers and/or receptors [155–159], polymodal C-receptors, unmyelinated free nerve endings [160] and the low threshold discriminative-spatial system, associated with Merkel's cell–neurite complex receptors and Ruffini corpuscle proprioceptors [47,137,161–165].
(d) The combination of attentional systems engaged in processing the location and quality of touch, particularly the midline fronto-parietal system activated by the task-positive network, an associative network with extensive bilateral connections with other areas of the brain [127,144,166];

In conclusion, there is significant support for the importance of integrating the orienting reflex in psychotherapy through both physical and non-physical cues. ORs appear to play a mediating role in the improved behavioral outcomes from Calatonia, by initially restoring psychophysical regulation and well-being—and eventually leading to a more positive sense of self. In patients with a history of trauma or attachment issues, this may mean establishing a context of safety within individual boundaries first, through dyadic regulation, before addressing psychological issues that may lead to more feelings of vulnerability [1,167].

Author Contributions: Conceptualization, A.R.B.; writing—original draft preparation, A.R.B.; writing—review and editing, W.E.C.; visualization, A.R.B and W.E.C.; supervision, W.E.C.; project administration, A.R.B. and W.E.C.; funding acquisition, N/A. All authors have read and agreed to the published version of the manuscript.

References

1. Fiskum, C. Psychotherapy Beyond All the Words: Dyadic Expansion, Vagal Regulation, and Biofeedback in Psychotherapy. *J. Psychother. Integr.* **2019**, *29*, 412–425. [CrossRef]
2. Knaster, M. *Discovering the Body's Wisdom: A Comprehensive Guide to more than Fifty Mind-Body Practices That Can Relieve Pain, Reduce Stress, and Foster Health, Spiritual Growth, and Inner Peace*; Bantam: New York, NY, USA, 1996.
3. Van der Kolk, B. *The Body Keeps the Score: Brain, Mind, and Body in the Healing of Trauma*; Penguin Books: New York, NY, USA, 2015.
4. Field, T. *Complementary and Alternative Therapies Research*; American Psychological Association: Washington, DC, USA, 2009.
5. Anderson, J.G.; Taylor, A.G. Effects of Healing Touch in Clinical Practice: A Systematic Review of Randomized Clinical Trials. *J. Holist. Nurs.* **2011**, *29*, 221–228. [CrossRef] [PubMed]
6. Tantia, J.F. Toward a Somatically-Informed Paradigm in Embodied Research. *Int. Body Psychother. J.* **2019**, *18*, 134–145.
7. Bradley, M.M. Natural selective attention: Orienting and emotion. *Psychophysiology* **2009**, *46*, 1–11. [CrossRef] [PubMed]
8. Miller, W. Motivational Interviewing: III. On the Ethics of Motivational Intervention. *Behav. Cogn. Psychother.* **1994**, *22*, 111–123. [CrossRef]
9. Bradley, M.M.; Codispoti, M.; Cuthbert, B.N.; Lang, P. Emotion and Motivation I: Defensive and Appetitive Reactions in Picture Processing. *Emotion* **2001**, *1*, 276–298. [CrossRef]

10. Harmon-Jones, E.; Harmon-Jones, C.; Summerell, E. On the Importance of Both Dimensional and Discrete Models of Emotion. *Behav. Sci.* **2017**, *7*, 66. [CrossRef]
11. Panksepp, J. Neurologizing the psychology of affects: How appraisal-based constructivism and basic emotion theory can coexist. *Perspect. Psychol. Sci.* **2007**, *2*, 281–296. [CrossRef]
12. Weiqi, Z.; Ye, L.; Hong, L.C.; Yu-Hsin, C.; Qian, C.; Xiaolan, F. The Influence of Event Valence and Emotional States on the Metaphorical Comprehension of Time. *Front. Psychol.* **2019**, *10*, 410.
13. Lang, P.J. Emotion and Motivation: Toward Consensus Definitions and a Common Research Purpose. *Emot. Rev.* **2010**, *2*, 229–233. [CrossRef]
14. Vrtička, P.; Vuilleumier, P. Neuroscience of human social interactions and adult attachment style. *Front. Hum. Neurosci.* **2012**, *6*, 212. [CrossRef] [PubMed]
15. Barrós-Loscertales, A.; Ventura-Campos, N.; Sanjuán-Tomás, A.; Belloch, V.; Parcet, M.A.; Avila, C. Behavioral activation system modulation on brain activation during appetitive and aversive stimulus processing. *Soc. Cogn. Affect. Neurosci.* **2010**, *5*, 18–28. [CrossRef] [PubMed]
16. Grossman, S.P. Motivation, Aversive, Biological Bases. In *States of Brain and Mind. Readings from the Encyclopedia of Neuroscience Series*; Hobson, J.A., Ed.; Birkhäuser: Boston, MA, USA, 1988; pp. 63–65.
17. Blanchard, A.R. Calatonia: Novel Insights from Neuroscience. In *Calatonia: A Therapeutic Approach that Promotes Somatic and Psychological Regulation*; Blanchard, A.R., Rios, A.M.G., Seixas, L.P., Eds.; Alma Street Enterprise: Miami, FL, USA, 2019; pp. 286–304.
18. Farah, R. *Calatonia: Subtle Touch in Psychotherapy*; Companhia Ilimitada: São Paulo, Brazil, 2017.
19. Sándor, P. Calatonia. *Bol. De Psicol.* **1969**, *XXI*, 92–100.
20. Sándor, P. Calatonia. In *Calatonia: A Therapeutic Approach that Promotes Somatic and Psychological Regulation*; Blanchard, A.R., Rios, A.M.G., Seixas, L.P., Eds.; Alma Street Enterprise: Miami, FL, USA, 2019; pp. 1–13.
21. Armando, M.D. Calatonia and Resillience. In *Calatonia: A Therapeutic Approach that Promotes Somatic and Psychological Regulation*; Blanchard, A.R., Rios, A.M.G., Seixas, L.P., Eds.; Alma Street Enterprise: Miami, FL, USA, 2019; pp. 263–285.
22. Insel, T.; Cuthbert, B.; Garvey, M.; Heinssen, R.; Pine, D.S.; Quinn, K.; Sanislow, C.; Wang, P. Research domain criteria (RDoC): Toward a new classification framework for research on mental disorders. *Am. J. Psychiatry* **2010**, *167*, 167–748. [CrossRef]
23. Gupta, A.; Love, A.; Kilpatrick, L.A.; Labus, J.S.; Bhatt, R.; Chang, L.; Tillisch, K.; Naliboff, B.; Mayer, E.A. Morphological Brain Measures of Cortico-Limbic Inhibition Related to Resilience. *J. Neurosci. Res.* **2017**, *95*, 1760–1775. [CrossRef]
24. Farah, R. The Academic Teaching of Calatonia. In *Calatonia: A Therapeutic Approach that Promotes Somatic and Psychological Regulation*; Blanchard, A.R., Rios, A.M.G., Seixas, L.P., Eds.; Alma Street Enterprise: Miami, FL, USA, 2019; pp. 26–45.
25. Machado Filho, P.T. The Legacy of Sándor. In *Calatonia: A Therapeutic Approach that Promotes Somatic and Psychological Regulation*; Blanchard, A.R., Rios, A.M.G., Seixas, L.P., Eds.; Alma Street Enterprise: Miami, FL, USA, 2019; pp. 14–25.
26. Kirsch, T. *The Jungians*; Routledge: London, UK, 2000.
27. Delmanto, S. *Subtle Touches: Calatonia, A Life Experience with Pethö Sándor's Work*; Summus: São Paulo, Brazil, 2008.
28. Gonçalves, M.I.C.; Pereira, M.A.; Ribeiro, A.J.; Rios, A.M.G. Subtle touch, calatonia and other somatic interventions with children and adolescents. *Int. Body Psychother. J.* **2007**, *6*, 33–47.
29. Rios, A.M.G.; Seixas, L.P.; Blanchard, A.R. The Body in Psychotherapy: Calatonia and Subtle Touch Techniques. In *Body, Mind, and Healing After Jung: A Space of Questions*; Jones, R., Ed.; Routledge: London, UK, 2010; pp. 228–250.
30. Blanchard, A.R.; Rios, A.M.G.; Seixas, L.P. (Eds.) *Calatonia: A Therapeutic Approach that Promotes Somatic and Psychological Regulation*; Alma Street Enterprise: Miami, FL, USA, 2019.
31. Morrison, I. Keep Calm and Cuddle on: Social Touch as a Stress Buffer. *Adapt. Hum. Behav. Physiol.* **2016**, *2*, 344–362. [CrossRef]
32. Greger Tavares, S.M.; Vannuchi, B.P.; Machado, F.P.T.; Andrade, A.L.M. Efeitos psicofisiológicos da Calatonia em adultos: Um estudo piloto na abordagem quanti-qualitativa. *Jung Corpo* **2015**, *15*, 17–33.

33. Lasaponari, E.F. A Utilização Da Calatonia No Período Pós-Operatório Imediato. Unpublished. Master's Thesis, Nursing School, University of São Paulo, São Paulo, Brazil, 2011. Available online: http://www.teses.usp.br/teses/disponiveis/7/7139/tde-21062011-152045/ (accessed on 6 February 2020).
34. Nossow, V.; Peniche, A.C.G. Paciente cirurgico ambulatorial: Calatonia e ansiedade. *Acta Paul. De Enferm.* **2007**, *20*, 161–167. [CrossRef]
35. Löken, L.S.; Olausson, H. The skin as a social organ. *Exp. Brain Res.* **2010**, *204*, 305–314.
36. Craig, A.D. How do you feel? Interoception: The sense of the physiological condition of the body. *Nat. Rev. Neurosci.* **2002**, *3*, 655–666. [CrossRef] [PubMed]
37. Craig, A.D. Interoception and emotion: A neuroanatomical perspective. In *Handbook of Emotions*; Lewis, M., Haviland-Jones, J.M., Feldman Barrett, L., Eds.; The Guildford Press: New York, NY, USA, 2008; pp. 272–288.
38. Löken, L.S.; Wessberg, J.; Morrison, I.; McGlone, F.; Olausson, H. Coding of pleasant touch by unmyelinated afferents in humans. *Nat. Neurosci.* **2009**, *12*, 547–548. [CrossRef] [PubMed]
39. Moehring, F.; Halder, P.; Seal, R.P.; Stucky, C.L. Uncovering the cells and circuits of touch in normal and pathological settings. *Neuron* **2018**, *100*, 349–360. [CrossRef] [PubMed]
40. Abraham, J.; Mathew, S. Merkel Cells: A Collective Review of Current Concepts. *Int. J. Appl. Basic Med. Res.* **2019**, *9*, 9–13.
41. Chang, W.; Kanda, H.; Ikeda, R.; Ling, J.; DeBerry, J.J.; Gu, J.G. Merkel disc is a serotonergic synapse in the epidermis for transmitting tactile signals in mammals. *Proc. Natl. Acad. Sci. USA* **2016**, *113*, E5491–E5500. [CrossRef] [PubMed]
42. Halata, Z.; Grim, M.; Baumann, K.I. Current understanding of Merkel cells, touch reception and the skin. *Expert Rev. Dermatol.* **2010**, *5*, 109–116. [CrossRef]
43. Johansson, R.S.; Vallbo, A.B. Tactile sensibility in the human hand: Relative and absolute densities of four types of mechanoreceptive units in glabrous skin. *J. Physiol.* **1979**, *286*, 283–300. [CrossRef]
44. Johansson, R.S.; Vallbo, Å.B. Tactile sensory coding in the glabrous skin of the human hand. *Trends Neurosci.* **1983**, *6*, 27–32. [CrossRef]
45. Maksimovic, S.; Baba, Y.; Lumpkin, E.A. Neurotransmitters and synaptic components in the Merkel cell-neurite complex, a gentle touch receptor. *Ann. N. Y. Acad. Sci.* **2013**, *1279*, 13–21. [CrossRef]
46. Maksimovic, S.; Nakatani, M.; Baba, Y.; Nelson, A.M.; Marshall, K.L.; Wellnitz, S.A.; Firozi, P.; Woo, S.H.; Ranade, S.; Patapoutian, A.; et al. Epidermal Merkel cells are mechanosensory cells that tune mammalian touch receptors. *Nature* **2014**, *509*, 617–621. [CrossRef]
47. McGlone, F.; Wessberg, J.; Olausson, H. Discriminative and Affective Touch: Sensing and Feeling. *Neuron* **2014**, *82*, 737–755. [CrossRef] [PubMed]
48. Rolls, E.T. The affective and cognitive processing of touch, oral texture, and temperature in the brain. *Neurosci. Biobehav. Rev.* **2010**, *34*, 237–245. [CrossRef] [PubMed]
49. Hayward, V. A Brief Overview of the Human Somatosensory System. In *Musical Haptics*; Papetti, S., Saitis, C., Eds.; Springer: Cham, Switzerland, 2018; pp. 29–48.
50. Millar, S. *Reading by Touch*; Routledge: New York, NY, USA, 1997.
51. Klooster, N.B.; Cook, S.W.; Uc, E.Y.; Duff, M.C. Gestures make memories, but what kind? Patients with impaired procedural memory display disruptions in gesture production and comprehension. *Front. Hum. Neurosci.* **2015**, *8*, 1054. [CrossRef] [PubMed]
52. Squire, L.R.; Dede, A.J. Conscious and unconscious memory systems. *Cold Spring Harb. Perspect. Biol.* **2015**, *7*, a021667. [CrossRef]
53. Allum, J.H.J.; Bloem, B.R.; Carpenter, M.G.; Hulliger, M.; Hadders-Algra, M. Proprioceptive control of posture: A review of new concepts. *Gait Posture* **1998**, *8*, 214–242. [CrossRef]
54. Drew, T.; Prentice, S.; Schepens, B. Cortical and brainstem control of locomotion. *Prog. Brain Res.* **2004**, *143*, 251–261.
55. Kennedy, P.M.; Inglis, J.T. Distribution and behaviour of glabrous cutaneous receptors in the human foot sole. *J. Physiol.* **2002**, *538*, 995–1002. [CrossRef]
56. Malcuit, G.; Bastien, C.; Pomerleau, A. Habituation of the orienting response to stimuli of different functional values in 4-month-old infants. *J. Exp. Child Psychol.* **1996**, *62*, 272–291. [CrossRef]
57. Buodo, G.; Sarlo, M.; Palomba, D. Attentional resources measured by reaction times highlight differences within pleasant and unpleasant, high arousing stimuli. *Motiv. Emot.* **2002**, *26*, 123–138. [CrossRef]

58. Fan, J.; McCandliss, B.D.; Fossella, J.; Flombaum, J.I.; Posner, M. The activation of attentional networks. *NeuroImage* **2005**, *26*, 471–479. [CrossRef]
59. Lang, P.J.; Bradley, M.M. Appetitive and Defensive Motivation: Goal-Directed or Goal-Determined? *Emot. Rev. J. Int. Soc. Res. Emot.* **2013**, *5*, 230–234. [CrossRef] [PubMed]
60. Posner, M.I.; Petersen, S.E. The Attention System of the Human Brain. *Annu. Rev. Neurosci.* **2003**, *13*, 25–42. [CrossRef] [PubMed]
61. Ross-Sheehy, S.; Schneegans, S.; Spencer, J.P. The Infant Orienting with Attention task: Assessing the neural basis of spatial attention in infancy. *Infancy Off. J. Int. Soc. Infant Stud.* **2015**, *20*, 467–506. [CrossRef] [PubMed]
62. Williams, L.M.; Brammer, M.J.; Skerrett, D.; Lagopolous, J.; Rennie, C.; Kozek, K.; Olivieri, G.; Peduto, T.; Gordon, E. The neural correlates of orienting: An integration of fMRI and skin conductance orienting. *Neuroreport* **2000**, *11*, 3011–3015. [CrossRef] [PubMed]
63. Geva, R.; Zivan, M.; Warsha, A.; Olchik, D. Alerting, orienting or executive attention networks: Differential patterns of pupil dilations. *Front. Behav. Neurosci.* **2013**, *7*, 145. [CrossRef]
64. Posner, M.I. *Attention in the Social World*; Oxford University Press: New York, NY, USA, 2012.
65. Posner, M.I. Attentional networks and consciousness. *Front. Psychol.* **2012**, *3*, 64. [CrossRef]
66. Pavlov, I.P. *Conditioned Reflexes*; Oxford University Press: Oxford, UK, 1927.
67. Loewenstein, G. The psychology of curiosity: A review and reinterpretation. *Psychol. Bull.* **1994**, *116*, 75–98. [CrossRef]
68. DeGangi, G.A. *The Dysregulated Adult: Integrated Treatment Approaches*; Academic Press: Cambridge, MA, USA, 2012.
69. DeGangi, G.A. *Pediatric Disorders of Regulation in Affect and Behavior: A Therapist's Guide to Assessment and Treatment*; Academic Press: Cambridge, MA, USA, 2017.
70. Sokolov, E.N. *Perception and the Conditioned Reflex*; Macmillan: New York, NY, USA, 1963.
71. Bradley, M.M.; Keil, A.; Lang, P.J. Orienting and Emotional Perception: Facilitation, Attenuation, and Interference. *Front. Psychol.* **2012**, *3*, 493. [CrossRef]
72. Graham, F.K.; Clifton, R.K. Heart-rate change as a component of the orienting response. *Psychol. Bull.* **1966**, *65*, 305–320. [CrossRef]
73. Bernstein, A.S. The Orienting Response as Novelty and Significance Detector: Reply to O'Gorman. *Psychophysiology* **1979**, *16*, 263–273. [CrossRef]
74. Sambo, C.F.; Forster, B. Sustained Spatial Attention in Touch: Modality-Specific and Multimodal Mechanisms. *Sci. World J.* **2011**, *11*, 199–213. [CrossRef] [PubMed]
75. Engbert, K.; Wohlschläger, A.; Haggard, P. Who is causing what? The sense of agency is relational and efferent-triggered. *Cognition* **2008**, *107*, 693–704. [CrossRef] [PubMed]
76. Mangalam, M.; Cutts, S.A.; Fragaszy, D.M. Sense of ownership and not the sense of agency is spatially bounded within the space reachable with the unaugmented hand. *Exp. Brain Res.* **2019**, *237*, 2911–2924. [CrossRef] [PubMed]
77. Tsakiris, M.; Schütz-Bosbach, S.; Gallagher, S. On agency and body-ownership: Phenomenological and neurocognitive reflections. *Conscious. Cogn.* **2007**, *16*, 645–660. [CrossRef]
78. Tomkins, S. *Affect Imagery Consciousness, Vol I: The Positive Affects*; Springer: New York, NY, USA, 1962.
79. Stevens, C.; Bavelier, D. The role of selective attention on academic foundations: A cognitive neuroscience perspective. *Dev. Cogn. Neurosci.* **2012**, *2*, S30–S48. [CrossRef] [PubMed]
80. Harjunen, V.J.; Spapé, M.; Ahmed, I.; Jacucci, G.; Ravaja, N. Individual differences in affective touch: Behavioral inhibition and gender define how an interpersonal touch is perceived. *Personal. Individ. Differ.* **2017**, *107*, 88–95. [CrossRef]
81. Parvizi, J.; Damasio, A. Consciousness and the brain-stem. *Cognition* **2001**, *79*, 135–160. [CrossRef]
82. Martins, I.; Tavares, I. Reticular Formation and Pain: The Past and the Future. *Front. Neuroanat.* **2017**, *11*, 51. [CrossRef]
83. Neugebauer, V. Chapter 15: Amygdala pain mechanisms. In *Handbook of Experimental Pharmacology*; Barrett, J.E., Ed.; Springer: New York, NY, USA, 2015; pp. 261–284.
84. Venkatraman, A.; Edlow, B.L.; Immordino-Yang, M.H. The Brainstem in Emotion: A Review. *Front. Neuroanat.* **2017**, *11*, 15. [CrossRef]

85. Youssef, A.M.; Macefield, V.G.; Henderson, L.A. Cortical influences on brainstem circuitry responsible for conditioned pain modulation in humans. *Hum. Brain Mapp.* **2016**, *37*, 2630–2644. [CrossRef]
86. Bremner, J.D. Traumatic stress: Effects on the brain. *Dialogues Clin. Neurosci.* **2006**, *8*, 445–461. [PubMed]
87. Jeewajee, A.; Lever, C.; Burton, S.; O'Keefe, J.; Burgess, N. Environmental novelty is signaled by reduction of the hippocampal theta frequency. *Hippocampus* **2008**, *18*, 340–348. [CrossRef] [PubMed]
88. Uddin, L.Q.; Nomi, J.S.; Hébert-Seropian, B.; Ghaziri, J.; Boucher, O. Structure and Function of the Human Insula. *J. Clin. Neurophysiol.* **2017**, *34*, 300–306. [CrossRef] [PubMed]
89. Howe, M.L.; Cicchetti, D.; Toth, S.L. Children's basic memory processes, stress, and maltreatment. *Dev. Psychopathol.* **2006**, *18*, 759–769. [CrossRef]
90. Balderston, N.L.; Schultz, D.H.; Helmstetter, F.J. The human amygdala plays a stimulus specific role in the detection of novelty. *NeuroImage* **2011**, *55*, 1889–1898. [CrossRef] [PubMed]
91. Bonnet, L.; Comte, A.; Tatu, L.; Millot, J.-L.; Moulin, T.; Medeiros de Bustos, E. The role of the amygdala in the perception of positive emotions: An "intensity detector". *Front. Behav. Neurosci.* **2015**, *9*, 178. [CrossRef]
92. Morrison, S.E.; Salzman, C.D. Revaluing the amygdala. *Curr. Opin. Neurobiol.* **2010**, *20*, 221–230. [CrossRef]
93. Murray, E.A. The amygdala, reward and emotion. *Trends Cogn. Sci.* **2007**, *11*, 489–497. [CrossRef]
94. Weymar, M.; Schwabe, L. Amygdala and Emotion: The Bright Side of It. *Front. Neurosci.* **2016**, *10*, 224. [CrossRef]
95. Phelps, E.A.; LeDoux, J.E. Contributions of the amygdala to emotion processing: From animal models to human behavior. *Neuron* **2005**, *48*, 175–187. [CrossRef]
96. Vasa, R.A.; Pine, D.S.; Thorn, J.M.; Nelson, T.E.; Spinelli, S.; Nelson, E.; Maheu, F.S.; Ernst, M.; Bruck, M.; Mostofsky, S.H. Enhanced Right Amygdala Activity in Adolescents during Encoding of Positively-Valenced Pictures. *Dev. Cogn. Neurosci.* **2011**, *1*, 88–99. [CrossRef] [PubMed]
97. Scherer, K.R. Emotions are emergent processes: They require a dynamic computational architecture. *Philos. Trans. R. Soc. B Biol. Sci.* **2009**, *364*, 3459–3474. [CrossRef] [PubMed]
98. Blackford, J.U.; Buckholtz, J.W.; Avery, S.N.; Zald, D.H. A unique role for the human amygdala in novelty detection. *NeuroImage* **2010**, *50*, 1188–1193. [CrossRef] [PubMed]
99. Vuilleumier, P. How brains beware: Neural mechanisms of emotional attention. *Trends Cogn. Sci.* **2005**, *9*, 585–594. [CrossRef]
100. Lang, P.J.; Bradley, M.M. Emotion and the motivational brain. *Biol. Psychol.* **2010**, *84*, 437–450. [CrossRef]
101. Schomaker, J.; Rangel-Gomez, M.; Meeter, M. Happier, faster: Developmental changes in the effects of mood and novelty on responses. *Q. J. Exp. Psychol.* **2016**, *69*, 37–47. [CrossRef]
102. Hammer, N.; Glätzner, J.; Feja, C.; Kühne, C.; Meixensberger, J.; Planitzer, U.; Schleifenbaum, S.; Tillmann, B.N.; Winkler, D. Human vagus nerve branching in the cervical region. *PLoS ONE* **2015**, *10*, e0118006. [CrossRef]
103. Keding, T.J.; Herringa, R.J. Paradoxical Prefrontal—Amygdala Recruitment to Angry and Happy Expressions in Pediatric Posttraumatic Stress Disorder. *Neuropsychopharmacology* **2016**, *41*, 2903–2912. [CrossRef]
104. Marusak, H.A.; Martin, K.R.; Etkin, A.; Thomason, M.E. Childhood Trauma Exposure Disrupts the Automatic Regulation of Emotional Processing. *Neuropsychopharmacology* **2015**, *40*, 1250–1258. [CrossRef]
105. White, S.F.; Costanzo, M.E.; Blair, J.R.; Roy, M.J. PTSD symptom severity is associated with increased recruitment of top-down attentional control in a trauma-exposed sample. *Neuroimage Clin.* **2015**, *7*, 19–27. [CrossRef]
106. Streeck-Fischer, A.; van der Kolk, B.A. Down will come baby, cradle and all: Diagnostic and therapeutic implications of chronic trauma on child development. *Aust. N. Z. J. Psychiatry* **2000**, *34*, 903–918. [CrossRef] [PubMed]
107. Block, S.R.; King, A.P.; Sripada, R.K.; Weissman, D.H.; Welsh, R.; Liberzon, I. Behavioral and neural correlates of disrupted orienting attention in posttraumatic stress disorder. *Cogn. Affect. Behav. Neurosci.* **2017**, *17*, 422–436. [CrossRef] [PubMed]
108. Teicher, M.H.; Alaptagin, K. Childhood maltreatment, cortical and amygdala morphometry, functional connectivity, laterality, and psychopathology. *Child Maltreat.* **2019**, *24*, 458–465. [CrossRef] [PubMed]
109. Butler, O.; Adolf, J.; Gleich, T.; Willmund, G.; Zimmermann, P.; Lindenberger, U.; Gallinat, J.; Kühn, S. Military deployment correlates with smaller prefrontal gray matter volume and psychological symptoms in a subclinical population. *Transl. Psychiatry* **2017**, *7*, e1031. [CrossRef]

110. Kim, S.; Kim, J.S.; Jin, M.J.; Im, C.-H.; Lee, S.-H. Dysfunctional frontal lobe activity during inhibitory tasks in individuals with childhood trauma: An event-related potential study. *Neuroimage Clin.* **2018**, *17*, 935–942. [CrossRef]
111. Sherin, J.E.; Nemeroff, C.B. Post-traumatic stress disorder: The neurobiological impact of psychological trauma. *Dialogues Clin. Neurosci.* **2011**, *13*, 263–278.
112. Herbert, C. Calatonia and Subtle Touch in the Healing of Trauma. In *Calatonia: A Therapeutic Approach that Promotes Somatic and Psychological Regulation*; Blanchard, A.R., Rios, A.M.G., Seixas, L.P., Eds.; Alma Street Enterprise: Miami, FL, USA, 2019; pp. 70–86.
113. Herbert, C. *Overcoming Traumatic Stress—A Self-Help Guide Using Cognitive Behavioural Techniques*; Robinson, Little Brown Book Group: London, UK, 2017.
114. Resick, P.A.; Monson, C.M.; Chard, K.M. *Cognitive Processing Therapy for PTSD: A Comprehensive Manual*; Guilford Press: New York, NY, USA, 2016.
115. Ogden, P.; Minton, K.; Pain, C. *Trauma and the Body: A Sensory Motor Approach to Therapy*; W.W. Norton: New York, NY, USA, 2006.
116. Payne, P.; Levine, P.A.; Crane-Godreau, M.A. Somatic experiencing: Using interoception and proprioception as core elements of trauma therapy. *Front. Psychol.* **2015**, *6*, 93.
117. Shapiro, F.; Forrest, M.S. *EMDR: The Break-Through Therapy for Overcoming Anxiety, Stress, and Trauma*; Basic Books: New York, NY, USA, 2004.
118. Seidler, G.H.; Wagner, F.E. Comparing the efficacy of EMDR and trauma-focused cognitive-behavioral therapy in the treatment of PTSD: A meta-analytic study. *Psychol. Med.* **2006**, *36*, 1515–1522. [CrossRef]
119. Patihis, L.; Cruz, C.S.; McNally, R.J. Eye Movement Desensitization and Reprocessing (EMDR). In *Encyclopedia of Personality & Individual Differences*; Zeigler-Hill, V., Shackelford, T.K., Eds.; Springer: New York, NY, USA, 2017.
120. Chamberlin, D.E. The Predictive Processing Model of EMDR. *Front. Psychol.* **2019**, *10*, 2267. [CrossRef]
121. Friston, K. The free-energy principle: A rough guide to the brain? *Trends Cogn. Sci.* **2009**, *13*, 293–301. [CrossRef]
122. Sokolov, E.N.; Spinks, J.A.; Naatanen, R.; Lyytinen, H. *The Orienting Response in Information Processing*; Lawrence Erlbaum: Mahwah, NJ, USA, 2002.
123. Torta, D.M.; Liang, M.; Valentini, E.; Mouraux, A.; Iannetti, G.D. Dishabituation of laser-evoked EEG responses: Dissecting the effect of certain and uncertain changes in stimulus spatial location. *Exp. Brain Res.* **2012**, *218*, 361–372. [CrossRef] [PubMed]
124. Schomaker, J.; Meeter, M. Short- and long-lasting consequences of novelty, deviance and surprise on brain and cognition. *Neurosci. Biobehav. Rev.* **2015**, *55*, 268–279. [CrossRef] [PubMed]
125. Harshaw, C. Interoceptive dysfunction: Toward an integrated framework for understanding somatic and affective disturbance in depression. *Psychol. Bull.* **2015**, *141*, 311–363. [CrossRef] [PubMed]
126. Kang, L.; Zhang, A.; Sun, N.; Liu, P.; Yang, C.; Li, G.; Liu, Z.; Wang, Y.; Zhang, K. Functional connectivity between the thalamus and the primary somatosensory cortex in major depressive disorder: A resting-state fMRI study. *BMC Psychiatry* **2018**, *18*, 339. [CrossRef] [PubMed]
127. Daffner, K.R.; Scinto, L.F.; Weitzman, A.M.; Faust, R.; Rentz, D.M.; Budson, A.E.; Holcomb, P.J. Frontal and parietal components of a cerebral network mediating voluntary attention to novel events. *J. Cogn. Neurosci.* **2003**, *15*, 294–313. [CrossRef]
128. Cacioppo, S.; Zhou, H.; Monteleone, G.; Majka, E.A.; Quinn, K.A.; Ball, A.B.; Norman, G.J.; Semin, G.R.; Cacioppo, J.T. You are in sync with me: Neural correlates of interpersonal synchrony with a partner. *Neuroscience* **2014**, *277*, 842–858. [CrossRef]
129. Dumas, G.; Nadel, J.; Soussignan, R.; Martinerie, J.; Garnero, L. Inter-brain synchronization during social interaction. *PLoS ONE* **2010**, *5*, e12166. [CrossRef]
130. Hove, M.J.; Risen, J.L. It's All in the Timing: Interpersonal Synchrony Increases Affiliation. *Soc. Cogn.* **2009**, *27*, 949–960. [CrossRef]
131. Hu, Y.; Hu, Y.; Li, X.; Pan, Y.; Cheng, X. Brain-to-brain synchronization across two persons predicts mutual prosociality. *Soc. Cogn. Affect. Neurosci.* **2017**, *12*, 1835–1844. [CrossRef]
132. Mu, Y.; Guo, C.; Han, S. Oxytocin enhances inter-brain synchrony during social coordination in male adults. *Soc. Cogn. Affect. Neurosci.* **2016**, *11*, 1882–1893. [CrossRef]

133. Koole, S.L.; Tschacher, W. Synchrony in Psychotherapy: A Review and an Integrative Framework for the Therapeutic Alliance. *Front. Psychol.* **2016**, *7*, 862. [CrossRef] [PubMed]
134. Schore, A.N. Relational trauma and the developing right brain: An interface of psychoanalytic self-psychology and neuroscience. *Ann. N. Y. Acad. Sci.* **2009**, *1159*, 189–203. [CrossRef] [PubMed]
135. Siegel, D.J. *The Developing Mind*; The Guilford Press: New York, NY, USA, 2012.
136. Jones, S.R. When brain rhythms aren't 'rhythmic': Implication for their mechanisms and meaning. *Curr. Opin. Neurobiol.* **2016**, *40*, 72–80. [CrossRef] [PubMed]
137. Ciaunica, A.; Fotopoulou, A. The touched self: Psychological and philosophical perspectives on proximal intersubjectivity and the self. In *Embodiment, Enaction, and Culture: Investigating the Constitution of the Shared World*; Durt, C., Fuchs, T., Tewes, C., Eds.; MIT Press: Cambridge, MA, USA, 2017; pp. 173–192.
138. Hallam, G.P.; Webb, T.L.; Sheeran, P.; Miles, E.; Niven, K.; Wilkinson, I.D.; Hunter, M.D.; Woodruff, P.W.; Totterdell, P.; Farrow, T.F. The neural correlates of regulating another person's emotions: An exploratory fMRI study. *Front. Hum. Neurosci.* **2014**, *8*, 376. [CrossRef] [PubMed]
139. Naruse, K.; Hirai, T. Effects of slow tempo exercise on respiration, heart rate, and mood state. *Percept. Mot. Ski.* **2000**, *91*, 729–740. [CrossRef]
140. Szirmai, I. How does the brain create rhythms? *Ideggyógy. Szle.* **2010**, *63*, 13–23.
141. Deco, G.; Kringelbach, M.L.; Jirsa, V.K.; Ritter, P. The dynamics of resting fluctuations in the brain: Metastability and its dynamical cortical core. *Sci. Rep.* **2017**, *7*, 1–14. [CrossRef]
142. Smallwood, J.; Schooler, J.W. The Science of Mind Wandering: Empirically Navigating the Stream of Consciousness. *Annu. Rev. Psychol.* **2015**, *66*, 487–518. [CrossRef]
143. Bell, P.T.; Shine, J.M. Subcortical contributions to large-scale network communication. *Neurosci. Biobehav. Rev.* **2016**, *71*, 313–322. [CrossRef]
144. Goldberg, I.I.; Harel, M.; Malach, R. When the Brain Loses Its Self: Prefrontal Inactivation during Sensorimotor Processing. *Neuron* **2006**, *50*, 329–339. [CrossRef]
145. Gollo, L.L.; Zalesky, A.; Hutchison, R.M.; van den Heuvel, M.; Breakspear, M. Dwelling quietly in the rich club: Brain network determinants of slow cortical fluctuations. *Philos. Trans. R. Soc. Lond. Ser. B Biol. Sci.* **2015**, *370*, 20140165. [CrossRef] [PubMed]
146. Hari, R.; Parkkonen, L. The brain timewise: How timing shapes and supports brain function. *Philos. Trans. R. Soc. Lond. Ser. B Biol. Sci.* **2015**, *370*, 20140170. [CrossRef] [PubMed]
147. Kaiser, R.H.; Andrews-Hanna, J.R.; Wager, T.D.; Pizzagalli, D.A. Large-Scale Network Dysfunction in Major Depressive Disorder: A Meta-analysis of Resting-State Functional Connectivity. *JAMA Psychiatry* **2015**, *72*, 603–611. [CrossRef] [PubMed]
148. Park, H.J.; Friston, K. Structural and functional brain networks: From connections to cognition. *Science* **2013**, *342*, 1238411. [CrossRef]
149. Santangelo, V. Large-Scale brain networks supporting divided attention across spatial locations and sensory modalities. *Front. Integr. Neurosci.* **2018**, *12*, 8. [CrossRef] [PubMed]
150. Compton, R.J.; Carp, J.; Chaddock, L.; Fineman, S.L.; Quandt, L.C.; Ratliff, J.B. Trouble Crossing the Bridge: Altered Interhemispheric Communication of Emotional Images in Anxiety. *Emotion* **2008**, *8*, 684–692. [CrossRef] [PubMed]
151. Compton, R.J.; Feigenson, K.; Widick, P. Take it to the bridge: An interhemispheric processing advantage for emotional faces. *Cogn. Brain Res.* **2005**, *24*, 66–72. [CrossRef] [PubMed]
152. Hearne, L.J.; Dean, R.J.; Robinson, G.A.; Richards, L.J.; Mattingley, J.B.; Cocchi, L. Increased cognitive complexity reveals abnormal brain network activity in individuals with corpus callosum dysgenesis. *Neuroimage Clin.* **2019**, *21*, 101595. [CrossRef] [PubMed]
153. Roland, J.L.; Snyder, A.Z.; Hacker, C.D.; Mitra, A.; Shimony, J.S.; Limbrick, D.D.; Raichle, M.E.; Smyth, M.D.; Leuthardt, E.C. On the role of the corpus callosum in interhemispheric functional connectivity in humans. *Proc. Natl. Acad. Sci. USA* **2017**, *114*, 13278–13283. [CrossRef]
154. Skumlien, M.; Sederevicius, D.; Fjell, A.M.; Walhovd, K.B.; Westerhausen, R. Parallel but independent reduction of emotional awareness and corpus callosum connectivity in older age. *PLoS ONE* **2018**, *13*, e0209915. [CrossRef]
155. Brauer, J.; Xiao, Y.; Poulain, T.; Friederici, A.D.; Schirmer, A. Frequency of Maternal Touch Predicts Resting Activity and Connectivity of the Developing Social Brain. *Cereb. Cortex* **2016**, *26*, 3544–3552. [CrossRef] [PubMed]

156. Iggo, A. Cutaneous mechanoreceptors with afferent C fibres. *J. Physiol.* **1960**, *152*, 337–353. [CrossRef] [PubMed]
157. Iggo, A.; Muir, A.R. The structure and function of a slowly adapting touch corpuscle in hairy skin. *J. Physiol.* **1969**, *200*, 763–796. [CrossRef] [PubMed]
158. Olausson, H.; Lamarre, Y.; Backlund, H.; Morin, C.; Wallin, B.G.; Starck, G.; Ekholm, S.; Strigo, I.; Worsley, K.; Vallbo, Å.B.; et al. Unmyelinated tactile afferents signal touch and project to insular cortex. *Nat. Neurosci.* **2002**, *5*, 900–904. [CrossRef]
159. Olausson, H.; Wessberg, J.; Morrison, I.; McGlone, F.; Vallbo, Å. The neurophysiology of unmyelinated tactile afferents. *Neurosci. Biobehav. Rev.* **2010**, *34*, 185–191. [CrossRef]
160. Monroe, C.M. The effects of therapeutic touch on pain. *J. Holist. Nurs. Off. J. Am. Holist. Nurses' Assoc.* **2009**, *27*, 85–92. [CrossRef]
161. Birznieks, I.; Macefield, V.G.; Westling, G.; Johansson, R.S. Slowly Adapting Mechanoreceptors in the Borders of the Human Fingernail Encode Fingertip Forces. *J. Neurosci.* **2009**, *29*, 9370–9379. [CrossRef]
162. Ebisch, S.J.; Salone, A.; Martinotti, G.; Carlucci, L.; Mantini, D.; Perrucci, M.G.; Saggino, A.; Romani, G.L.; Di Giannantonio, M.; Northoff, G.; et al. Integrative Processing of Touch and Affect in Social Perception: An fMRI Study. *Front. Hum. Neurosci.* **2016**, *10*, 209. [CrossRef]
163. Grion, N.; Akrami, A.; Zuo, Y.; Stella, F.; Diamond, M.E. Coherence between Rat sensorimotor system and hippocampus is enhanced during tactile discrimination. *PLoS Biol.* **2016**, *14*, e1002384. [CrossRef]
164. Macefield, V.G. Physiological characteristics of lowthreshold mechanoreceptors in joints, muscle and skin in human subjects. *Clin. Exp. Pharmacol. Physiol.* **2005**, *32*, 135–144. [CrossRef]
165. Mountcastle, V.C. *The Sensory Hand: Neural Mechanisms of Somatic Sensation*; Harvard University Press: Harvard, MA, USA, 2005.
166. Rushworth, M.F.S.; Paus, T.; Sipila, P.K. Attention systems and the organization of the human parietal cortex. *NeuroImage* **2001**, *13*, 353. [CrossRef]
167. O'Brien, K.M.; Afzal, K.; Tronick, E. Relational psychophysiology and mutual regulation during dyadic therapeutic and developmental relating. In *Interdisciplinary Handbook of the Person-Centered Approach*; Cornelius-White, J., Motschnig-Pitrik, R., Lux, M., Eds.; Springer: New York, NY, USA, 2013; pp. 183–197.

3

Suicide in Schizophrenia: An Educational Overview

Leo Sher [1,2,*] **and René S. Kahn** [1,2]

1 James J. Peters Veterans' Administration Medical Center, Bronx, New York, NY 10468, USA
2 Icahn School of Medicine at Mount Sinai, New York, NY 10029, USA
* Correspondence: Leo.Sher@mssm.edu;

Abstract: Suicide is an important public health problem. The most frequent psychiatric illnesses associated with suicide or severe suicide attempt are mood and psychotic disorders. The purpose of this paper is to provide an educational overview of suicidal behavior in individuals with schizophrenia. A lifetime suicide rate in individuals with schizophrenia is approximately 10%. Suicide is the largest contributor to the decreased life expectancy in individuals with schizophrenia. Demographic and psychosocial factors that increase a risk of suicide in individuals with schizophrenia include younger age, being male, being unmarried, living alone, being unemployed, being intelligent, being well-educated, good premorbid adjustment or functioning, having high personal expectations and hopes, having an understanding that life's expectations and hopes are not likely to be met, having had recent (i.e., within past 3 months) life events, having poor work functioning, and having access to lethal means, such as firearms. Throughout the first decade of their disorder, patients with schizophrenia are at substantially elevated suicide risk, although they continue to be at elevated suicide risk during their lives with times of worsening or improvement. Having awareness of symptoms, especially, awareness of delusions, anhedonia, asociality, and blunted affect, having a negative feeling about, or non-adherence with, treatment are associated with greater suicide risk in patients with schizophrenia. Comorbid depression and a history of suicidal behavior are important contributors to suicide risk in patients with schizophrenia. The only reliable protective factor for suicide in patients with schizophrenia is provision of and compliance with comprehensive treatment. Prevention of suicidal behavior in schizophrenia should include recognizing patients at risk, delivering the best possible therapy for psychotic symptoms, and managing comorbid depression and substance misuse.

Keywords: suicide; schizophrenia; antipsychotics; depression

---

1. Suicide as a Medical and Social Problem

Suicide is an important public health problem [1,2]. According to the World health Organization (WHO), each year, about one million people die by suicide across the world [1]. It implies that every 40 s, an individual dies by suicide someplace on the globe and many more people make non-lethal suicide attempts. It has been proposed that the number of persons who make non-lethal suicide attempts is about 10–15 times the amount of people who die by suicide. Deaths by suicide and non-lethal suicide attempts greatly affect families, communities, and societies. In the United States, the expenses of managing suicide attempters and examining deaths by suicide have been assessed as being $190 million per year [3]. A recent study showed that non-lethal suicide attempts are associated with decreased life span [4]. It is worth noting that this study found that most additional deaths are attributable to physical/medical conditions.

Rates of suicide death are very significant in many countries across the world [1]. A report issued in November 2018 by the United States Centers for Disease Control and Prevention indicates that from 1999 through 2017, the age-adjusted rate of suicide in the United States rose 33% from 10.5 to 14.0 per 100,000 [5]. It is possible that suicide rates are underestimated. A lot of suicide deaths may be wrongly recorded as 'unnatural' or 'undetermined' deaths. Actual suicide rates may well be 10%–50% higher than reported.

Globally, men die by suicide 3–7 times more often than women [1,6]. The sex dissimilarities in suicide rates are particularly substantial in Eastern European nations [1,6]. In the United States, in 2017, the age-adjusted suicide rate for men (22.4 per 100,000) was 3.67 times larger than for women (6.1 per 100,000) [5].

Studies in the U.S. suggest that more than 90% of victims of suicide have a psychiatric disorder [2,7–9]. Furthermore, most people who attempt suicide have a psychiatric disorder. The most frequent psychiatric illnesses associated with suicide or severe suicide attempt are mood and psychotic disorders [2,7–10]. A 5-year follow-up study of 1065 patients with psychotic disorders conducted by the World Health Organization (WHO) found that "the risk for suicide in schizophrenia is as great, if not greater, than the risk of suicide associated with affective disorders" [11]. Alcohol and drug abuse, anxiety and personality disorders are also associated with an elevated suicide risk [12–15].

Medical disorders, particularly illnesses associated with chronic pain, significantly increase suicide risk [16–20]. While many deaths due to opioid overdoses are accidental, an increasing amount of data indicates that the presence of pain plays a role in the decision to end life via opioid overdoses [19]. Neurological conditions such as stroke, epilepsy, head injury, or Huntington's disease also confer greater suicide risk [20,21]. Obstacles to preventing suicidal behavior include inadequate rates of detection of persons with psychiatric illnesses, insufficient dissemination of evidence-based methods among community providers, and enormous complexity in detecting imminent suicide risk, even in persons who are being cared for psychiatric conditions [22,23].

Adolescence is a period of transition from childhood to adulthood and also, a time of increased vulnerability to psychiatric disorders including psychotic disorders [24]. A systematic review suggests that the number of adversities or negative life events experienced by adolescents appear to have a positive dose–response relationship with youth suicidal behavior [25]. Hence, traumatic experiences during adolescence may contribute to the pathophysiology of both psychotic disorders and suicidal behavior.

The purpose of this paper is to provide an educational overview of suicidal behavior in individuals with schizophrenia. Most literature searches were performed using the PubMed database.

2. Epidemiology of Suicidal Behavior in Schizophrenia

As early as 1911, E. Bleuler characterized "the suicidal drive" as the "most serious of all schizophrenic symptoms" [26]. In 1919, Kraepelin stated that suicide happened in both acute and chronic stages of schizophrenia [27]. In 1939, before contemporary treatments became available, Rennie [28] observed that 11 percent of 500 patients with schizophrenia had died by suicide throughout a 20-year follow-up period.

Contemporary research studies indicate that a lifetime rate of suicide in individuals with schizophrenia is between 4% and 13%, while the modal rate is about 10% [29]. The reported rates of suicide attempts in patients with schizophrenia vary between from 18% to 55% [29–31].

Considerable evidence suggests that schizophrenia decreases the longevity by about 10 years [32]. Suicide is the largest contributor to the decreased life expectancy in individuals with schizophrenia. Recognition of suicide risk factors in patients with schizophrenia is vital in order to enhance patient treatment and advance approaches to decrease the incidence of suicide in patients with schizophrenia.

3. Demographic and Psychosocial Risk Factors

Studies and observations suggest that the following demographic and psychosocial factors increase the risk of suicide in individuals with schizophrenia [10,29,33–36]:

- Younger age
- Being male

- Being unmarried
- Living alone
- Being unemployed
- Being intelligent
- Being well-educated
- Good premorbid adjustment or functioning
- Having high personal expectations and hopes
- Having an understanding that life's expectations and hopes are not likely to be met
- Having had recent (i.e., within past 3 months) life events
- Having poor work functioning
- Having access to lethal means, such as firearms

Studies have demonstrated that suicidal behavior takes place when patients with schizophrenia are younger than age 45 years [37–39]. However, this association is probably more related to the onset of schizophrenia than to age itself.

Similar to the general population and patients with other psychiatric disorders, males with schizophrenia die by suicide more frequently than females with schizophrenia, but the gender difference among suicide victims with schizophrenia is considerably less (60% vs. 40%) [40–42]. Unlike the general population in which females usually make more non-lethal suicide acts than do men, rates of suicide attempts among individuals with schizophrenia have not been found to differ by gender [42–44].

Being single and being unemployed are suicide risk factors for individuals with schizophrenia [29,33,34,42,45]. Some researchers believe that there is a problem with interpreting these findings because most persons with schizophrenia are single and unemployed.

4. Risk Factors Related to Symptomatology and the Course of Illness

Throughout the first decade of their disorder, patients with schizophrenia are at substantially elevated suicide risk, although they continue to be at elevated suicide risk during their lives, with times of worsening or improvement [33,42,46]. Excess mortality due to suicide during the 40-year follow up of 200 patients with schizophrenia was as follows: 44 percent of the patients with schizophrenia who died by suicide committed suicide during the first decade of observation, 22 percent during the second decade, and another 22 percent during the third decade [47].

Studies indicate that suicide risk is significantly elevated during the first psychotic break [29,46,48–50]. Research of first-episode patients usually has higher estimations of suicide rates than studies with lengthier follow up periods. It has been noted that during early stages of schizophrenia, limited suicidal ideation may quickly intensify to a suicide attempt. A delay in getting psychiatric treatment may substantially contribute to elevated suicide risk early in the course of schizophrenia. Other suicide risk factors early in the course of schizophrenia include earlier age of the onset of psychotic symptoms, female sex, suicidal plans, a history of suicide attempt, seriousness of psychiatric pathology, a history of emotional trauma, and decent insight. Suicidality during the first psychotic episode is associated with a good understanding of the situation and beliefs about bad outcomes for psychotic conditions.

Having had an earlier age of onset, being in an early part of the course of illness, having awareness of symptoms, especially, awareness of delusions, anhedonia, asociality, and blunted affect, having a negative feeling about, or non-adherence with, treatment are associated with greater suicide risk in patients with schizophrenia [33,51–53]. In addition, a number of psychiatric admissions is an important suicide risk factor in both inpatients and outpatients with schizophrenia [35,51].

Recurrent relapses, a significant severity of the disease, a descending shift in societal and occupational functioning, and a true and realistic understanding of the harmful influence of the disorder are regarded as schizophrenia-specific suicide risk factors [10]. Patients with the paranoid subtype of schizophrenia are eight times more likely to die by suicide in comparison with patients with the deficit subtype of schizophrenia [54]. Delusions are associated with more suicidal behavior in individuals with schizophrenia [53]. A research report indicates that hostility at hospital admission is linked with long-term suicidal risk [54].

Lack of adherence to antipsychotic drugs may increase suicide risk [53,55]. For example, a large follow-up study of patients released from hospitals after a hospitalization related to the first episode of schizophrenia showed that not getting antipsychotic drugs led to a 12-fold rise in the relative risk of all-cause mortality and a 37-fold rise in suicide mortality [55].

It is important to note that as a result of psychotic disorganization, an individual with schizophrenia may be involved in very unsafe, risky behavior without understanding otherwise predictable threats [29]. Such behavior may look like suicidal behavior.

5. Risk Factors Related to Comorbid Disorders

Comorbid depression and a history of suicidal behavior are important contributors to suicide risk in patients with schizophrenia [33,53,56]. One study showed that depressive symptoms, suicidal ideation and plans and a history of suicide attempts are amongst the most important forecasters of suicidal behavior in the early phases of schizophrenia [57]. Two studies suggest that patients with schizophrenia who were hospitalized after a suicide attempt had the greatest risk, of all variables examined, of dying by suicide [58,59]. Other works also indicate that suicide risk in individuals with schizophrenia is associated with mood syndromes, especially depressed mood, hopelessness and demoralization [29,33,53,60]. Panic symptoms may also contribute to suicidal behavior in patients with schizophrenia [61].

A systematic review indicates that four investigations recognized alcohol abuse as a predisposing aspect to suicidal behavior amongst individuals with schizophrenia, while three investigations recognized substance use disorders and one research investigation recognized smoking only [53]. However, one study has shown that neither alcohol nor drug abuse elevates suicide risk in individuals with schizophrenia [62]. Furthermore, a research group observed that abuse of stimulants, such as cocaine or amphetamine increases the risk of suicidal behavior in schizophrenia [63]. As noted above, the presence of medical and/or neurological disorders may increase suicide risk [16–21].

6. Risk Factors Related to Antipsychotic Medications

Some observations suggest that the side effects of antipsychotic medications may contribute to suicidality in individuals with schizophrenia [64–66]. It has been suggested that antipsychotics-induced akathisia, akinesia, tardive dyskinesia and depressogenic effects of antipsychotic medications may increase suicide risk. For example, it has been observed that there is a significant association among akathisia and suicidality in first-episode psychosis [65,66].

It is important to note that one study observed a lower suicide risk among patients with extrapyramidal symptoms [67]. The authors believe that this finding could potentially reflect greater adherence to antipsychotic treatment, exposure to higher doses, or polypharmacy in this patient group.

7. Neurobiological Aspects of Suicidal Behavior in Schizophrenia

Some lines of evidence suggest that suicidal behavior in schizophrenia has a neurobiological basis [68–73]. Dexamethasone suppression test (DST) deviations have been observed in patients with schizophrenia who attempted suicide [68,69]. For example, it has been observed that dexamethasone non-suppression may be associated with a history of suicide attempts among medication-free persons with schizophrenia [68]. Hypothalamic-pituitary-adrenal axis (HPA) hyperactivity leading to glucocorticoid neurotoxicity may be the primary way through which tissue injury occurs in several parts of the brain, as observed in neuroimaging investigations of suicide attempters with schizophrenia [70].

Some studies found lower 5-hydroxy acetic acid (5-HIAAA) levels in the cerebrospinal fluid (CSF) of suicidal patients in comparison to the CSF levels of non-suicidal individuals with schizophrenia [71,74], while other studies did not detect this difference [75–77]. One research group found that a blunted prolactin response to a D-fenfluramine administration was associated with suicidal behavior in individuals with a history of schizophrenia [78]. A significant link was found between single nucleotide polymorphisms ADRA2B rs1018351 and SLC6A3 rs403636 and a history of suicidal behavior in schizophrenia patients [73].

8. Prevention of Suicide in Patients with Schizophrenia

Suicide prevention in patients with schizophrenia is a complex task. Clinicians need to be trained in how to identify patients who are at high suicide risk. Careful management of psychotic symptoms, comorbid depression and substance use disorders is necessary to prevent suicide in individuals with schizophrenia.

Efforts in suicide prevention should focus on enhancing compliance with medications. Studies suggest that antipsychotic medications, including clozapine, risperidone, olanzapine, and quetiapine may reduce suicide risk [33,79–83].

Several studies demonstrated efficacy of clozapine for the management of suicidality in schizophrenia [81,82]. It has been proposed that this decline in suicidal behavior can be ascribed to reduction in depressive symptomatology [84]. In December 2002, the U.S. Food and Drug Administration (FDA) granted indication for clozapine to decrease the risk of recurring suicidal behavior in individuals with schizophrenia/schizoaffective disorder [50]. Potentially, early use of clozapine may significantly reduce risk of suicide in patients with schizophrenia [53]. A recent study indicates that clozapine should be administered after patients with schizophrenia fail a single antipsychotic medication trial—not until two antipsychotic drugs have been attempted, as is the existing guideline [85]. Such an approach may reduce suicidality in individuals with schizophrenia.

Other second-generation antipsychotics may also have anti-suicidal properties [33,80,86]. For example, a retrospective study of the influences of atypical antipsychotic drugs on suicidal behavior in individuals with schizophrenia or schizoaffective disorder showed that among persons who made a suicide attempt, 16.1% took second-generation antipsychotic medications, whereas in the non-suicidal group 37% took second-generation antipsychotics [80]. Another study has shown a fourfold rise in suicide attempts among individuals with schizophrenia who stopped taking olanzapine or risperidone [86].

Long-acting injections are frequently used for the treatment of psychotic disorders [87]. Observations of the effect of depot antipsychotic medications on suicide risk have produced inconsistent results. For example, Battaglia et al. [87] showed that monthly intramuscular injections of fluphenazine decanoate reduce self-harm behavior in outpatients with histories of multiple suicide attempts. Shear et al. [88] reported suicides in two young men who developed severe akathisia after treatment with depot fluphenazine. A Cochrane review by Adams and Eisenbruch [89] compared depot fluphenazine medication to oral fluphenazine for treatment of schizophrenia and found no difference between fluphenazine hydrochloride and its depot form for outcomes such as depressed mood or suicide. A meta-analysis showed that pooled long-acting antipsychotics (aripiprazole, fluphenazine, haloperidol, olanzapine, paliperidone, risperidone, and zuclopenthixol) did not differ from pooled oral antipsychotics regarding all-cause death or death due to suicide [90]. Pompilli et al. [91] suggest that long-acting injections of second-generation antipsychotics can be an effective treatment strategy to improve adherence and may result in suicide prevention by targeting modifiable suicide risk factors.

Concurrent depression is a significant risk factor for suicidal behavior in individuals with schizophrenia [29,33,34]. Studies suggest a relation between a decrease in suicide risk and the use of antidepressants [92,93]. The use of antidepressants has been associated with a decrease in all-cause mortality when used together with antipsychotic drugs [94]. Psychiatrists should consider the addition of antidepressant medications for concurrent depression in patients with schizophrenia [29,33,34]. Furthermore, medications that reduce substance abuse (e.g., naltrexone or acamprosate) should be prescribed for patients with comorbid schizophrenia/schizoaffective disorder and substance use disorder.

Non-pharmacological approaches are also important in decreasing suicidal behavior in schizophrenia [33,34,95]. Psychosocial interventions play an important role in the treatment of suicidal patients with schizophrenia. It is vital to educate mental health providers about suicidology [34]. They need to be prepared to deal with the depression, anxiety, anguish, and hopelessness of suicidal individuals with schizophrenia. Empathic care and support are critical for decreasing suicidal risk [33,34,95]. Clinicians should recognize the patient's distress, talk to the patient about his/her daily problems, and assist patients in establishing realistic goals.

Supportive, reality-orientated therapies are important in the management of patients with psychotic disorders [34]. Individual and group sessions can help patients to learn how to handle difficulties. Psychosocial interventions including cognitive-behavioral therapy, cognitive remediation, supportive therapy, supported education, training, and employment are important for successful management of schizophrenia [34,96]. One study found that cognitive therapy decreases suicidal ideation in individuals with schizophrenia [97]. Interventions such as vocational rehabilitation, social skill training, and supported employment may reduce social isolation and feeling of hopelessness, and consequently, decrease suicidality in schizophrenia patients.

Family interventions may reduce the risk of suicidal behavior, and therefore, should be a necessary component of a treatment plan of each patient with schizophrenia [98,99]. Such interventions considerably lessen rates of readmission and relapse in individuals with psychotic disorders and enhance their social and vocational performance [98,99]. Family interventions usually increase adherence to pharmacological therapy [99]. Relatives of patients with schizophrenia sometimes display excessive emotional reactions and convey intolerant, judgmental, and/or emotionally overinvolved attitudes toward patients [100–102]. Family members high in expressed emotion may cause suicidal behavior in patients with schizophrenia [100]. One of the goals of family interventions is to reduce psychological distress among family members and to decrease expressed emotion in families of patients with schizophrenia. Hence, it is essential to help families of persons with schizophrenia and to explain to patients' families that their attitude towards the patient can aid or impede recovery. It is necessary to educate families that they need to assist mental health providers to make sure that pharmacological and non-pharmacological treatments are being followed, especially after discharge from inpatient hospitalization. Families of individuals with schizophrenia need to be informed regarding manifestations of suicidality and what needs to be done if an individual with schizophrenia develops suicidal ideation, intent, or plan.

In summary, the only reliable protective factor for suicide in patients with schizophrenia is provision of and compliance with comprehensive treatment. Prevention of suicidal behavior in schizophrenia should include recognizing patients at risk, delivering the best possible therapy for psychotic symptoms, and managing comorbid depression and substance misuse. It is imperative to educate mental health and non-mental health providers about suicide prevention strategies.

Author Contributions: Conceptualization, L.S. and R.S.K.; Writing-Original Draft Preparation, L.S. and R.S.K.; Writing-Review & Editing, L.S.

References

1. World Health Organization. Preventing Suicide. A Global Imperative. WHO, 2014. Available online: http://www.who.int/mental_health/suicide-prevention/world_report_2014/en/ (accessed on 14 January 2019).
2. Hawton, K.; van Heeringen, K. Suicide. *Lancet* **2009**, *373*, 1372–1381. [CrossRef]
3. Wyatt, R.J.; Henter, I.; Leary, M.C.; Taylor, E. An economic evaluation of schizophrenia-1991. *Soc. Psychiatry Psychiatr. Epidemiol.* **1995**, *30*, 196–205. [PubMed]

4. Jokinen, J.; Talbäck, M.; Feychting, M.; Ahlbom, A.; Ljung, R. Life expectancy after the first suicide attempt. *Acta Psychiatr. Scand.* **2018**, *137*, 287–295. [CrossRef] [PubMed]
5. Hedegaard, H.; Curtin, S.C.; Warner, M. Suicide mortality in the United States, 1999–2017. *NCHS Data Brief.* **2018**, *330*, 1–8.
6. Rutz, W.; Rihmer, Z. Suicidality in men—Practical issues, challenges, solutions. *J. Men's Health Gender* **2007**, *4*, 393–401. [CrossRef]
7. Mann, J.J. A current perspective of suicide and attempted suicide. *Ann. Intern. Med.* **2002**, *136*, 302–311. [CrossRef] [PubMed]
8. Sher, L.; Oquendo, M.A.; Mann, J.J. Risk of suicide in mood disorders. *Clin. Neurosci. Res.* **2001**, *1*, 337–344. [CrossRef]
9. Brådvik, L. Suicide risk and mental disorders. *Int. J. Environ. Res. Public Health* **2018**, *15*, 2028. [CrossRef]
10. Caldwell, C.B.; Gottesman, I.I. Schizophrenics kill themselves too: A review of risk factors for suicide. *Schizophr. Bull.* **1990**, *16*, 571–589. [CrossRef]
11. Sartorius, N.; Jablensky, A.; Korten, A.; Ernberg, G.; Anker, M.; Cooper, J.E.; Day, R. Early manifestations and first-contact incidence of schizophrenia in different cultures. A preliminary report on the initial evaluation phase of the WHO Collaborative Study on determinants of outcome of severe mental disorders. *Psychol. Med.* **1986**, *16*, 909–928. [CrossRef]
12. Sher, L. Alcohol and suicide: Neurobiological and clinical aspects. *Sci. World J.* **2006**, *21*, 700–706. [CrossRef] [PubMed]
13. Ho, R.C.; Ho, E.C.; Tai, B.C.; Ng, W.Y.; Chia, B.H. Elderly suicide with and without a history of suicidal behavior: Implications for suicide prevention and management. *Arch. Suicide Res.* **2014**, *18*, 363–375. [CrossRef]
14. Krysinska, K.; Heller, T.S.; De Leo, D. Suicide and deliberate self-harm in personality disorders. *Curr. Opin. Psychiatry* **2006**, *19*, 95–101. [CrossRef] [PubMed]
15. Choo, C.; Diederich, J.; Song, I.; Ho, R. Cluster analysis reveals risk factors for repeated suicide attempts in a multi-ethnic Asian population. *Asian J. Psychiatr.* **2014**, *8*, 38–42. [CrossRef] [PubMed]
16. Ahmedani, B.K.; Peterson, E.L.; Hu, Y.; Rossom, R.C.; Lynch, F.; Lu, C.Y.; Waitzfelder, B.E.; Owen-Smith, A.A.; Hubley, S.; Prabhakar, D.; et al. Major physical health conditions and risk of suicide. *Am. J. Prev. Med.* **2017**, *53*, 308–315. [CrossRef]
17. Elman, I.; Borsook, D.; Volkow, N.D. Pain and suicidality: Insights from reward and addiction neuroscience. *Prog. Neurobiol.* **2013**, *109*, 1–27. [CrossRef] [PubMed]
18. Rogers, M.L.; Joiner, T.E. Interactive effects of acute suicidal affective disturbance and pain persistence on suicide attempt frequency and lethality. *Crisis* **2019**, in press. [CrossRef]
19. King, S.A. Opioids, Suicide, Mental Disorders, and Pain. *Psychiatr. Times* **2018**, *35*, 11. Available online: https://www.psychiatrictimes.com/psychopharmacology/opioids-suicide-mental-disorders-and-pain (accessed on 24 April 2019).
20. Coughlin, S.S.; Sher, L. Suicidal behavior and neurological illnesses. *J. Depress. Anxiety* **2013**, *9*, 12443.
21. Oquendo, M.A.; Friedman, J.H.; Grunebaum, M.F.; Burke, A.; Silver, J.M.; Mann, J.J. Suicidal behavior and mild traumatic brain injury in major depression. *J. Nerv. Ment. Dis.* **2004**, *192*, 430–434. [CrossRef]
22. Brent, D. Prevention programs to augment family and child resilience can have lasting effects on suicidal risk. *Suicide Life Threat. Behav.* **2016**, *46*, S39–S47. [CrossRef] [PubMed]
23. Sher, L. Is it possible to predict suicide? *Aust. N. Z. J. Psychiatry* **2011**, *45*, 341. [CrossRef]
24. Varese, F.; Smeets, F.; Drukker, M.; Lieverse, R.; Lataster, T.; Viechtbauer, W.; Read, J.; van Os, J.; Bentall, R.P. Childhood adversities increase the risk of psychosis: A meta-analysis of patient-control, prospective-and cross-sectional cohort studies. *Schizophr. Bull.* **2012**, *38*, 661–671. [CrossRef] [PubMed]
25. Serafini, G.; Muzio, C.; Piccinini, G.; Flouri, E.; Ferrigno, G.; Pompili, M.; Girardi, P.; Amore, M. Life adversities and suicidal behavior in young individuals: A systematic review. *Eur. Child. Adolesc. Psychiatry* **2015**, *24*, 1423–1446. [CrossRef] [PubMed]
26. Bleuler, E. *Dementia Praecox: oder Gruppe der Schizophrenien*; Franz Deuticke: Leipzig, Germany, 1911.
27. Kraepelin, E. Psychiatrische Randbemerkungen zur Zeitgeschichte. *Suddeutsch. Monatshefte* **1919**, *2*, 171–183. [CrossRef]
28. Rennie, T.A.C. Follow-up study of five hundred patients with schizophrenia admitted to the hospital from 1913 to 1923. *Arch. Neurol. Psychiatry* **1939**, *42*, 877–891. [CrossRef]

29. Siris, S.G. Suicide and schizophrenia. *J. Psychopharmacol.* **2001**, *15*, 127–135. [CrossRef] [PubMed]
30. Cohen, S.; Lavelle, J.; Rich, C.L.; Bromet, E. Rates and correlates of suicide attempts in first-admission psychotic patients. *Acta Psychiatr. Scand.* **1994**, *90*, 167–171. [CrossRef]
31. Gupta, S.; Black, D.W.; Arndt, S.; Hubbard, W.C.; Andreasen, N.C. Factors associated with suicide attempts among patients with schizophrenia. *Psychiatr. Serv.* **1998**, *49*, 1353–1355. [CrossRef]
32. White, J.; Gray, R.; Jones, M. The development of the serious mental illness physical Health Improvement Profile. *J. Psychiatr. Ment. Health Nurs.* **2009**, *16*, 493–498. [CrossRef]
33. Balhara, Y.P.; Verma, R. Schizophrenia and suicide. *East. Asian Arch. Psychiatry* **2012**, *22*, 126–133. [PubMed]
34. Roy, A.; Pompili, M. Management of schizophrenia with suicide risk. *Psychiatr. Clin. N. Am.* **2009**, *32*, 863–883. [CrossRef] [PubMed]
35. Popovic, D.; Benabarre, A.; Crespo, J.M.; Goikolea, J.M.; González-Pinto, A.; Gutiérrez-Rojas, L.; Montes, J.M.; Vieta, E. Risk factors for suicide in schizophrenia: Systematic review and clinical recommendations. *Acta Psychiatr. Scand.* **2014**, *130*, 418–426. [CrossRef] [PubMed]
36. Verma, D.; Srivastava, M.K.; Singh, S.K.; Bhatia, T.; Deshpande, S.N. Lifetime suicide intent, executive function and insight in schizophrenia and schizoaffective disorders. *Schizophr. Res.* **2016**, *178*, 12–16. [CrossRef] [PubMed]
37. Black, D.W.; Winokur, G.; Warrack, G. Suicide in schizophrenia: The Iowa Record Linkage Study. *J. Clin. Psychiatry* **1985**, *46*, 14–17. [PubMed]
38. Copas, J.B.; Robin, A. Suicide in psychiatric in-patients. *Br. J. Psychiatry* **1982**, *141*, 503–511. [CrossRef] [PubMed]
39. Newman, S.C.; Bland, R.C. Mortality in a cohort of patients with schizophrenia: A record linkage study. *Can. J. Psychiatry* **1991**, *36*, 239–245. [CrossRef] [PubMed]
40. Breier, A.; Astrachan, B.M. Characterization of schizophrenic patients who commit suicide. *Am. J. Psychiatry* **1984**, *141*, 206–209.
41. Roy, A. Suicide in chronic schizophrenia. *Br. J. Psychiatry* **1982**, *141*, 171–177. [CrossRef]
42. Harkavy-Friedman, J.M.; Nelson, E. Management of the suicidal patient with schizophrenia. *Psychiatr. Clin. North. Am.* **1997**, *20*, 625–640. [CrossRef]
43. Inamdar, S.C.; Lewis, D.O.; Siomopoulos, G.; Shanok, S.S.; Lamela, M. Violent and suicidal behavior in psychotic adolescents. *Am. J. Psychiatry* **1982**, *139*, 932–935. [PubMed]
44. Roy, A.; Mazonson, A.; Pickar, D. Attempted suicide in chronic schizophrenia. *Br. J. Psychiatry* **1984**, *144*, 303–306. [CrossRef] [PubMed]
45. Niskanen, P. Treatment results achieved in psychiatric day hospital care: A follow-up of 100 patients. *Acta Psychiatr. Scand.* **1974**, *50*, 401–409. [CrossRef] [PubMed]
46. Nordentoft, M.; Madsen, T.; Fedyszyn, I. Suicidal behavior and mortality in first-episode psychosis. *J. Nerv. Ment. Dis.* **2015**, *203*, 387–392. [CrossRef] [PubMed]
47. Tsuang, M.T.; Woolson, R.F. Excess mortality in schizophrenia and affective disorders. Do suicides and accidental deaths solely account for this excess? *Arch. Gen. Psychiatry* **1978**, *35*, 1181–1185. [CrossRef] [PubMed]
48. Barrett, E.A.; Sundet, K.; Faerden, A.; Nesvåg, R.; Agartz, I.; Fosse, R.; Mork, E.; Steen, N.E.; Andreassen, O.A.; Melle, I. Suicidality before and in the early phases of first episode psychosis. *Schizophr. Res.* **2010**, *119*, 11–17. [CrossRef]
49. Chan, S.K.W.; Chan, S.W.Y.; Pang, H.H.; Yan, K.K.; Hui, C.L.M.; Chang, W.C.; Lee, E.H.M.; Chen, E.Y.H. Association of an early intervention service for psychosis with suicide rate among patients with first-episode schizophrenia-spectrum disorders. *JAMA Psychiatry* **2018**, *75*, 458–464. [CrossRef]
50. Ventriglio, A.; Gentile, A.; Bonfitto, I.; Stella, E.; Mari, M.; Steardo, L.; Bellomo, A. Suicide in the early stage of schizophrenia. *Front. Psychiatry* **2016**, *7*, 116. [CrossRef]
51. Carlborg, A.; Winnerbäck, K.; Jönsson, E.G.; Jokinen, J.; Nordström, P. Suicide in schizophrenia. *Expert Rev. Neurother.* **2010**, *10*, 1153–1164. [CrossRef]
52. Hawton, K.; Sutton, L.; Haw, C.; Sinclair, J.; Deeks, J.J. Schizophrenia and suicide: Systematic review of risk factors. *Br. J. Psychiatry* **2005**, *187*, 9–20. [CrossRef]
53. Hor, K.; Taylor, M. Suicide and schizophrenia: A systematic review of rates and risk factors. *J. Psychopharmacol.* **2010**, *24*, 81–90. [CrossRef]

54. Fenton, W.S.; McGlashan, T.H.; Victor, B.J.; Blyler, C.R. Symptoms, subtype, and suicidality in patients with schizophrenia spectrum disorders. *Am. J. Psychiatry* **1997**, *154*, 199–204. [PubMed]
55. Tiihonen, J.; Wahlbeck, K.; Lönnqvist, J.; Klaukka, T.; Ioannidis, J.P.; Volavka, J.; Haukka, J. Effectiveness of antipsychotic treatments in a nationwide cohort of patients in community care after first hospitalisation due to schizophrenia and schizoaffective disorder: Observational follow-up study. *BMJ* **2006**, *333*, 224. [CrossRef] [PubMed]
56. Hettige, N.C.; Bani-Fatemi, A.; Sakinofsky, I.; De Luca, V. A biopsychosocial evaluation of the risk for suicide in schizophrenia. *CNS Spectr.* **2018**, *23*, 253–263. [CrossRef] [PubMed]
57. Bertelsen, M.; Jeppesen, P.; Petersen, L.; Thorup, A.; Øhlenschlaeger, J.; le Quach, P.; Christensen, T.Ø.; Krarup, G.; Jørgensen, P.; Nordentoft, M. Suicidal behaviour and mortality in first-episode psychosis: The OPUS trial. *Br. J. Psychiatry* **2007**, *51*, s140–s146. [CrossRef]
58. Reutfors, J.; Brandt, L.; Jönsson, E.G.; Ekbom, A.; Sparén, P.; Osby, U. Risk factors for suicide in schizophrenia: Findings from a Swedish population-based case-control study. *Schizophr. Res.* **2009**, *108*, 231–237. [CrossRef] [PubMed]
59. Sinclair, J.M.; Mullee, M.A.; King, E.A.; Baldwin, DS. Suicide in schizophrenia: A retrospective case-control study of 51 suicides. *Schizophr. Bull.* **2004**, *30*, 803–811. [CrossRef]
60. Saarinen, P.I.; Lehtonen, J.; Lönnqvist, J. Suicide risk in schizophrenia: An analysis of 17 consecutive suicides. *Schizophr. Bull.* **1999**, *25*, 533–542. [CrossRef]
61. Goodwin, R.; Lyons, J.S.; McNally, R.J. Panic attacks in schizophrenia. *Schizophr. Res.* **2002**, *58*, 213–220. [CrossRef]
62. McGirr, A.; Turecki, G. What is specific to suicide in schizophrenia disorder? Demographic, clinical and behavioural dimensions. *Schizophr. Res.* **2008**, *98*, 217–224. [CrossRef]
63. González-Pinto, A.; Aldama, A.; González, C.; Mosquera, F.; Arrasate, M.; Vieta, E. Predictors of suicide in first-episode affective and nonaffective psychotic inpatients: Five-year follow-up of patients from a catchment area in Vitoria, Spain. *J. Clin. Psychiatry* **2007**, *68*, 242–247. [CrossRef] [PubMed]
64. Aguilar, E.J.; Siris, S.G. Do antipsychotic drugs influence suicidal behavior in schizophrenia? *Psychopharmacol. Bull.* **2007**, *40*, 128–142. [PubMed]
65. Seemüller, F.; Schennach, R.; Mayr, A.; Musil, R.; Jäger, M.; Maier, W.; Klingenberg, S.; Heuser, I.; Klosterkötter, J.; Gastpar, M.; et al. German Study Group on First-Episode Schizophrenia. Akathisia and suicidal ideation in first-episode schizophrenia. *J. Clin. Psychopharmacol.* **2012**, *32*, 694–698. [CrossRef] [PubMed]
66. Seemüller, F.; Lewitzka, U.; Bauer, M.; Meyer, S.; Musil, R.; Schennach, R.; Riedel, M.; Doucette, S.; Möller, H.J. The relationship of Akathisia with treatment emergent suicidality among patients with first-episode schizophrenia treated with haloperidol or risperidone. *Pharmacopsychiatry* **2012**, *45*, 292–296. [CrossRef] [PubMed]
67. Reutfors, J.; Clapham, E.; Bahmanyar, S.; Brandt, L.; Jönsson, E.G.; Ekbom, A.; Bodén, R.; Ösby, U. Suicide risk and antipsychotic side effects in schizophrenia: Nested case-control study. *Hum. Psychopharmacol.* **2016**, *31*, 341–345. [CrossRef] [PubMed]
68. Jones, J.S.; Stein, D.J.; Stanley, B.; Guido, J.R.; Winchel, R.; Stanley, M. Negative and depressive symptoms in suicidal schizophrenics. *Acta Psychiatr. Scand.* **1994**, *89*, 81–87. [CrossRef]
69. Płocka-Lewandowska, M.; Araszkiewicz, A.; Rybakowski, J.K. Dexamethasone suppression test and suicide attempts in schizophrenic patients. *Eur. Psychiatry* **2001**, *16*, 428–431. [CrossRef]
70. Bradley, A.J.; Dinan, T.G. A systematic review of hypothalamic-pituitary-adrenal axis function in schizophrenia: Implications for mortality. *J. Psychopharmacol.* **2010**, *24*, 91–118. [CrossRef]
71. Cooper, S.J.; Kelly, C.B.; King, D.J. 5-Hydroxyindoleacetic acid in cerebrospinal fluid and prediction of suicidal behaviour in schizophrenia. *Lancet* **1992**, *340*, 940–941. [CrossRef]
72. Kim, S.; Choi, K.H.; Baykiz, A.F.; Gershenfeld, H.K. Suicide candidate genes associated with bipolar disorder and schizophrenia: An exploratory gene expression profiling analysis of post-mortem prefrontal cortex. *BMC Genom.* **2007**, *8*, 413. [CrossRef]
73. Molnar, S.; Mihanović, M.; Grah, M.; Kezić, S.; Filaković, P.; Degmecić, D. Comparative study on gene tags of the neurotransmission system in schizophrenic and suicidal subjects. *Coll. Antropol.* **2010**, *34*, 1427–1432. [PubMed]

74. Neider, D.; Lindström, L.H.; Bodén, R. Risk factors for suicide among patients with schizophrenia: A cohort study focused on cerebrospinal fluid levels of homovanillic acid and 5-hydroxyindoleacetic acid. *Neuropsychiatr. Dis. Treat.* **2016**, *12*, 1711–1714. [CrossRef] [PubMed]
75. Roy, A.; Ninan, P.; Mazonson, A.; Pickar, D.; Van Kammen, D.; Linnoila, M.; Paul, S.M. CSF monoamine metabolites in chronic schizophrenic patients who attempt suicide. *Psychol. Med.* **1985**, *15*, 335–340. [CrossRef] [PubMed]
76. Lemus, C.Z.; Lieberman, J.A.; Johns, C.A.; Pollack, S.; Bookstein, P.; Cooper, T.B. CSF 5-hydroxyindoleacetic acid levels and suicide attempts in schizophrenia. *Biol. Psychiatry* **1990**, *27*, 926–929. [CrossRef]
77. Carlborg, A.; Jokinen, J.; Nordström, A.L.; Jönsson, E.G.; Nordström, P. CSF 5-HIAA, attempted suicide and suicide risk in schizophrenia spectrum psychosis. *Schizophr. Res.* **2009**, *112*, 80–85. [CrossRef]
78. Corrêa, H.; Duval, F.; Mokrani, M.C.; Bailey, P.; Trémeau, F.; Staner, L.; Diep, T.S.; Crocq, M.A.; Macher, J.P. Serotonergic function and suicidal behavior in schizophrenia. *Schizophr. Res.* **2002**, *56*, 75–85. [CrossRef]
79. Keck, P.E., Jr.; Strakowski, S.M.; McElroy, S.L. The efficacy of atypical antipsychotics in the treatment of depressive symptoms, hostility, and suicidality in patients with schizophrenia. *J. Clin. Psychiatry* **2000**, *61*, 4–9.
80. Barak, Y.; Mirecki, I.; Knobler, H.Y.; Natan, Z.; Aizenberg, D. Suicidality and second generation antipsychotics in schizophrenia patients: A case-controlled retrospective study during a 5-year period. *Psychopharmacology* **2004**, *175*, 215–219. [CrossRef]
81. Meltzer, H.Y.; Alphs, L.; Green, A.I.; Altamura, A.C.; Anand, R.; Bertoldi, A.; Bourgeois, M.; Chouinard, G.; Islam, M.Z.; Kane, J.; et al. International Suicide Prevention Trial Study Group. Clozapine treatment for suicidality in schizophrenia: International Suicide Prevention Trial (InterSePT). *Arch. Gen. Psychiatry* **2003**, *60*, 82–91. [CrossRef]
82. Sernyak, M.J.; Desai, R.; Stolar, M.; Rosenheck, R. Impact of clozapine on completed suicide. *Am. J. Psychiatry* **2001**, *158*, 931–937. [CrossRef]
83. Tiihonen, J.; Mittendorfer-Rutz, E.; Majak, M.; Mehtälä, J.; Hoti, F.; Jedenius, E.; Enkusson, D.; Leval, A.; Sermon, J.; Tanskanen, A.; et al. Real-world effectiveness of antipsychotic treatments in a Nationwide Cohort of 29,823 patients with schizophrenia. *JAMA Psychiatry* **2017**, *74*, 686–693. [CrossRef] [PubMed]
84. Saunders, K.E.; Hawton, K. The role of psychopharmacology in suicide prevention. *Epidemiol. Psichiatr. Soc.* **2009**, *18*, 172–178. [CrossRef] [PubMed]
85. Kahn, R.S.; Winter van Rossum, I.; Leucht, S.; McGuire, P.; Lewis, S.W.; Leboyer, M.; Arango, C.; Dazzan, P.; Drake, R.; Heres, S.; et al. Amisulpride and olanzapine followed by open-label treatment with clozapine in first-episode schizophrenia and schizophreniform disorder (OPTiMiSE): A three-phase switching study. *Lancet Psychiatry* **2018**, *5*, 797–807. [CrossRef]
86. Herings, R.M.; Erkens, J.A. Increased suicide attempt rate among patients interrupting use of atypical antipsychotics. *Pharmacoepidemiol. Drug Saf.* **2003**, *12*, 423–424. [CrossRef] [PubMed]
87. Battaglia, J.; Wolff, T.K.; Wagner-Johnson, D.S.; Rush, A.J.; Carmody, T.J.; Basco, M.R. Structured diagnostic assessment and depot fluphenazine treatment of multiple suicide attempters in the emergency department. *Int. Clin. Psychopharmacol.* **1999**, *14*, 361–372. [CrossRef] [PubMed]
88. Shear, M.K.; Frances, A.; Weiden, P. Suicide associated with akathisia and depot fluphenazine treatment. *J. Clin. Psychopharmacol.* **1983**, *3*, 235–236. [CrossRef]
89. Adams, C.E.; Eisenbruch, M. Depot fluphenazine for schizophrenia. *Cochrane Database Syst. Rev.* **2000**, *2*, CD000307.
90. Kishi, T.; Matsunaga, S.; Iwata, N. Mortality risk associated with long-acting injectable antipsychotics: A systematic review and meta-analyses of randomized controlled trials. *Schizophr. Bull.* **2016**, *42*, 1438–1445. [CrossRef]
91. Pompili, M.; Orsolini, L.; Lamis, D.A.; Goldsmith, D.R.; Nardella, A.; Falcone, G.; Corigliano, V.; Luciano, M.; Fiorillo, A. Suicide prevention in schizophrenia: Do long-acting injectable antipsychotics (LAIs) have a role? *CNS Neurol. Disord. Drug Targets* **2017**, *16*, 454–462. [CrossRef]
92. Henriksson, S.; Isacsson, G. Increased antidepressant use and fewer suicides in Jämtland county, Sweden, after a primary care educational programme on the treatment of depression. *Acta Psychiatr. Scand.* **2006**, *114*, 159–167. [CrossRef]
93. Isacsson, G.; Rich, C.L. Antidepressant drug use and suicide prevention. *Int. Rev. Psychiatry* **2005**, *17*, 153–162. [CrossRef] [PubMed]

94. Haukka, J.; Tiihonen, J.; Härkänen, T.; Lönnqvist, J. Association between medication and risk of suicide, attempted suicide and death in nationwide cohort of suicidal patients with schizophrenia. *Pharmacoepidemiol. Drug Saf.* **2008**, *17*, 686–696. [CrossRef] [PubMed]
95. Cotton, P.G.; Drake, R.E.; Gates, C. Critical treatment issues in suicide among schizophrenics. *Hosp. Community Psychiatry* **1985**, *36*, 534–536. [CrossRef] [PubMed]
96. Kahn, R.S.; Sommer, I.E.; Murray, R.M.; Meyer-Lindenberg, A.; Weinberger, D.R.; Cannon, T.D.; O'Donovan, M.; Correll, C.U.; Kane, J.M.; van Os, J.; et al. Schizophrenia. *Nat. Rev. Dis. Primers* **2015**, *1*, 15067. [CrossRef] [PubMed]
97. Bateman, K.; Hansen, L.; Turkington, D.; Kingdon, D. Cognitive behavioral therapy reduces suicidal ideation in schizophrenia: Results from a randomized controlled trial. *Suicide Life Threat. Behav.* **2007**, *37*, 284–290. [CrossRef] [PubMed]
98. McFarlane, W.R.; Dixon, L.; Lukens, E.; Lucksted, A. Family psychoeducation and schizophrenia: A review of the literature. *J. Marital Fam. Ther.* **2003**, *29*, 223–245. [CrossRef] [PubMed]
99. Onwumere, J.; Bebbington, P.; Kuipers, E. Family interventions in early psychosis: Specificity and effectiveness. *Epidemiol. Psychiatr. Sci.* **2011**, *20*, 113–119. [CrossRef]
100. Demir, S. The relationship between expressed emotion and the probability of suicide among Turkish psychiatric outpatients: A descriptive cross-sectional survey. *Fam. Community Health* **2018**, *41*, 111–116. [CrossRef]
101. Napa, W.; Tungpunkom, P.; Pothimas, N. Effectiveness of family interventions on psychological distress and expressed emotion in family members of individuals diagnosed with first-episode psychosis: A systematic review. *JBI Database Syst. Rev. Implement. Rep.* **2017**, *15*, 1057–1079. [CrossRef]
102. Amaresha, A.C.; Venkatasubramanian, G. Expressed emotion in schizophrenia: An overview. *Indian J. Psychol. Med.* **2012**, *34*, 12–20.

4

Psychotherapy with Suicidal Patients: The Integrative Psychodynamic Approach of the Boston Suicide Study Group

Mark Schechter [1,2,*], Elsa Ronningstam [2,3], Benjamin Herbstman [2,3] and Mark J. Goldblatt [2,3]

1 North Shore Medical Center, 81 Highland Avenue, Salem, MA 01970, USA
2 Harvard Medical School, 25 Shattuck Street, Boston, MA 02115, USA; ronningstam@email.com (E.R.); bherbstman@mclean.harvard.edu (B.H.); mark_goldblatt@hms.harvard.edu (M.J.G.)
3 McLean Hospital, 115 Mill Street, Belmont, MA 02478, USA
* Correspondence: mschechter@partners.org;

Abstract: Psychotherapy with suicidal patients is inherently challenging. Psychodynamic psychotherapy focuses attention on the patient's internal experience through the creation of a therapeutic space for an open-ended exploration of thoughts, fears, and fantasies as they emerge through interactive dialogue with an empathic therapist. The Boston Suicide Study Group (M.S., M.J.G., E.R., B.H.), has developed an integrative psychodynamic approach to psychotherapy with suicidal patients based on the authors' extensive clinical work with suicidal patients (over 100 years combined). It is fundamentally psychodynamic in nature, with an emphasis on the therapeutic alliance, unconscious and implicit relational processes, and the power of the therapeutic relationship to facilitate change in a long-term exploratory treatment. It is also integrative, however, drawing extensively on ideas and techniques described in Dialectical Behavioral Therapy (DBT), Mentalization Based Treatment (MBT), Cognitive-Behavioral Therapy (CBT), as well on developmental and social psychology research. This is not meant to be a comprehensive review of psychodynamic treatment of suicidal patients, but rather a description of an integrative approach that synthesizes clinical experience and relevant theoretical contributions from the literature that support the authors' reasoning. There are ten key aspects of this integrative psychodynamic treatment: 1. Approach to the patient in crisis; 2, instilling hope; 3. a focus on the patient's internal affective experience; 4. attention to conscious and unconscious beliefs and fantasies; 5. improving affect tolerance; 6. development of narrative identity and modification of "relational scripts"; 7. facilitation of the emergence of the patient's genuine capacities; 8. improving a sense of continuity and coherence; 9 attention to the therapeutic alliance; 10. attention to countertransference. The elements of treatment are overlapping and not meant to be sequential, but each is discussed separately as an essential aspect of the psychotherapeutic work. This integrative psychodynamic approach is a useful method for suicide prevention as it helps to instill hope, provides relational contact and engages the suicidal patient in a process that leads to positive internal change. The benefits of the psychotherapy go beyond crisis intervention, and include the potential for improved affect tolerance, more fulfilling relational experiences, emergence of previously warded off experience of genuine capacities, and a positive change in narrative identity.

Keywords: psychodynamic psychotherapy; integrative; suicide; therapeutic alliance; countertransference; hope

---

1. Introduction

Psychodynamic psychotherapy focuses attention on the patient's internal experience through the creation of a therapeutic space for an open-ended exploration of thoughts, fears, and fantasies as they emerge through interactive dialogue with an empathic therapist. The Boston Suicide Study Group (M.S., M.J.G., E.R., B.H.) has developed an integrative psychodynamic approach to psychotherapy with suicidal patients based on the authors' extensive clinical work with suicidal patients. It is fundamentally psychodynamic in nature, with an emphasis on the therapeutic alliance, unconscious and implicit relational processes, and the power of the therapeutic relationship to facilitate change in a long-term exploratory treatment. However, this is also an integrative approach, drawing extensively on DBT, MBT, CBT, and developmental and social psychology research. The authors have identified ten key aspects of their treatment approach: approach to the patient in crisis; instilling hope; a focus on the patient's internal affective experience; attention to conscious and unconscious beliefs and fantasies; improving affect tolerance; development of narrative identity and modification of "relational scripts"; facilitation of the emergence of the patient's genuine capacities that have been thwarted in the course of development; improving a sense of continuity and coherence; attention to the therapeutic alliance; and attention to countertransference. These elements of treatment are overlapping and are not meant to be sequential. In fact, the therapist and patient may at times be engaged in working in multiple areas fluidly and simultaneously in the course of treatment. This paper discusses each of these areas, making use of relevant literature and clinical examples to support the authors' reasoning.

Psychotherapy with suicidal patients is inherently extremely challenging. First, the therapist must accept that despite his or her best efforts there is no way to definitively control the outcome, and a patient may complete suicide. Suicidal patients are suffering terribly, and therapists are generally highly motivated to help but often lack any tools to alleviate the suffering (at least in the immediate term). Hopelessness can be particularly difficult to bear, and the therapist may feel worn down over time, beginning to accede to the patient's often stated belief that nothing can possibly be of help. In order to instill hope the therapist must have his or her own roadmap for how psychotherapy can help the patient to improve. It is our hope that this paper will help psychotherapists to understand our integrative psychodynamic approach and the ways in which it can help the patient move from suicidal despair to a life that feels worth living.

2. Background

The authors of this paper represent the Boston Suicide Study Group. We are all psychoanalysts with extensive experience in clinical work with suicidal patients (over 100 years combined) and an interest in what can be learned from integrating ideas and techniques from other psychotherapeutic approaches. We have studied and treated many psychiatric patients who have presented with suicidal ideation and plans, among them many who have made serious suicide attempts as well as some completed suicides. We have also studied the literature on psychotherapies for suicidal patients and on psychodynamic psychotherapy. This paper has been written with the intent to synthesize what we have found to be the key elements and successful treatment with suicidal patients, and to support our reasoning with relevant literature and clinical examples. It is not meant to be a comprehensive, systematic review of the literature on psychodynamic psychotherapy with suicidal patients, but rather an opportunity for us to share our integrative psychodynamic approach.

3. Elements of the Integrative Psychodynamic Approach

3.1. Approach to the Patient in Crisis

A thorough safety evaluation is essential when a patient is in an acute suicidal crisis. The therapist needs to assess the degree of imminent risk and to determine whether measures beyond psychotherapy are required to keep the patient safe (e.g., emergency department, psychiatric hospitalization, etc.). Reviews of evidence-based treatments of chronic suicidality have found that all recommend a clear frame for the treatment and a defined strategy for managing suicidal crises (i.e., a crisis plan) [1,2]. Early establishment of a treatment alliance is facilitated by the therapist's attitude of non-judgmental acceptance and validation of the patient's experience [3–5].

Patients generally enter to the clinical encounter feeling terrible about themselves, with feelings of shame, harsh self-criticism/self-attack, and a sense of hopelessness and/or failure. The therapist's empathic ability to communicate an understanding of the ways in which the patient's crisis and suicidality are understandable, given his or her situation, past experiences and current internal state, forms the foundation of the alliance. Validation helps to mitigate the experience of loneliness and aloneness, decreases self-blame and harsh self-attack, and models a hopeful attitude about the possibility that the patient can be understood and ultimately helped.

The therapist is interested in the patient's "reasons for living" [6–8], including the patient's important relationships such as family (in particularly children), to get a sense of what the patient feels there is in life to live *for*. The therapist is in a unique position to engage into a respectful dialogue with the patient, not necessarily accepting the patient's automatic defenses as the final answer. It is not uncommon, for example, for patients to say that they believe that their children "will be better off without me", as well as describe themselves as "a burden" to loved ones. With gentle confrontation and exploration, one finds that some patients actually hold more conflicted feelings and beliefs but are locked in on these explanations because it protects them from bearing the pain of their conflict and from the genuine consequences that their suicide would engender. An iterative dialogue with the therapist, in which the therapist explores and questions the patient's expressed beliefs, opens up the possibility of modification. The therapist's interest in what the patient thinks and feels about suicide and death can also be experienced as a validation, that the patient is worth the therapist's interest and engagement. The goal is not to try to control the patient's beliefs, but rather to enable the patient to experience suicidal behavior as less desirable, acceptable, and effective than the alternative of working on coping and managing distress. This can help to tip the balance away from self-destructive action [8,9].

3.2. Instilling Hope

Patients who struggle with despair and suicidality often come to the therapeutic encounter with feelings of shame, discouragement, and hopelessness. They have no "road map," of how they could possibly get from where they are feeling now to building a life worth living. The therapist can help to provide such a "road map", based on an understanding of the gains that can be achieved in the psychotherapeutic process. The patient sustains hope through the therapeutic relationship, symptom management and validation of a core identity [10], and this facilitates a gradual change in perspective on life and living.

Snyder [11] described hope as requiring both a sense of agency (sense that one has some capacity to affect positive change) and pathways (a sense of some possible routes for moving forward). The therapist holds both of these components of hope and communicates them both implicitly and directly to the patient. This helps the patient to begin to experience a sense of agency, and to have some glimmer of how he or she can survive the current feelings and go on to have a life worth living. Helping to sustain the therapist's hope is the data that suicidal behavior is often a transient phenomenon. Studies have found that the vast majority of people who survive even the most severe suicide attempts actually do not go on to kill themselves [12,13]. Psychotherapy has been found to reduce the risk of recurrent suicide attempts and self-injury [14].

Psychotherapy can help support the patient who is engaging in an internal process that can gradually lead to a changed perspective and greater hope for the future. One aspect of this process is a genuine acceptance of the actual conditions that precipitated the suicidal crisis. This is especially important for patients who have faced drastic changes in life (e.g., losses, humiliations, etc.), or are coming to a realization that life is not going to turn out as expected or envisioned. Related to this is a person's ability to tolerate and accept loss, sadness, and disappointment. This involves a process of grief and mourning for what one had and will never have again, and/or what could have been but will not be. It requires engagement of the patient's self-reflective capacity, which is facilitated in psychotherapy by validation of the patient's pain, modeling reflection, affective engagement and modulation of the patient's harsh self-criticism/self-attack and feelings of failure.

Over time, the therapist can support the patient in moving from a fixation on what is ideal, to recognizing the possibility of what can be good enough. Early in the process, the "good enough" is often devalued and depicted as not worth living for, but with ongoing reflection, mourning, and support, the patient can learn that it is possible to find meaning and even joy in life with goals and expectations that have shifted in line with what is possible. This includes a re-engagement in relationships and a greater sense of belonging. At the same time, mobilization of the patient's sense of agency and instilling of hope for the future can lead to actions on the patient's part that can have a positive impact on relationships and circumstances. This can create a positive feedback loop that can lead to actual achievements beyond what the patient could have envisioned in a prior state of hopelessness.

3.3. Focus on Internal Experience and Affect

A distinguishing aspect of psychodynamic psychotherapy is the close attention to the patient's internal experience. Shneidman eloquently described suicide as 'a combined movement toward cessation and away from intolerable, unendurable, unacceptable anguish' ([15], p. 6). Multiple other terms have been used in the literature to describe this affective state by many differing theoretical orientations, trying to capture essentially the same experience: It has been variously referred to as "desperation" [16], "mental pain" [17], "psychache" [18], "emotional dysregulation" [3], and "annihilation anxiety" [19]. Hendin et al. [16] found that therapists reported a higher number of intense, agonizing affective states in patients who completed suicide in the course of psychotherapy, as compared with a severely depressed, non-suicidal comparison group. The most frequently cited affect was desperation, defined as a state of anguish accompanied by an urgent need for relief. More recently, Galynker [20] has focused on "entrapment", an emotional experience of desperation with no perceived way out.

The state of "aloneness" has been described as an unbearable experience that makes people feel desperate and puts them at risk for suicidal behavior [21,22]. Joiner and colleagues have studied a closely related experience, that of "thwarted belongingness", and found it to be a key factor in making completion of suicide possible [23,24]. Maltsberger [22] described aloneness as "an experience beyond hope .... This anxiety is the anxiety of annihilation—panic and terror. People will do anything to escape from this experience" (p. 50). The experience can feel timeless, as though once it has started it will continue for every, which adds to the sense of desperation. Aloneness is qualitatively different from loneliness, which is contingent and time limited. It is the loss of capacity to *experience* the closeness and caring of others, even if they are present and available.

In the face of an unrelenting, unbearable affective experience, cognition changes in a way that makes rational problem solving much more difficult. Baumeister [25] described the suicidal patient as moving into a state of cognitive "deconstruction" (pp. 92–93), characterized by rigidity, increasingly concrete thinking. a narrowing of sense of time to the present and an exclusive focus on immediate goals, and a lack of integration and meaning. Linehan [3] has observed that in states of severe emotional dysregulation, patients often lose certain capacities that they have in a calmer state of mind. Thinking becomes much more concrete and constricted; when the patient sees no alternative, no endpoint or escape, the risk of suicidal behavior is increased. Maltsberger [26] described the traumatic state of disintegration that accompanies a suicidal state.

An unbearable affective experience is distinct from depression. For vulnerable patients, it can come on suddenly, in response to a stressor, at times without the patient making the connection between stress and response. It can also be relieved transiently if the patient is suddenly provided a respite, such as by psychiatric hospitalization. The relief, however, can be suddenly and overwhelmingly reversed when the patient is re-exposed to overwhelming stressors at discharge, which is probably a major factor in the high rate of post-discharge suicide [27]. Ideally, psychotherapeutic efforts in the hospital can be targeted toward helping the patient to anticipate and problem-solve for upcoming crises, and to develop a usable and well-practiced crisis plan. It is important for the therapist to be aware that the immediate period post-discharge is very high risk for the patient, and to intervene accordingly.

3.4. Attention to Patients Conscious and Unconscious Beliefs and Fantasies

Psychodynamic psychotherapy provides an opportunity to explore the patient's conscious and unconscious beliefs and fantasies about suicide. These fantasies are often not rational and in contradiction with the patient's known reality. The idea of suicide can have very different meanings and can be facilitated or mitigated by different sets of fantasies. Some may be conscious, and others may be out of their awareness. These beliefs and fantasies can be wide ranging, and at times in contradiction with each other and/or with reality. Some patients believe they deserve punishment; others long for a fantasized reunion with lost parents or a loved one; some have a fantasy that they will get to "see" the reaction of others to the suicide, and even that they will experience pleasure in doing so, even while knowing rationally that this is not the case; some experience their body as hateful and want to destroy it, perhaps because it is identified with a past abuser (see [28]).

The patient's fantasies about suicide and death can influence the likelihood of suicidal action. Articulating and exploring these fantasies enables a therapeutic dialogue which gives the therapist the opportunity to respectfully challenge certain automatic assumptions. For example, perhaps the mother who states the belief that her child would be better off without her, is in fact able and willing to consider the possibility that she might be misreading the situation because of her depression and despair. A man who is experiencing aloneness and has a fantasy of rejoining his deceased wife in heaven may be willing to consider the possibility that suicide might *not* mean a blissful reunion, and that there are other consequences that he is not letting himself think through. The therapist's interest in exploring the patient's fantasies demonstrates his or her wish to get a full understanding of the patient's experience, and in this way may bolster the patient's sense that he or she matters. It also provides an opportunity for gradual modification of these beliefs in the context of an iterative dialogue over time.

Some suicidal contemplation and fantasy can be "self-sustaining". Rather than facilitating action, these thoughts can help to calm people down and help them regulate affect in a way that helps preclude the need to act on suicide [29]. These are often patients for whom the idea that they could complete suicide has served as a psychological "out" which gives them a feeling of *potential* escape from their distress; as long as they hold onto suicide as an option, they do not need to act. This kind of suicidal contemplation is "a self-soothing measure and an aid to narcissistic cohesion" (p. 612). Patients often do not understand this distinction and may be very troubled by their suicidal thoughts even as it serves an important function for them. The therapist can reassure the patient about the role of suicidal fantasy, and that thoughts do not equate with action. In fact, in the general population the ratio of those who harbor suicidal thoughts to those who kill themselves is over 200:1 [30].

3.5. Improving Affect Tolerance

Increasing affect tolerance is central to psychotherapy with patients with emotional dysregulation. Affect tolerance might roughly be defined as increasing one's capacity to think in the presence of strong emotions, and to bear feelings without having to suppress, dissociate, or act impulsively. In Dialectical Behavior Therapy (DBT), emotion regulation and distress tolerance skills are targeted to increase affect tolerance [3]. The therapist may integrate teaching the patient these skills in a psychodynamic treatment frame.

Perhaps unique to psychodynamic therapy is the opportunity to work with the patient on unconscious fears and avoidances that have a profound effect on the patient's sense of self, transferences, core beliefs, and relationships. The patient brings his or her sense of shame, humiliation, and feelings of despair to the treatment, often unconsciously fearing negative reaction on the part of the therapist that comes from a template of past relationships. Ideally with validation and support, these feelings can gradually extinguish, giving the patient more flexibility and choice. People are unaware of automatic avoidance defenses and are highly motivated to continue to use them to ward off anxiety provoking and conflictual thoughts and feelings. This keeps such material out of consciousness, and unavailable to be worked on in therapy. When the therapist gently notices avoidant defenses (e.g., "when I said that, I noticed you averted your eyes and started to change the subject ... what was going on there?"), it offers the patient an opportunity to consider what he or she is warding off. At times, the therapist may use explicit exposure techniques (e.g., "can you try saying that again while looking me in the eye, and just sit with what you are feeling?") in order to facilitate the patient's exposure to underlying uncomfortable feelings that are being warded off. With ongoing therapy, the need for these automatic avoidant defenses gradually begins to lessen. The extinguishing of shame, fear, expectancies of harsh attacks/blame, etc., allows for greater tolerance of affect, increasing the patient's flexibility and freedom of expression. This work is closely related to work on narrative identity (described below), with the working through of the patient's "relational scripts" that have led to recurrent experiences that sustain negative ideas/beliefs/conclusions about self.

3.6. Narrative Identity and "Relational Scripts"

The development of personal "narratives" has been found to be critical to the establishment and ongoing development of identity [31–37] People tell themselves stories to link experiences, make meaning from events, establish a sense of continuity of experience, and articulate ways in which they have changed [38]. In this way, people develop a "life story," described as "an internalized and evolving narrative of the self that selectively reconstructs the past and anticipates the future in such a way as to provide a life with an overall sense of coherence and purpose" ([36], p. 1372). The personal narratives of the depressed or suicidal patient's self-narrative are generally harshly self-critical and negative (e.g., "Everything I try to do fails I never get things right"). Galynker described the "suicidal narrative" as telling the story of "a present that is so intolerable that the future becomes unimaginable" ([20], p. 31).

Personal narratives are actually co-constructed, with the listener influencing whether and how the story is told, and meanings that can be derived from it [33,39,40]. Sharing one's personal stories with others helps to make meaning from experiences, and to try out ways of understanding oneself. Psychodynamic psychotherapy provides an opportunity for the patient to engage with a new "listener," an active participant who engages in the development of the patient's narrative [37]. The therapist notices and takes up the harsh self-criticism and self-attack embedded in the patient's story, and in so doing begins a process of modification.

Patients often begin treatment with a narrative that does not "connect the dots" between past experience and current despair. A patient might tell a story of severe neglect and/or abuse that clearly would lead to problems with self-esteem and trust but not make this connection. Together, therapist and patient engage in an iterative dialogue in which the patient's narrative is reworked and co-constructed. Not all patients come into treatment with the capacity to share a coherent narrative, particularly in the context of neglectful and abusive early experiences. Problems may occur at the "pre-narrative" and "proto-narrative" levels at which mental images are generated and linked to emotions, which eventually become the building blocks for higher level, verbal, narrative construction [41]. Early trauma and neglect can lead to a lack of emotional marking of mental images and an inability to recruit these images into meaningful sequences that integrate cognition and emotion. As a result, narratives are disorganized, impoverished, and sometimes frankly incoherent, and "the therapist finds it difficult to comprehend the patient's mental state" (p. 236). This leads to problems with self-cohesion and emotion regulation. Psychotherapy can help the patient to link emotions, mental images narrative fragments, and behavior with a goal of increasing self-coherence.

Early attachment and caregiver experiences form the foundation for development of Identity and sense of self in relation to others. The infant/child requires recognition and marking of mental and emotional states in order to develop their own capacity to recognize, label, and ultimately modulate emotions [42–44]. This is foundational for the development of mentalization, the ability to appreciate and reflect on the mental states of others. The child who is not recognized and "kept in mind" is bound to have difficulties in self-recognition at multiple levels, and to be more vulnerable to states of disorganization, overwhelming affect, and experiences of aloneness. The individual develops the "inner working models" [45] or "implicit relational scripts" [46–48] from the relational experiences with early caregivers. These models define how one experiences oneself, and therefore how one acts, in relation to others. "These are the automatic procedural relationship rules that one lives by, generally without awareness: "This is how people experience me; this is how I am valued, or not valued, by others; this is how I tend to be treated; this is how my relationships go; this is what happens when I make my wishes and needs known; this is who I am" ([37], p. 29).

Implicit beliefs about self and relational patterns tend to be tenacious and resistant to change. Studies in social psychology have found that people tend to "self-verify," seeking and selectively attending to feedback that confirms and reinforces the way that they already see themselves [49–51]. From an analytic perspective, Wachtel [52] described how people actively (although non-consciously) elicit confirmation of their self-concept by acting in ways that tend to evoke confirmatory responses; thus, the patient receives ongoing reinforcement that sustains his or her self-concept, even if that experience is terribly painful. The therapist engages the patient and disrupts the patient's nonconscious relational scripts by behaving differently than was unconsciously expected, thus offering the possibility that the therapeutic relationship has the potential to facilitate change. The therapist also attends to the myriad of relational experiences that continue to reinforce and sustain the patient's self-beliefs and behaviors. This means actively helping the patient to create new relational experiences that disrupt the repetitive elicitation of social feedback that confirms and sustains the patient's maladaptive beliefs about self.

The therapist's activity may include what are traditionally thought of as cognitive-behavioral strategies (e.g., problem-solving, modeling alternative ways of relating, exposure, role playing) to help the patient navigate difficult relational situations with the best possible chance to have positive and 'script disrupting' experiences. This is an iterative process, with repeated discrepant experiences with the therapist and with others gradually modifying the underlying dysfunctional relational scripts. It is especially critical in the psychotherapy of those who are vulnerable to suicidal states, for whom the repeated nonconscious evocation of confirmatory negative interpersonal experiences can quickly lead to turmoil and despair, making suicidal behavior more likely. This will be discussed further in the discussion below about the therapeutic alliance.

3.7. The Emergence and Recognition of the Patient's Genuine Capacities

The emerging recognition and appreciation of one's genuine capacities is a developmental process that can be derailed through trauma or other negative developmental experiences [37,53]. Loewald [54] described the importance of the analyst in this regard, holding and communicating a vision of the patient as who he or she is, as well as the "more" that he or she can come to be. Patients who are vulnerable to suicidal states often have anxiety associated with experiencing themselves positively, with harsh self-attack and automatic avoidant defenses that keep them from fully taking in positive relational and other experiences. The therapist, by noticing this nonconscious avoidance, calls attention to and thereby disrupts these defenses in a way that gives the patient an opportunity to bear the anxiety and conflict associated with experiencing oneself more fully. At times, this can mean integrating more formal exposure into the treatment (e.g., "I noticed when you talked about the 'A' that you got in class, you looked away and started to mumble ... What were you feeling? Maybe you can say it again but try to look right at me and use a strong voice. Let's see if you can sit with the feelings that this brings up."). Over time, the anxiety begins to diminish, and the patient gradually begins to feel more comfortable with a more complete experience of himself or herself. This creates a positive feedback loop as the patient also begins to act in a way that is consistent with his or her emerging identity and thus is more likely to elicit, and attend to, confirmatory feedback (53), which has been described as a renegotiation of identity [50].

3.8. Continuity and Coherence

Continuity is the sense of being the same person with linked experiences over time; coherence has to do with linking experiences, roles and beliefs as part of an integrated whole [35]. Patients with Borderline Personality Disorder (BPD) have been described as being vulnerable to a sudden loss of continuity—the loss of evocative memory—that leaves them unable to evoke soothing introjects and acutely vulnerable to experiences of aloneness and suicidal desperation [21]. Maltsberger [27] envisioned the "descent into suicide" as an overwhelming, unbearable flooding of negative affect that leads to a breakup of self-cohesion, to which those who do not have a strong base of continuity of self are particularly vulnerable.

Severe distress becomes unbearable when one loses the capacity to experience connection with others, a state of excruciating aloneness. This becomes even more dire "with the loss of a continuous thread of being that mitigates the sense that now is all there is, that pain will be forever, that there is no hope of moving forward because there is no forward, and that suicide might be the only option" ([37], p. 34). Recurrent affective dysregulation, mood changes and psychotic experiences can themselves be experienced as traumatic and are disruptive to developing and sustaining continuity and coherence [19].

What this means is that the therapist should consider a sense of continuity and coherence a treatment goal rather than an expectation [37]. The therapist, at times, may need to painstakingly help the patient link experiences with each other, reminding the patient that aspects of the past continue to influence the present, and even helping the patient to link dissociated experiences day-to-day. Some patients are vulnerable to feeling suddenly disconnected, alone and desperate, without any sense that something may have happened to cause their change in mental state, and the timeless sense that they will never feel better again. At these moments, the therapist may help the patient through these experiences by inter-session contact of some kind (e.g., phone, email, voice mail), and also by helping the patient to connect feelings with experiences to begin to understand the transient vulnerability to these dissociated states.

3.9. Attention to the Therapeutic Alliance

Building and maintaining a strong therapeutic alliance is a cornerstone of psychotherapy with suicidal patients, but it is fraught with significant challenges (see [55,56]). Psychotherapy often involves strong transference–countertransference reactions to which both patient and therapist contribute. Patients often come to the encounter with intense affects, and negative relational expectations. Negative therapeutic reactions and treatment crises are common, and often inculcate a fear of catastrophic consequences. Dealing with these inherent difficulties is a challenge for both patient and therapist and is critical to the success of the therapy [57–59].

A related challenge for the therapist is the need to move flexibly between empathic listening and an ongoing suicide risk assessment [55,56]. The therapist shifts between creating a psychotherapeutic space and observing the patient objectively. When there is a change in the patient's emotional state or degree of relatedness, the therapist begins an assessment of the patient's safety, the strength of the alliance, and whether there is a need for other safety interventions. Anxiety about the patient's safety can paradoxically take the therapist away from a stance of empathic attunement.

Suicidal patients generally have a harshly self-critical internal narrative, and an underlying expectation of negative interpersonal experiences that confirm their bad sense of self. In this context, the therapist needs to be actively affirmative and validating in order to achieve "functional neutrality" [60]. One issue on which psychodynamics differ is how to conceptualize and to manage the patient's aggression and negative transference. Transference Focused Psychotherapy (TFP), for example, prioritizes interpreting aggressive, split off, unintegrated parts, and considers this an essential element even early in the course of treatment [61]. Our approach prioritizes attunement to the patient's internal experience (as experienced by the patient), which we see as essential to strengthening the alliance and helping the patient with the experience of aloneness. We conceptualize aggression as most often a secondary response to the patient's internal state of desperation. A metaphor that we find helpful is that of a person who is drowning, unable to breathe, and who desperately grasps for a life raft, pushing past and inadvertently injuring another person. One could take up the aggression as primary, but we do not feel that this is closest to the patient's experience, for whom the lashing out came from a desperate effort to breathe and to stay alive. This is very much akin to the suicidal patient's desperate experience of aloneness, abandonment, and other unbearable emotional experiences, which leads to an urgent need for relief/escape. We do not ignore aggression and take it up as needed to preserve the treatment and the frame. However, in our view, interpreting the negative transference, especially for early in treatment, can be experienced as distant and critical, which is antithetical to our goal of the early attunement and validation. In this way, we are very much aligned with the approach in Mentalization Based Therapy (MBT), with an emphasis on validation of the patient's transference feeling, avoiding genetic interpretations that might be experienced as distancing and invalidating, exploring the transference, attending closely to the therapist's contribution to the patient's transference experience, and collaborative exploration [62].

The strength of the therapeutic alliance, including rupture and successful repair of the alliance, is a critical factor in the success of any psychotherapy (see [56–58]). In working with emotionally dysregulated patients, ruptures in the alliance can be particularly abrupt and severe—sometimes in response to something that occurs in the therapy, sometimes related to external stressors—with a risk of affective turmoil and potential for suicidal behavior. These ruptures can be extremely difficult for the therapist as well as for the patient, but if they can be repaired, they offer an opportunity for implicit relational learning and growth. In this context:

> ... the patient has the chance to discover experientially that an old relational pattern does not have to be repeated, and that the therapeutic relationship holds the promise of trying out, practicing and even solidifying something new. The patient also has the chance to learn that the therapist, and the relationship, can survive the intensity of the patient's sudden withdrawal or affective storm. These moments are essential in gradually building trust, in strengthening the emotional bond between patient and therapist and in holding out the hope that the relationship might actually be of help ([56], p. 319).

In this reworking of the script, the patient has an opportunity to experience the therapist as caring, and himself or herself as being worthy of being cared about. Working through ruptures often requires that the patient experience something different from the therapist, in some way above and beyond what the patient expected. This might be in the form of a self-disclosure (e.g., the therapist might acknowledge an unempathetic reaction, and share that something about what the patient had said reminded him or her of a troubling experience), an action (e.g., having the patient stay a few minutes beyond the hour because of the importance of the patient's association), or some other spontaneous and genuine way of relating to the patient.

Stern et al. [46] described the therapeutic importance of "moments of meeting," in which "the therapist must use a specific aspect of his or her individuality that carries a personal signature. The two are meeting as persons relatively unhidden by their usual therapeutic roles, for that moment" (p. 913). Linehan [4] used the term "radical genuineness" to capture the same experience. Hoffman [63], writing about psychoanalysis, captured the implicit meaning in the therapist's doing something that is experienced as different in response to the patient's need:

> When the patient senses that the analyst, in becoming more personally expressive and involved, is departing from an internalized convention of some kind, the patient has reason to feel recognized in a special way, the deviation, whatever its content and whatever the nature of the pressure from the patient, may reflect an emotional engagement on the analyst's part that is responsive in a unique way to this particular patient ... there is something about the deviation itself, regardless of content, that has therapeutic potential (pp. 187–193).

Similarly, the patient may require measures that go beyond the traditional frame of the psychotherapy session to maintain or regain an empathic connection [64]. Interventions such as between session contact, offering additional sessions, and intermittent telephone, email or text support can help the patient cope with affective intensity when in crisis. These actions may also have internal meaning for the patient, serving to enhance internalization of the therapist as a positive introject and strengthen the therapeutic alliance [56]. Thoughtful flexibility regarding the treatment frame can be experienced as validating by the patient (i.e., the therapist cares enough to be flexible and is willing to prioritize the patient's perceived needs) and often helps to strengthen and solidify the therapeutic alliance. In cases of severe personality disorders such as antisocial and severely narcissistic personality disorders, it may at times be beneficial to set and adhere to a more rigid frame (such as that advocated in TFP) [61]. On the other hand, a strict requirement for adherence to a set frame may evoke feelings of being controlled and entrapped, and in some circumstances can hinder the development of the alliance. In our view, it is important that the patient experiences agency in the treatment and feels that the therapist is listening and taking seriously his or her concerns, with some degree of flexibility. This is best accomplished through a sensitive and proactive collaborative negotiation with the patient around frame issues, with attention to the patient's wishes and perceived needs, therapeutic goals, and the therapist's personal limits.

Patients who have experienced traumatic affective experiences (not just overt trauma and neglect, but also truly overwhelming and unbearable affective experiences and psychotic states) are vulnerable to an erosion of the capacity to fully engage with sustaining relationships [19]. In this context, it can be too hard for the patient to sustain hope, and too easy to begin to give up on the ties to loved ones that are life-sustaining. If the patient can experience the therapist's genuine affective involvement—at both a cognitive and implicit relational level—this can be the first step to regaining some hope for change. The therapist's effort at repair, experienced as genuine and emotionally resonant by the patient, "is inviting the patient to hang on, to turn towards the relationship instead of away from it and to use the therapist's help to find ways to cope without resorting to suicide" ([56], p. 320).

3.10. *Attention to Countertransference*

Psychotherapy with suicidal patients is inherently extremely challenging. First, the therapist must accept that despite his or her best efforts there is no way to definitively control the outcome, and a patient may complete suicide. The lack of control about a potentially catastrophic outcome for which the therapist may feel blamed engenders anxiety, fear, and other emotions that are inescapable. In addition, repeatedly sitting with a patient who is in terrible emotional pain, without the means to provide relief, is a very difficult emotional task for the therapist.

Hopelessness can be particularly difficult to bear, and the therapist may feel worn down over time, beginning to accede to the patient's often stated belief that nothing can possibly be of help [55]. In most cases, this is a "countertransference hopelessness" which can unconsciously be communicated to the patient in verbal interaction and also in non-verbal cues. This then invites feelings of aloneness and abandonment in the patient, increasing hopelessness. The therapist can use his or her own reflective capacity, internal sustaining resources, knowledge about psychotherapeutic potential for change, and clinical experience to balance these reactions to the patient and to maintain hope. Consultation with a colleague or supervisor or a colleague can be effective in helping the therapist to regain balance and re-engage with the patient.

Suicidal patients are suffering terribly, and therapists are highly motivated to help, but often lack any tools to alleviate the suffering (at least in the immediate term). This can activate multiple affects in the therapist and trigger unconscious defense mechanisms. The therapist may feel suddenly anxious, overwhelmed, frustrated, and hopeless. The therapist's automatic defenses against such feelings may include avoidance of affect; exclusive focus on symptoms rather than feelings; efforts to control the patient's behavior, or an opposite lack of engagement in the patient's decision-making; and denial about the seriousness of the patient's distress. In their classic paper, Maltsberger and Buie [65] discuss the "countertransference hate" that can arise in the therapist. They describe two components: "malice" which is a more overt experience leading to expression of irritation or anger towards the patient, and the even more concerning "aversion", which represents unconscious emotional withdrawal. It is the latter, aversion, that is most scary in terms of increasing potential suicide risk, as patients tend to be exquisitely attuned to the therapist's emotional state and level of engagement. Unconscious withdrawal by the therapist may be experienced with an increase in aloneness and a sense of abandonment, which can put the patient at risk for despair and suicidal behavior. Again, discussion with colleagues and formal consultation can be extremely helpful for the therapist to get out of the intensity of the dyad and to explore his or her feelings about the patient and the treatment.

4. Conclusions

In this paper, the Boston Suicide Study Group has presented a theoretical and clinical approach to psychotherapy with suicidal patients. It is fundamentally a psychodynamic treatment, with an emphasis on the therapeutic alliance, unconscious and implicit relational processes, and the power of the therapeutic relationship to facilitate change in a long-term exploratory treatment. It is also integrative, incorporating ideas from DBT, MBT, and CBT, developmental and social psychology in a psychodynamic frame. There are ten key aspects of this integrative psychodynamic treatment: 1. approach to the patient in crisis; 2, instilling hope; 3. a focus on the patient's internal affective experience; 4. attention to conscious and unconscious beliefs and fantasies; 5. improving affect tolerance; 6. development of narrative identity and modification of "relational scripts"; 7. facilitation of the emergence of the patient's genuine capacities; 8. improving a sense of continuity and coherence; 9 attention to the therapeutic alliance; 10. attention to countertransference. These elements of treatment are overlapping and are not meant to be sequential, but they provide a "road map" of the various ways in which this psychotherapy facilitates a patient's move from despair and suicidality to a more satisfying relational experience with others.

Engagement with an empathic therapist provides a secure environment for exploration of the suicidal patient's internal subjective experience. The therapist helps to instill hope by bearing the patient's pain while helping the patient to discover and mobilize a sense of agency, mourn what truly is not possible, re-engage in relationships, and begin to envision a life that is worth living. The therapist notices and disrupts the patient's non-conscious defenses, leading to exposure to previously warded off feelings and greater affect tolerance. In listening to and engaging in the patient's narrative, the therapist helps to co-construct a new narrative that is more empathic and less self-attacking, renegotiating narrative identity in a more realistic and positive way. The therapist facilitates the gradual emergence of the patient's genuine capacities, modulating self-attack and disrupting avoidant defenses, and providing the patient an opportunity to bear the anxiety and conflict associated with experiencing oneself more fully. Great attention is paid to the therapeutic alliance and the therapist's countertransference.

The therapist engages with and disrupts the patient's nonconscious relational scripts by behaving differently than unconsciously expected, thus offering the possibility that the therapeutic relationship has the potential to facilitate change. At the same time, the therapist actively supports the patient in creating new relational experiences that begin to elicit feedback that is discrepant with maladaptive core beliefs about self. Ruptures in the therapeutic alliance can be extremely painful, but repair of the alliance offers a further opportunity for implicit relational learning and growth.

Author Contributions: Writing—original draft, M.S.; Writing—review and editing, E.R., B.H. and M.G.

Acknowledgments: The authors wish to acknowledge John T. (Terry) Maltsberger, who was a mentor to all of us and the leader of the Boston Suicide Study Group. While Terry was not with us for the preparation of this manuscript, he was ever present in our hearts and minds. We are forever grateful for his wisdom and friendship.

References

1. Weinberg, I.; Ronningstam, E.; Goldblatt, M.J.; Schechter, M.; Wheelis, J.; Maltsberger, J.T. Strategies in Treatment of Suicidality: Identification of Common and Treatment-Specific Interventions in Empirically Supported Treatment Manuals. *J. Clin. Psychiatry* **2010**, *71*, 699–706. [CrossRef] [PubMed]
2. Sledge, W.; Plakun, E.M.; Bauer, S.; Brodsky, B.; Caligor, E.; Clemens, N.A.; Deen, S.; Kay, J.; Lazar, S.; Mellman, L.A.; et al. Psychotherapy for suicidal patients with borderline personality disorder: An expert consensus review of common factors across five therapies. *Bord. Personal. Disord. Emot. Dysregul.* **2014**, *1*, 16. [CrossRef] [PubMed]
3. Linehan, M. *Cognitive-Behavioral Treatment of Borderline Personality Disorder*; Diagnosis and Treatment of Mental Disorders; Guilford Press: New York, NY, USA, 1993; ISBN 978-0-89862-183-9.
4. Linehan, M.M. Validation and psychotherapy. In *Empathy Reconsidered: New Directions in Psychotherapy*; Bohart, A.C., Greenberg, L.S., Eds.; American Psychological Association: Washington, DC, USA, 1997; pp. 353–392. ISBN 978-1-55798-410-4.
5. Schechter, M. The Patient's Experience of Validation in Psychoanalytic Treatment. *J. Am. Psychoanal. Assoc.* **2007**, *55*, 105–130. [CrossRef] [PubMed]
6. Linehan, M.M.; Goodstein, J.L.; Nielsen, S.L.; Chiles, J.A. Reasons for staying alive when you are thinking of killing yourself: The reasons for living inventory. *J. Consult. Clin. Psychol.* **1983**, *51*, 276–286. [CrossRef] [PubMed]
7. Strosahl, K.; Chiles, J.A.; Linehan, M. Prediction of suicide intent in hospitalized parasuicides: Reasons for living, hopelessness, and depression. *Compr. Psychiatry* **1992**, *33*, 366–373. [CrossRef]
8. Malone, K.M.; Oquendo, M.A.; Haas, G.L.; Ellis, S.P.; Li, S.; Mann, J.J. Protective Factors Against Suicidal Acts in Major Depression: Reasons for Living. *Am. J. Psychiatry* **2000**, *157*, 1084–1088. [CrossRef]
9. Chiles, J.A.; Strosahl, K.D.; McMurtray, L.; Linehan, M.M. Modeling effects on suicidal behavior. *J. Nerv. Ment. Dis.* **1985**, *173*, 477–481. [CrossRef]
10. Goldblatt, M.J. The psychodynamics of hope in suicidal despair. *Scand. Psychoanal. Rev.* **2017**, *40*, 54–62. [CrossRef]
11. Snyder, C.R. TARGET ARTICLE: Hope Theory: Rainbows in the Mind. *Psychol. Inq.* **2002**, *13*, 249–275. [CrossRef]
12. Seiden, R.H. Where are they now? A follow-up study of suicide attempters from the Golden Gate Bridge. *Suicide Life Threat. Behav.* **1978**, *8*, 203–216.
13. Suominen, K.; Isometsä, E.; Suokas, J.; Haukka, J.; Achte, K.; Lönnqvist, J. Completed Suicide After a Suicide Attempt: A 37-Year Follow-Up Study. *Am. J. Psychiatry* **2004**, *161*, 562–563. [CrossRef] [PubMed]
14. Calati, R.; Courtet, P. Is psychotherapy effective for reducing suicide attempt and non-suicidal self-injury rates? Meta-analysis and meta-regression of literature data. *J. Psychiatr. Res.* **2016**, *79*, 8–20. [CrossRef] [PubMed]
15. Shneidman, E. What do suicides have in common? Summary of the psychological approach. In *Suicide: Guidelines for Assessment, Management, and Treatment*; Bongar, B.M., Ed.; Oxford University Press: New York, NY, USA, 1992; pp. 3–15. ISBN 978-0-19-506846-7.
16. Hendin, H.; Maltsberger, J.T.; Haas, A.P.; Szanto, K.; Rabinowicz, H. Desperation and Other Affective States in Suicidal Patients. *Suicide Life Threat. Behav.* **2004**, *34*, 386–394. [CrossRef] [PubMed]
17. Orbach, I.; Mikulincer, M.; Gilboa-Schechtman, E.; Sirota, P. Mental Pain and Its Relationship to Suicidality and Life Meaning. *Suicide Life Threat. Behav.* **2003**, *33*, 231–241. [CrossRef] [PubMed]
18. Shneidman, E.S. Commentary: Suicide as Psychache. *J. Nerv. Ment. Dis.* **1993**, *181*, 145–147. [CrossRef]
19. Maltsberger, J.T.; Goldblatt, M.J.; Ronningstam, E.; Weinberg, I.; Schechter, M. Traumatic Subjective Experiences Invite Suicide. *J. Am. Acad. Psychoanal. Dyn. Psychiatry* **2011**, *39*, 671–693. [CrossRef] [PubMed]
20. Galynker, I.I. *The Suicidal Crisis: Clinical Guide to the Assessment of Imminent Suicide Risk*; Oxford University Press: New York, NY, USA, 2018; ISBN 978-0-19-026085-9.
21. Adler, G.; Buie, D.H. Aloneness and borderline psychopathology: The possible relevance of child development issues. *Int. J. Psychoanal.* **1979**, *60*, 83–96. [PubMed]
22. Maltsberger, J.T. Suicide Danger: Clinical Estimation and Decision. *Suicide Life Threat. Behav.* **1988**, *18*, 47–54. [CrossRef] [PubMed]

23. Joiner, T.E. *Why People Die by Suicide*; Harvard University Press: Cambridge, MA, USA, 2005; ISBN 978-0-674-01901-0.
24. Van Orden, K.A.; Witte, T.K.; Cukrowicz, K.C.; Braithwaite, S.R.; Selby, E.A.; Joiner, T.E. The interpersonal theory of suicide. *Psychol. Rev.* **2010**, *117*, 575–600. [CrossRef]
25. Baumeister, R.F. Suicide as escape from self. *Psychol. Rev.* **1990**, *97*, 90–113. [CrossRef]
26. Maltsberger, J.T. The descent into suicide. *Int. J. Psychoanal.* **2004**, *85*, 653–668. [CrossRef] [PubMed]
27. Schechter, M.; Goldblatt, M.J.; Ronningstam, E.; Herbstman, B.; Maltsberger, J.T. Postdischarge suicide: A psychodynamic understanding of subjective experience and its importance in suicide prevention. *Bull. Menn. Clin.* **2016**, *80*, 80–96. [CrossRef] [PubMed]
28. Maltsberger, J.T.; Buie, D.H. The devices of suicide. Revenge, riddance, and rebirth. *Int. Rev. Psychoanal.* **1980**, *7*, 61–72.
29. Maltsberger, J.T.; Ronningstam, E.; Weinberg, I.; Schechter, M.; Goldblatt, M.J. Suicide fantasy as a life-sustaining recourse. *J. Am. Acad Psychoanal. Dyn. Psychiatry* **2010**, *38*, 611–623. [CrossRef] [PubMed]
30. Baldessarini, R.J. *Suicide Risks: Rates & Predictors in Major Mood Disorders and Post-Discharge*; McLean Hospital Grand Rounds: Belmont, MA, USA, 2019.
31. McAdams, D.P. Personality, Modernity, and the Storied Self: A Contemporary Framework for Studying Persons. *Psychol. Inq.* **1996**, *7*, 295–321. [CrossRef]
32. McAdams, D.P. The psychology of life stories. *Rev. Gen. Psychol.* **2001**, *5*, 100–122. [CrossRef]
33. Thorne, A. Personal memory telling and personality development. *Pers. Soc. Psychol. Rev.* **2000**, *4*, 45–56. [CrossRef]
34. Pasupathi, M. The social construction of the personal past and its implications for adult development. *Psychol. Bull.* **2001**, *127*, 651–672. [CrossRef]
35. Pasupathi, M. Identity: Commentary: Identity Development: Dialogue Between Normative and Pathological Developmental Approaches. *J. Personal. Disord.* **2014**, *28*, 113–120. [CrossRef]
36. McAdams, D.P.; Bauer, J.J.; Sakaeda, A.R.; Anyidoho, N.A.; Machado, M.A.; Magrino-Failla, K.; White, K.W.; Pals, J.L. Continuity and Change in the Life Story: A Longitudinal Study of Autobiographical Memories in Emerging Adulthood. *J. Personal.* **2006**, *74*, 1371–1400. [CrossRef]
37. Schechter, M.; Herbstman, B.; Ronningstam, E.; Goldblatt, M.J. Emerging Adults, Identity Development, and Suicidality: Implications for Psychoanalytic Psychotherapy. *Psychoanal. Study Child.* **2018**, *71*, 20–39. [CrossRef]
38. Pasupathi, M.; Weeks, T.L. Integrating self and experience in narrative as a route to adolescent identity construction. *New Dir. Child. Adolesc. Dev.* **2011**, *2011*, 31–43. [CrossRef] [PubMed]
39. Pasupathi, M.; Hoyt, T. The development of narrative identity in late adolescence and emergent adulthood: The continued importance of listeners. *Dev. Psychol.* **2009**, *45*, 558–574. [CrossRef] [PubMed]
40. McLean, K.C.; Mansfield, C.D. The co-construction of adolescent narrative identity: Narrative processing as a function of adolescent age, gender, and maternal scaffolding. *Dev. Psychol.* **2012**, *48*, 436–447. [CrossRef]
41. Salvatore, G.; Dimaggio, G.; Semerari, A. A model of narrative development: Implications for understanding psychopathology and guiding therapy. *Psychol. Psychother. Theory Res. Pract.* **2004**, *77*, 231–254. [CrossRef] [PubMed]
42. Fonagy, P.; Steele, M.; Steele, H.; Moran, G.S.; Higgitt, A.C. The capacity for understanding mental states: The reflective self in parent and child and its significance for security of attachment. *Infant Ment. Health J.* **1991**, *12*, 201–218. [CrossRef]
43. Fonagy, P.; Target, M. Attachment and reflective function: Their role in self-organization. *Dev. Psychopathol.* **1997**, *9*, 679–700. [CrossRef] [PubMed]
44. Fonagy, P.; Target, M.; Gergely, G.; Allen, J.G.; Bateman, A.W. The Developmental Roots of Borderline Personality Disorder in Early Attachment Relationships: A Theory and Some Evidence. *Psychoanal. Inq.* **2003**, *23*, 412–459. [CrossRef]
45. Bowlby, J. *Attachment and Loss: Attachment*; Basic Books: New York, NY, USA, 1969; Volume I.
46. Stern, D.N.; Sander, L.W.; Nahum, J.P.; Harrison, A.M.; Lyons-Ruth, K.; Morgan, A.C.; Bruschweiler-Stern, N.; Tronick, E.Z. Non-interpretive mechanisms in psychoanalytic therapy. The "something more" than interpretation. The Process of Change Study Group. *Int. J. Psychoanal.* **1998**, *79*, 903–921.
47. Lyons-Ruth, K. The two-person unconscious: Intersubjective dialogue, enactive relational representation, and the emergence of new forms of relational organization. *Psychoanal. Inq.* **1999**, *19*, 576–617. [CrossRef]

48. Lyons-Ruth, K. The Interface Between Attachment and Intersubjectivity: Perspective from the Longitudinal Study of Disorganized Attachment. *Psychoanal. Inq.* **2007**, *26*, 595–616. [CrossRef]
49. Swann, W.B.; Read, S.J. Acquiring self-knowledge: The search for feedback that fits. *J. Personal. Soc. Psychol.* **1981**, *41*, 1119–1128. [CrossRef]
50. Swann, W.B. Identity negotiation: Where two roads meet. *J. Personal. Soc. Psychol.* **1987**, *53*, 1038–1051. [CrossRef]
51. Swann, W.B.; Bosson, J.K. Self and identity. In *Handbook of Social Psychology*; Fiske, S.T., Gilbert, D.T., Lindzey, G., Jongsma, A.E., Eds.; Wiley: Hoboken, NJ, USA, 2010; pp. 589–628. ISBN 978-0-470-13747-5.
52. Wachtel, P.L. Knowing oneself from the inside out, knowing oneself from the outside in: The "inner" and "outer" worlds and their link through action. *Psychoanal. Psychol.* **2009**, *26*, 158–170. [CrossRef]
53. Buie, D.H. Core Issues in the Treatment of Personality-Disordered Patients. *J. Am. Psychoanal. Assoc.* **2013**, *61*, 10–23. [CrossRef] [PubMed]
54. Loewald, H.W. On the therapeutic action of psycho-analysis. *Int. J. Psychoanal.* **1960**, *41*, 16–33. [PubMed]
55. Schechter, M.; Goldblatt, M. Psychodynamic therapy and the therapeutic alliance: Validation, empathy, and genuine relatedness. In *Building a Therapeutic Alliance with the Suicidal Patient*; Michel, K., Jobes, D.A., Eds.; American Psychological Association: Washington, DC, USA, 2011; pp. 93–107. ISBN 978-1-4338-0907-1.
56. Schechter, M.; Goldblatt, M.; Maltsberger, J.T. The Therapeutic Alliance and Suicide: When Words Are Not Enough: The Therapeutic Alliance and Suicide. *Br. J. Psychother.* **2013**, *29*, 315–328. [CrossRef]
57. Safran, J.D.; Crocker, P.; McMain, S.; Murray, P. Therapeutic alliance rupture as a therapy event for empirical investigation. *Psychother. Theory Res. Pract. Train.* **1990**, *27*, 154–165. [CrossRef]
58. Safran, J.D.; Muran, J.C. The resolution of ruptures in the therapeutic alliance. *J. Consult. Clin. Psychol.* **1996**, *64*, 447–458. [CrossRef]
59. Safran, J.D.; Muran, J.C.; Samstag, L.W.; Stevens, C. Repairing alliance ruptures. *Psychother. Theory Res. Pract. Train.* **2001**, *38*, 406–412. [CrossRef]
60. Kris, A.O. Helping Patients by Analyzing Self-Criticism. *J. Am. Psychoanal. Assoc.* **1990**, *38*, 605–636. [CrossRef] [PubMed]
61. Yeomans, F.E.; Clarkin, J.F.; Kernberg, O.F. *A Primer on Transference-Focused Psychotherapy for the Borderline Patient*; J. Aronson: Northvale, NJ, USA, 2002; ISBN 978-0-7657-0355-2.
62. Bateman, A.; Fonagy, P. Mentalization based treatment for borderline personality disorder. *World Psychiatry* **2010**, *9*, 11–15. [CrossRef] [PubMed]
63. Hoffman, I.Z. Dialectical thinking and therapeutic action in the psychoanalytic process. *Psychoanal. Q.* **1994**, *63*, 187–218. [CrossRef] [PubMed]
64. Goldblatt, M.J. Hostility and Suicide: The experience of aggression from within and without. In *Relating to Self-Harm and Suicide*; Briggs, S., Lemma, A., Crouch, W., Eds.; Routledge: New York, NY, USA, 2008.
65. Maltsberger, J.T.; Buie, D.H. Countertransference hate in the treatment of suicidal patients. *Arch. Gen. Psychiatry* **1974**, *30*, 625–633. [CrossRef] [PubMed]

5

Effect of Psycho-Regulatory Massage Therapy on Pain and Depression in Women with Chronic and/or Somatoform Back Pain

Sabine B.-E. Baumgart [1,*], Anja Baumbach-Kraft [2] and Juergen Lorenz [3]

1 Faculty of Medicine, Institute for Health and Nursing Sciences, Martin Luther University Halle-Wittenberg, 06108 Halle, Germany
2 M.Sc. Public Health, 24105 Kiel, Germany; baumbach.anja@gmail.com
3 Department of Biomedical Engineering, Faculty of Life Science, University of Applied Sciences, 21033 Hamburg, Germany; juergen.lorenz@haw-hamburg.de
* Correspondence: edelbaumgart@web.de

Abstract: Chronic unspecific back pain (cBP) is often associated with depressive symptoms, negative body perception, and abnormal interoception. Given the general failure of surgery in cBP, treatment guidelines focus on conservative therapies. Neurophysiological evidence indicates that C-tactile fibers associated with the oxytonergic system can be activated by slow superficial stroking of the skin in the back, shoulder, neck, and dorsal limb areas. We hypothesize that, through recruitment of C-tactile fibers, psycho-regulatory massage therapy (PRMT) can reduce pain in patients with cBP. In our study, 66 patients were randomized to PRMT or CMT (classical massage therapy) over a 12-week period and tested by questionnaires regarding pain (HSAL= Hamburger Schmerz Adjektiv Liste; Hamburg Pain adjective list), depression (BDI-II = Beck depression inventory), and disability (ODI = Oswestry Disability Index). In all outcome measures, patients receiving PRMT improved significantly more than did those receiving CMT. The mean values of the HSAL sensory subscale decreased by −51.5% in the PRMT group compared to −6.7% in the CMT group. Depressive symptoms were reduced by −55.69% (PRMT) and −3.1% (CMT), respectively. The results suggest that the superiority of PRMT over CMT may rely on its ability to activate the C-tactile fibers of superficial skin layers, recruiting the oxytonergic system.

Keywords: massage therapy; chronic back pain; depression; oxytocin; C-tactile fibers; somatoform pain (ICD 10); somatic symptom disorder (DSM-5)

---

1. Introduction

Chronic back pain (cBP) has a leading position worldwide in disease-related disability and loss of quality of life [1]. It represents a common health problem, especially among women. According to a GEDA ("Gesundheit in Deutschland Aktuell", current state of health in Germany) survey from 2009/2010, one in four women reported suffering cBP (lasting >3 months) within the last 12 months [2]. Modern recommendations by national and international health organizations focus on non-drug therapy options in the treatment of chronic (non-specific) back pain. A variety of treatment modalities are suggested, including physical and rehabilitation interventions [3] and instrument-based techniques such as transcutaneous electrical nerve stimulation (TENS) [4], acupuncture [5], low-level laser therapy (LLLT) [6], and shock wave therapy [7]. Additional treatment with pain-relieving medication is recommended. Surgery is not recommended because there is little evidence of its effectiveness [5,8,9]. Chou et al. [10] underlined these recommendations and showed that psychological impairments, e.g., sleep disorders, mood fluctuation, depression, and listlessness, are frequent co-morbidities of chronic pain. A central characteristic of patients with chronic pain is their negative body perception [11], inhibiting cognitive access to therapy [12–14].

In the 1980s, Groddek and Dogs integrated massage therapy as a form of body therapy into the treatment of chronic pain to gain direct access to the patient's emotions via their skin and its nervous system, thus facilitating positive body perception and cognitive-behavioral treatment [15,16]. Berg et al. and Listing et al. [17,18] showed how professional therapeutic touch in the form of massage can reduce the physical and psychological symptoms of patients with pain and/or depression. A reduction in pain, mood disorders, and listlessness and fatigue was reported. Furthermore, general psychological tension was reduced, and well-being was increased. Baumgart et al. reviewed randomized controlled trials (RCTs) published from 1996 to 2009 that investigated the effectiveness of massage for patients with depression both as the main diagnosis and a co-morbidity [16]. The authors concluded that the effectiveness of massage therapy depends on the design of the parameters of (a) pressure, (b) speed, (c) direction, and (d) rhythm [14,18–22]. Studies on the effects of oxytocin and its interactions with the neuro-physiological system have provided possible explanations for the effect of touch or massage therapy in chronic pain (with and without depression) [23]. In their study, Walker and McGlone illustrated the connection between the type of touch (effect parameters: pressure and time), its neurological transmission of stimuli via C-tactile fibers, and the significance of oxytocin with regard to pain-relieving effects [24]. C-tactile afferent fibers mediate pleasantness of touch and serve a fundamental role in the hedonic function of tactile sensation [25]. Kane and Terrel emphasized the role of touch for child development and propagated the integration of touch into the treatment of developmental trauma [26]. Experimental evidence indicates that activation of C-tactile fibers can significantly alleviate muscle pain [27]. The stimulus of a gentle or moderate touch, transduced in the skin by C-tactile fibers, is transmitted via ascending spinothalamic pathways to the insular cortex, an area of the limbic system. Through connections with the paraventricular nucleus, the thalamus stimulates the synthesis of oxytocin when a touch is perceived as pleasant [23,28,29].

Based on these considerations, we hypothesize that pain experience and depressive symptoms can be reduced and physical capacity can be improved by gentle massage that is optimized to activate C-tactile skin afferents. The aim of this study is to examine the effect of both classical and psycho-regulatory massage in patients with cBP on pain experience, depressive symptoms, and physical capacity.

2. Materials and Methods

The study was conducted as a double-blind RCT. The study is registered in the German Registry for Clinical Studies (DRKS00006876), and the protocol was approved by the ethics committee of the University of Halle (Saale), Germany (Nr. 2014-22).

2.1. Eligibility Criteria

The eligibility criteria and baseline data were assessed prior to randomization. The inclusion and exclusion criteria can be found in Table 1 and were defined via extensive literature research. The diagnosis M54 in the ICD-10 (International Statistical Classification of Diseases and Related Health Problems) represents a composite of diagnoses related to back pain.

Table 1. List of eligibility criteria for study participation.

Inclusion Criteria	Exclusion Criteria
• Back pain diagnosis according to the ICD-10 code: M54 and F45, medically certified • Pain duration of >6 months • Patient age 18–75 years • Voluntary participation in the study • Sufficient knowledge of German to understand the questionnaires	• Limited ability for consent to study participation • Inflammatory disorders • Open wounds • Ongoing application for pension

Clear diagnosis of chronic pain is difficult, since 90% of the diagnoses do not reveal any apparent clinical findings [30,31]; thus, chronic pain is primarily defined by the duration of the pain [32,33]. Since chronic pain can lead to psychological co-morbidity [34], the diagnostic group of somatoform disorders (ICD-10, F45) was also included. These disorders are generally defined by the occurrence of physical problems without a clear somatic diagnosis.

2.2. Participants

We conducted 107 recruitment interviews. Of these, 41 patients did not participate for the following reasons: n = 16 did not meet eligibility criteria, n = 3 stated that the number of interventions was too high, n = 11 were not comfortable with the nudity required for massage therapy, n = 8 found that the questionnaires were too complicated, and n = 3 did not want to use massage oil. Overall, n = 66 patients were randomized into either the intervention or control group using hidden lots covered in envelopes. One patient was excluded prior to the first treatment due to acute illness; 61 patients completed the treatment. Two patients in each treatment group discontinued the treatments without giving any reason (see Figure 1).

2.3. Interventions

Interventions took place in the physiotherapy practice operated by the principle investigator (SB). The outpatient setting was chosen to maximize external validity. The intervention group received psycho-regulatory massage therapy (PRMT) and the control group received classical massage therapy (CMT). Patients were blinded towards the type of massage they received. However, they were aware of the study's aim to compare the two types of massage. Data analysis was blind towards a patient's treatment method. All therapists employed in the practice participated in the study (n = 7). The design of effect parameters differed between the intervention and control groups in terms of pressure, speed, direction, and rhythm [12,14], as shown in Table 2. The interventions also differed in respect to the target organ and body areas treated. PRMT targets the skin and the superficial fascia, whereas CMT targets all layers of the tissue, including the periosteum. The PRMT unfolds from three partial massages to a full body massage. It is applied with warm oil in both supine and prone body positions and involves soft to moderate intensities of continuous slow strokes. They are uninterrupted throughout the entire session except during the change from supine to prone body position. The therapist does not touch the different body parts in separate sequences, but moves in harmonious transitions from limbs to trunk to create a whole-body experience. An extended description of the PRMT technique is added as supplemental material. In contrast, CMT is applied to the back alone and extends from the sacrum to the neck.

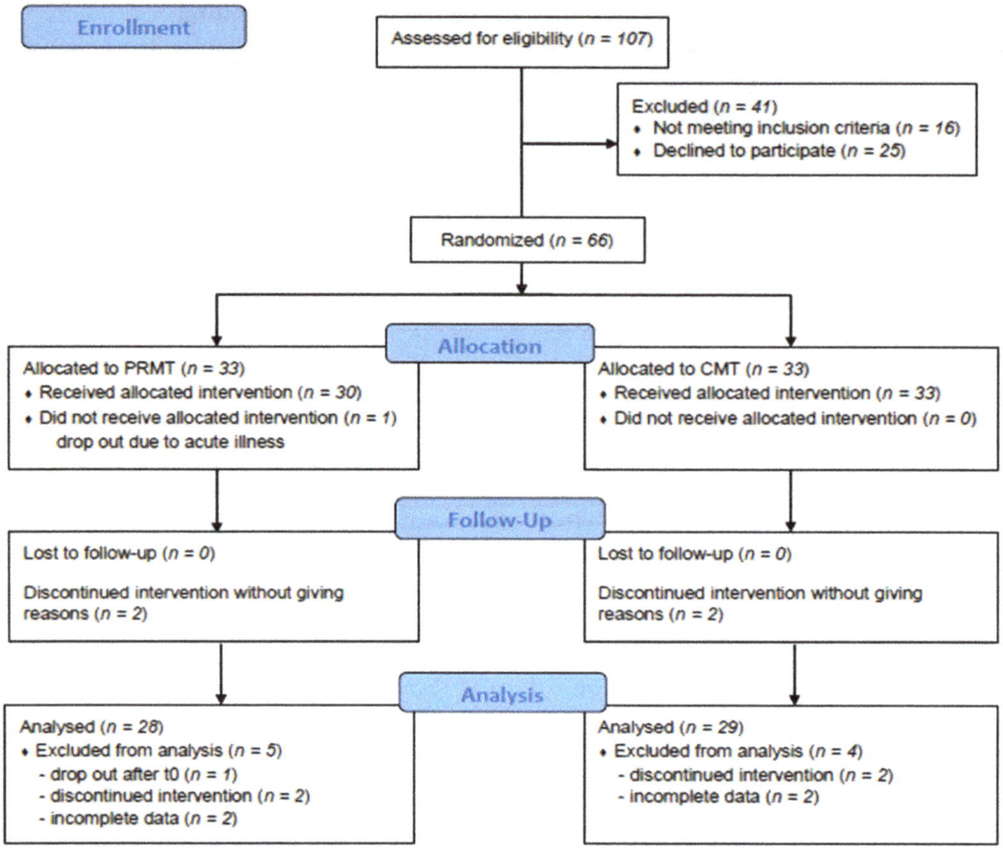

Figure 1. CONSORT (Consolidated Standards of Reporting Trials) flow chart of participants in this study comparing PRMT (psycho-regulatory massage therapy) and CMT (classical massage therapy).

Table 2. Effect parameters of the interventions.

Parameters	PRMT	CMT
Pressure	• soft to moderate	• soft to strong
Speed	• continuously decreasing to a speed of 10–3 cm per second	• a slow speed is recommended for pain reduction • not clearly defined, depends on training and individual therapist
Direction	• Body areas are connected • ending with cranial to caudal strokes	• depends on therapist's training • from the origin to the beginning of a muscle
Rhythm	• harmonious and constant contact with the patients until the end of the treatment	• not defined

PRMT, psychregulatory massage therapy; CMT, classical massage therapy.

The intervention group was treated by seven therapists who received professional training to standardize the performance of PRMT, which was applied for 30 to 60 min [35,36]. The control group received 20 min of CMT, which was not standardized but applied individually, reflecting standard care within the German statutory health insurance scheme. All treatments were applied non-verbally in a closed therapy room with only the patient and therapist present. Patients were treated by the same therapist during the whole study period, for optimal therapeutic effectiveness [18,21]. Each group received 10 treatments overall, which were scheduled twice a week.

2.4. Data collection

After 3 months, follow-up data were collected. Figure 2 shows the structure and course of the study. Data were collected via questionnaires, handed out by the therapists and filled by the patients themselves. Baseline data (T0) were collected prior to randomization and the first intervention. At T1 (5th treatment), T2 (10th treatment), and at follow-up (T3), data were collected after the interventions.

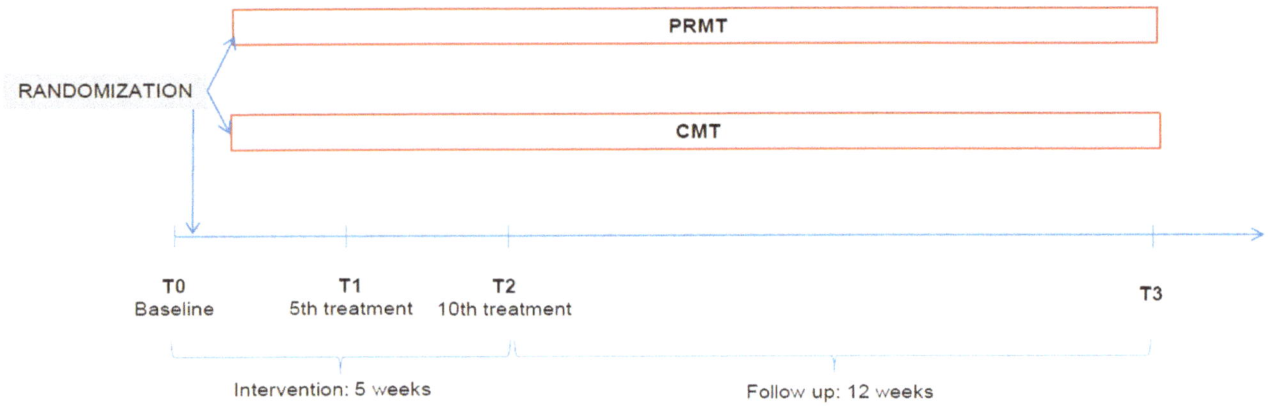

Figure 2. Study timeline (T, time of measurement; PRMT, psychoregulatory massage therapy; CMT, classical massage therapy).

Pain was assessed using the Hamburg Pain Adjective List (Hamburger Schmerz Adjektiv Liste, HSAL), a multi-dimensional questionnaire for pain experience in adults with acute or chronic pain. The HSAL consists of 37 adjectives, 21 of those describing the affective experience of pain (pain suffering + pain anxiety) and 16 describing the sensory experience of pain (pain rhythm + pain acuity). Each item can be answered on a scale from 0 (not correct at all) to 6 (completely correct), and the answers are added up to create a total score (maximum of 222, corresponding to a maximum of pain) [37]. The validity of the HSAL has been assessed by several studies in different clinical situations (Cronbach's alpha of the primary scales is between 0.80 and 0.90) [38]. The HSAL questionnaire is especially suitable in connection with psychiatric scales (depression, anxiety) and also has good applicability for monitoring patient health.

Depressiveness was measured using the Beck Depression Inventory (BDI-II), scaling 0–3 for each item; the maximum overall score is 63 points [39,40]. The severity of depression is categorized into five groups:

0–8 no depression;
9–13 minimal depression;
14–19 mild depression;
20–28 moderate depression;
29–63 severe depression [41].

The clinical relevance of the respective changes in depression was assessed according to the criteria of Hiroe et al. [42]. Accordingly, a 5-point change in BDI-II score indicates minimal relevance, 10–19 points is moderate, and more than 20 points corresponds to a strong effect.

Quality of life was measured using the Oswestry Disability Index (ODI), a self-rating questionnaire about disability in patients with back pain [43]. The questionnaire consists of 10 items, which are categorized into (1) physical complaints (or disability), (2) activity, and (3) participation according to the International Classification of Functioning, Disability and Health (ICF). A maximum score of 50 indicates maximum impairment. The scores are then converted into percentages depending on the number of questions answered. Mannion et al. [44,45] and Hooff et al. [46] investigated the validity of the German version. Their results showed that the ODI is a good measurement tool for assessing a patient's disability due to back pain (Cronbach's alpha = 0.90). The total ODI score represents a percentage and is interpreted as follows:

0–2 minimal disability (all activities of daily living (ADL) are mostly possible, often no therapy necessary, activation of life is enough);

21–40 moderate disability (participation is already limited and incapacity to work often occurs, conservative treatment);

41–60 severe disability (pain is the main problem and ADL are affected, intensive diagnostics are necessary);

61–80 crippled (all areas of life are affected);

81–100 bedridden or the patient exaggerates [47,48].

2.5. Sample Size and Randomization

For sample size calculation on the basis of overall pain experience as the primary outcome, alpha was set to 5%, statistical power should be at least 90% (SD 2.0), and the drop-out rate was expected to be 20%, resulting in a group size of $n = 33$. Block randomization was carried out with a block size of 10 by an independent statistician from University of Halle, Saale (Germany).

2.6. Statistical Analysis

Given the ordinal data type of all questionnaires (HSAL-total, HSAL-affective, HSAL-sensory, BDI-II-score, and ODI (%)) that were, in at least one session, not normally distributed, as tested with the Kolmogorov–Smirnov test, we applied the Wilcoxon rank-sum test for two independent samples to analyze group differences (CMT vs. PRMT) at baseline (T0) and to test the magnitude of change from baseline to the T1, T2, and T3 time points (SPSS, Version 26). A significant difference (two-tailed test) was accepted at p-values below 0.05. To test the effect of sessions, we applied the Friedmann ANOVA test separately for CMT and PRMT. In case of significance, we used the Wilcoxon test for paired samples. According to the total of six comparisons, we used Bonferroni correction, resulting in a p-value of 0.008 as the threshold for significance.

3. Results

The results of the non-parametric comparison using the Wilcoxon rank-sum test for two independent samples are summarized in Table 3 for all study parameters. The baseline condition (T0) yielded non-significant differences for all questionnaire scores.

HSAL total, affective, and sensory scores for pain: The total scores and the affective and sensory subscores of HSAL were significantly smaller in the T2 and T3 sessions in the PRMT group compared to the CMT group. No difference appeared in session T1. The Friedmann ANOVA yielded a non-significant effect of treatment session for CMT in HSAL-Total ($p = 0.56$), weak significance for HSAL-Affective that failed to reach the significance criterion in any of the six comparisons, and an absence of significance for HSAL-Sensory ($p = 0.127$). In contrast, all HSAL parameters were statistically significant for the effect of treatment session in PRMT ($p < 0.001$). Post hoc Wilcoxon testing revealed significant decreases in all HSAL parameters for comparisons T3 vs. T0, T4 vs. T0, T3 vs. T2, and T4 vs. T2 ($p < 0.001$; Bonferroni-corrected).

BDI-II score for depression: PRMT reduced the intensity of depression more than CMT already during T1, but more strongly during sessions T2 and T3. The Friedman ANOVA resulted in a significant session effect in CMT ($p = 0.03$); however, no post hoc comparison reached the Bonferroni-corrected threshold criterion. In contrast, PRMT had a significant effect of session with statistically significant post hoc Wilcoxon testing in all six comparisons ($p < 0.001$): T0 vs. T1, T0 vs. T2, T0 vs. T3, T1 vs. T2, T1 vs. T3, and T2 vs. T3. Thus, the BDI-II score continuously decreased over the three months of treatment. Overall, the severity of depression decreased by 55.69% with PRMT, from a moderate to minimal level of severity on average [45]. Under CMT, the mean BDI-II score changed by −3.1% over the whole study period.

Table 3. Results (mean and SD) for pain experience (HSAL total score and affective and sensory subscales), depressive symptoms (BDI-II), and disability (ODI); results of the Wilcoxon rank-sum test for independent samples tested for effect of treatment (PRMT vs. CMT) and *p*-values for two-tailed comparisons.

		T0	T1	T2	T3
	CMT	108.72	113.34	104.76	102.62
	SD	51.86	61.75	62	61.92
	PRMT	124.82	115.04	72.14	67.32
	SD	57.81	51.38	36.16	32.86
HSAL-Total	Wilcoxon_Z	−1.76	−1.04	−4.47	−3.65
	p	n.s.	n.s.	<0.001	<0.001
	CMT	66.38	67.03	61.79	60.86
	SD	34.79	38.7	38.28	38.49
	PRMT	75.86	70.39	44.75	43.93
	SD	33.13	30.68	23.3	21.83
HSAL-Affective	Wilcoxon Z	−0.84	−1.763	−3.54	−3.38
	p	n.s.	n.s.	<0.001	<0.001
	CMT	44.66	46.31	42.97	41.69
	SD	23.73	26.34	26.41	26.45
	PRMT	48.93	44.29	27.39	23.75
HSAL-Sensory	SD	26.91	23.72	16.17	15.8
	Wilcoxon Z	−0.61	−1.91	−3.86	−3.94
	p	n.s.	n.s.	<0.001	<0.001
	CMT	19.3	20.52	19.59	18.69
	SD	9.64	10.61	11.4	10.36
BDI-II score	PRMT	23.29	20.46	12.25	10.32
	SD	11.58	10.7	7.62	5.9
	Wilcoxon Z	−0.6	−2.35	−4.21	−4.41
	p	n.s.	<0.05	<0.001	0.001
	CMT	39.9	39.73	39.09	38.52
	SD	14.1	16.23	16.86	16.42
ODI (%)	PRMT	38.26	36.12	25.95	23.82
	SD	12.5	14.06	10.49	11.6
	Wilcoxon Z	−0.09	−2.09	−4.19	−4.2
	p	n.s.	<0.05	<0.001	<0.001

BDI-II: Beck Depression Inventory, 2nd version; ODI: Oswestry Disability Index; PRMT: Psycho-regulatory massage therapy; CMT: classical massage therapy; n.s.: not significant.

ODI (%) score for disability: The progression of improvement in functional status achieved by PRMT in comparison to CMT is quite similar to that for depression. A weak, yet significantly better improvement in PRMT than in CMT occurred in T1, but much greater treatment differences appeared in T2 and T3. The Friedmann ANOVA showed non-significant change by CMT ($p = 0.56$). In contrast, there was a significant change in ODI (%) by PRMT ($p < 0.001$) with significant post hoc differences in all comparisons, except for T3 vs. T2. Table 4 shows the distribution of patients within the different levels of disability (reflecting limitations in quality of life, daily activities, and participation) at baseline and follow-up measurements. Before intervention, the vast majority (90.62%) of the PRMT group had a moderate to severe level of disability. At follow-up, 86.66% of the patients had minimal to moderate levels of disability. On average, the degree of disability improved by at least one level in 90% of the PRMT group, while CMT did not lead to any substantial change. The effect size according to Cohen, $f = 0.47$, corresponds to a strong effect.

Table 4. Distribution of patients at baseline (T0) and follow-up (T3) according to the respective levels of disability.

Level of Disability	PRMT n = 28		CMT n = 29	
	T0	T3	T0	T3
Minimal	6.25%	43.33%	9.09%	10.34%
Moderate	46.87%	43.33%	45.45%	51.73%
Severe	43.75%	13.34%	33.34%	20.69%
Crippled	3.12%	0%	12.12%	17.24%
Bedridden	0%	0%	0%	0%

4. Discussion

The primary aim of this study was to examine the effect of two forms of massage therapy in patients with chronic back pain (cBP). According to the general consensus about pain as a multidimensional experience [49,50] pain was assessed via HSAL (the Hamburg Pain Adjective List). In the group receiving PRMT, the decrease in the HSAL total score was statistically significant (−57.7 points), relating to an improvement of 46%. In contrast, the HSAL total score improved only by 5.6% in the group receiving CMT, failing to reach statistical significance and indicating no clinical relevance. In terms of decrease in symptoms of affective and sensory pain experience, PRMT thus shows strong superiority over CMT. Consistent with our results, Cherkin et al. [51] investigated 10 massage applications with a duration of 50–60 min and compared "structural" massages with relaxing massages. Relaxing massages were superior to structural massages, the latter being comparable to CMT. The follow-up at 10 weeks showed that the results persisted in both groups; thus, a long-term effect analogous to the results of the present study could also be observed. Without emphasizing different techniques, Wallach et al. [52] observed a sustained long-term effect of CMT after three months involving 10 applications of massage therapy of 20 min each over 10 weeks. Hamre et al. [53] investigated the effect of rhythmic massage therapy in a four-year prospective cohort study. They examined 85 chronically ill patients, 45 of whom suffered from chronic back or neck pain. Eighteen of the patients also suffered from depression and fatigue. The disease and symptom scores used in that study, each on a scale of 0 to 10, improved significantly. The disease score decreased from 6.3 to 2.77 points, and the symptom score decreased from 5.76 to 3.13 points. The SF-36 questionnaire also showed an improvement in the physical component score and the mental score. Thus, the symptoms of chronic disease were reduced, and at the same time, the quality of life of the patients improved.

Models from neuro-biological research might explain the positive effects of massage and the role of their specific techniques. Studies using microneurography have indicated the existence of low-threshold slowly conducting C-fibers in superficial skin layers that are predominantly activated by soft and low-velocity (3 cm/s) stroking stimuli [27]. In contrast, stronger pressure stimuli penetrating into deeper subepidermal skin layers activate rapidly conducting A-tactile afferents. A-tactile and C-tactile afferents are regarded as important for discriminant and affective dimensions of touch perception, respectively [28]. Accordingly, A-tactile fibers are predominantly abundant in the glabrous skin of the hands, whereas C-tactile fibers predominate in the hairy skin of the limbs and back. Several authors have pointed to the importance of the type of touch to be applied: slow, harmonic, and rhythmic with moderate pressure [24,54–57].

Boehme et al. compared patients suffering from fibromyalgia with healthy controls by using functional magnetic resonance imaging (fMRI) imaging of brain activity in response to selective C-tactile stimuli and additionally analyzed the voxel-based morphometry in areas of the limbic cortex [58]. They observed an abnormal pattern of deactivation and activation within the posterior insula during pleasantness and pain ratings, respectively, and a reduced grey matter density in the hippocampus and anterior insula. The authors interpreted their results as indications of anhedonia to gentle touch in fibromyalgia. Notably, classical massage is reported to worsen pain, whereas soft skin stroking, lymphatic drainage, and superficial vacuum massage alleviate pain in fibromyalgia patients [59]. Liljencrantz and Olausson [56] also reported anxiety-reducing effects of stimulating C-tactile afferents.

Craig [60] and Devue et al. [61] identified a functional network between the anterior insula and the cingulate gyrus, which serves primarily for self-recognition and awareness of one's own body. External impulses like touch and their subjective processing are thus integrated into emotional experiences. Older studies identified interoceptive afferents of primates as correlates of a so-called "gut feeling", which represents a complex integration of sensory perceptions and corresponding emotional responses. In the early 1990s, Damasio demonstrated that emotional and mental responses to stimuli mediate spino-thalamic and insular impulses that are integrated into body perception [62]. Paulsen and Stein reported that patients with depression and/or anxiety disorders experience significantly altered interoceptive signal processing. Signals are passed on blurred and amplified, so that homeostatic states are difficult to predict [63].

Several studies have shown an interaction of C-tactile afferents with the oxytonergic system in reducing pain and improving body perception [24,54,55]. Pfeifer et al. [64] and Uvnäs-Moberg and Peterson [23] postulated a positive influence on pain memory via the limbic system and activation of the oxytonergic system. This hypothesis was confirmed by follow-up data. A long-term effect was shown in both groups at three months post-intervention. This is coherent with the neuro-biologic findings by Lund et al. [65], who reported a long-term pain-reducing effect of soft massage-like touch through interaction of the oxytonergic system with the opioid system and activation of periaqueductal grey neurons. Miranda-Cardenaz et al. [66] and DeLaTorre [67] detected oxytocin receptors in the laminae of the dorsal horns. By micro-stimulation of the paraventricular nucleus and intrathecal administration of oxytocin, they were able to demonstrate an inhibited stimulus response of the wide dynamic-range neurons in the spinal horn in chronic pain syndrome. The authors considered this to be a descending oxytonergic control mechanism that influences chronic pain perception. Oxytocin also plays an antagonistic role in the glutamatergic spinal sensory conduction of acute pain stimuli [68]. Oxytocin inhibits the conduction of pain in the protopathic ascending pathways and plays a role in the function of the opioid system and gate control mechanism [64,65]. Thus, oxytocin can inhibit acute and chronic pain stimuli at different levels of the central nervous system (CNS).

The results on depression severity in our study, as measured by the BDI-II questionnaire, lend further strong support for the importance of C-tactile stimulation underlying the superior efficacy of PRMT over CMT. In the PRMT group, improvements on the BDI-II correspond to a moderate clinical effect [46]. In contrast, the severity of depression did not change significantly following CMT. These results support findings from a systematic review by Baumgart et al. that found massage therapy to be effective for depression and anxiety as a primary diagnosis and a co-morbidity, respectively [16]. Finally, disability and activity improved significantly within the PRMT group. Inter-group analysis also showed a significant effect in favor of PRMT compared to CMT. The PRMT group showed an improvement rate of 37.76%—the CMT group, only 3.46%. Changes of at least 18% are considered clinically relevant [46]. In this study, an important aim of chronic pain treatment (increase in function and activity) was achieved with PRMT [61]. Positive psycho-emotional effects, including a decrease in depressive symptoms, increase the motivation to maintain physical integrity, which is associated with an increase in personal activity [20,69,70]. Perceiving the back as a pleasant body part might reduce negative self-referential processing and open the patients towards treatments aiming at cognitive emotion regulation, e.g., mindfulness training [71].

There are limitations of our study. Since this study was conducted in the outpatient setting of a physiotherapy practice, the level of treatment standardization was low. Factors such as the patient's daily routine; sleep, waking, and eating rhythm; and time of intervention were not standardized to increase external validity. Treatment prescription was done by private orthopedic surgeons and general practitioners using the ICD-10 codes M54 and F45, which qualified the patients for study inclusion. There might have been variability among doctors in the use of these diagnoses. Yet, no patient had indication of specific back diseases causing their pain. Use of the term "somatoform" might be debatable, and it differs between the DSM (Diagnostic and Statistical Manual of Mental Disorders) and ICD classifications. During the update to DSM-5, the class of "somatoform disorders" was changed to "somatic symptom disorder", whereas the term is still used in the ICD-10. Furthermore, patients were allowed to use their pain medication as usual and receive other therapies, introducing a certain risk of bias to our results. Future studies could examine how the use of analgesics can be reduced by PRMT. Standard regulations of health care insurances allow 20 to 30 min of treatment duration for CMT, but 60 min for PRMT, because the latter involves a whole-body massage. Thus, longer treatment sessions might have contributed to the superiority of PRMT over CMT. The follow-up period of our study was three months, to increase comparability with other studies [16]. However, future studies could choose a longer follow-up period to better assess the long-term effects of PRMT intervention. Although the BDI-II score yielded no significant group differences at baseline, there was no stratification of patients according to the severity of depressive symptoms by an expert in psychiatry. Our results strongly suggest that patients with indications of depressive comorbidity benefit the most from PRMT. Although our a priori concept and conduct of PRMT aimed at an optimization of recruiting C-tactile afferent activity, we have no physiological proof of its importance in our study. Heart rate variability analysis has been found to be sensitive to the pleasantness of C-tactile stimulation [72] and appears to be compatible with study designs such as the one presented here.

5. Conclusions

Our results indicate that psycho-regulatory massage therapy (PRMT) is more effective than classical massage therapy (CMT) in reducing pain and depression and enhancing physical capacity and activity in patients suffering from chronic unspecific back pain. Unlike CMT, PRMT characterizes a massage technique by which the therapist applies soft and slow strokes upon the skin of the back, neck, shoulders, and upper arms that specifically activate C-tactile fibers. Future studies should examine the importance of individual differences of co-morbidity with depression in patients suffering from chronic unspecific back pain for the superiority of PRMT over CMT. This knowledge would improve the selection of individualized physical therapy options for these patients.

Author Contributions: S.B.-E.B.: Conceptualization, formal analysis, resources, writing—original draft. A.B.-K.: writing—review and editing, visualization. J.L.: Supervision, statistical analysis, writing—review and editing. All authors have read and agreed to the published version of the manuscript.

References

1. Vos, T.; Barber, R.M.; Bell, B.; Bertozzi-Villa, A.; Biryukov, S.; Bolliger, I.; Charlson, F.; Davis, A.; Degenhardt, L.; Dicker, D.; et al. Global, regional, and national incidence, prevalence, and years lived with disability for 301 acute and chronic diseases and injuries in 188 countries, 1990–2013: A systematic analysis for the Global Burden of Disease Study 2013. *Lancet* **2015**, *386*, 743–800. [CrossRef]
2. Schneider, S.; Randoll, D.; Buchner, M. Why do women have back pain more than men? *Clin. J. Pain* **2006**, *22*, 738–747. [CrossRef] [PubMed]
3. Van Middelkoop, M.; Rubinstein, S.M.; Kuijpers, T.; Verhagen, A.P.; Ostelo, R.W.; Koes, B.W.; van Tulder, M. A systematic review on the effectiveness of physical and rehabilitation interventions for chronic non-specific low back pain. *Eur. Spine J.* **2010**, *20*, 19–39. [CrossRef] [PubMed]
4. Khadilkar, A.; Milne, S.; Brosseau, L.; Wells, G.; Tugwell, P.; Robinson, V.; Shea, B.; Saginur, M. Transcutaneous electrical nerve stimulation for the treatment of chronic low back pain: A systematic review. *Spine* **2005**, *30*, 2657–2666. [CrossRef] [PubMed]
5. Xu, M.; Yan, S.; Yin, X.; Li, X.; Gao, S.; Han, R.; Wei, L.; Luo, W.; Lei, G. Acupuncture for chronic low back pain in long-term follow-up: A meta-analysis of 13 randomized controlled trials. *Am. J. Chin. Med.* **2013**, *41*, 1–19. [CrossRef]

6. Glazov, G.; Yelland, M.; Emery, J. Low-level laser therapy for chronic non-specific low back pain: A meta-analysis of randomised controlled trials. *Acupunct. Med.* **2016**, *34*, 328–341. [CrossRef] [PubMed]
7. Seco-Calvo, J.; Kovacs, F.M.; Urrútia, G. The efficacy, safety, effectiveness, and cost-effectiveness of ultrasound and shock wave therapies for low back pain: A systematic review. *Spine J.* **2011**, *11*, 966–977. [CrossRef]
8. Oliveira, C.B.; Maher, C.G.; Pinto, R.Z.; Traeger, A.C.; Lin, C.-W.C.; Chenot, J.-F.; van Tulder, M.; Koes, B.W. Clinical practice guidelines for the management of non-specific low back pain in primary care: An updated overview. *Eur. Spine J.* **2018**, *27*, 2791–2803. [CrossRef]
9. Airaksinen, O.; Brox, J.I.; Cedraschi, C.; Hildebrandt, J.; Klaber-Moffett, J.; Kovacs, F.; Mannion, A.F.; Reis, S.; Staal, J.B.; Ursin, H.; et al. Chapter 4 European guidelines for the management of chronic nonspecific low back pain. *Eur. Spine J.* **2006**, *15*, 192–300. [CrossRef]
10. Chou, R. Nonpharmacologic therapies for low back pain. *Ann. Intern. Med.* **2017**, *167*, 606–607. [CrossRef]
11. Levenig, C.G.; Kellmann, M.; Kleinert, J.; Belz, J.; Hesselmann, T.; Hasenbring, M.I. Body image is more negative in patients with chronic low back pain than in patients with subacute low back pain and healthy controls. *Scand. J. Pain* **2019**, *19*, 147–156. [CrossRef] [PubMed]
12. Rohricht, F.; Beyer, W.; Priebe, S. Disturbances of body-experience in acute anxiety and depressive disorders neuroticism or somatization? *Psychother. Psych. Med.* **2002**, *52*, 205–213.
13. Field, T. Massage therapy. *Med. Clin. North Am.* **2002**, *86*, 163–171. [CrossRef]
14. Baumgart, S. Psychoaktive massage und atemtherapie-konzept und fallbericht. *Phys. Ther. Theor. Prax.* **2008**, *6*, 277–281.
15. Dogs, W. Psychomotorik der massage. *Phys. Ther.* **1988**, *1*, 12–14.
16. Baumgart, S.; Müller-Oerlinghausen, B.; Schendera, C.F.G. Wirksamkeit der massagetherapie bei depression und angsterkrankungen sowie bei depressivität und angst als komorbidität—eine systematische übersicht kontrollierter studien. *Phys. Med. Rehabil. Kurortmed.* **2011**, *21*, 167–182. [CrossRef]
17. Müller-Oerlinghausen, B.; Berg, C.; Droll, W. Die Slow Stroke®massage als ein körpertherapeutischer ansatz bei depression. *Psychiatr. Prax.* **2007**, *34*, 305–308. [CrossRef]
18. Listing, M.; Reißhauer, A.; Krohn, M.; Voigt, B.; Tjahono, G.; Becker, J.; Klapp, B.F.; Rauchfuß, M. Massage therapy reduces physical discomfort and improves mood disturbances in women with breast cancer. *Psychol. Oncol.* **2009**, *18*, 1290–1299. [CrossRef]
19. Diego, M.A.; Field, T.; Sanders, C.; Hernandez-Reif, M. Massage therapy of moderate and light pressure and vibration effects on EEG and heart rate. *Int. J. Neurosci.* **2004**, *114*, 31–44. [CrossRef]
20. Olausson, H.W.; Wessberg, J.; Morrison, I.; McGlone, F.; Vallbo, Å. The neurophysiology of unmyelinated tactile afferents. *Neurosci. Biobehav. Rev.* **2010**, *34*, 185–191. [CrossRef]
21. Moyer, C.A. Massage therapy: An examination of the contextual model. *Diss. Abstr. Int. Sect. B Sci. Eng.* **2008**, *69*, 1337.
22. Kolster, B.C. Wirkprinzipien der massage. In *Massage*; Springer: Berlin/Heidelberg, Germany, 2003; pp. 22–34.
23. Uvnas-Moberg, K.; Petersson, M. Oxytocin, a mediator of anti-stress, well-being, social interaction, growth and healing. *Z Psychosom. Med. Psychother.* **2005**, *51*, 57–80. [PubMed]
24. Walker, S.C.; McGlone, F.P. The social brain: Neurobiological basis of affiliative behaviours and psychological well-being. *Neuropeptides* **2013**, *47*, 379–393. [CrossRef] [PubMed]
25. McGlone, F.; Wessberg, J.; Olausson, H. Discriminative and affective touch: Sensing and feeling. *Neuron* **2014**, *82*, 737–755. [CrossRef] [PubMed]
26. Kain, K.L.; Levine, P.A.; Terrell, S.J. *Nurturing Resilience: Helping Clients Move Forward from Developmental Trauma*; North Atlantic Books: Berkeley, CA, USA, 2018.
27. Shaikh, S.; Nagi, S.S.; McGlone, F.; Mahns, D.A. Psychophysical Investigations into the role of low-threshold C fibres in non-painful affective processing and pain modulation. *PLoS ONE* **2015**, *10*, e0138299. [CrossRef] [PubMed]
28. Okabe, S.; Yoshida, M.; Takayanagi, Y.; Onaka, T. Activation of hypothalamic oxytocin neurons following tactile stimuli in rats. *Neurosci. Lett.* **2015**, *600*, 22–27. [CrossRef] [PubMed]
29. Richard, P.; Moos, F.; Freund-Mercier, M.J. Central effects of oxytocin. *Physiol. Rev.* **1991**, *71*, 331–370. [CrossRef]
30. Dworkin, R.H.; Turk, D.C.; Peirce-Sandner, S.; Baron, R.; Bellamy, N.; Burke, L.B.; Chappell, A.; Chartier, K.; Cleeland, C.S.; Costello, A.; et al. Research design considerations for confirmatory chronic pain clinical trials: IMMPACT recommendations. *Pain* **2010**, *149*, 177–193. [CrossRef]

31. Henningsen, P. The psychosomatics of chronic back pain. Classification, aetiology and therapy. *Orthopäde* **2004**, *33*, 558–567. [CrossRef]
32. Abraham, I.; Killackey-Jones, B. Lack of evidence-based research for idiopathic low back pain. *Arch. Intern. Med.* **2002**, *162*, 1442–1444. [CrossRef]
33. Deyo, R.A. Diagnostic Evaluation of LBP. *Arch. Intern. Med.* **2002**, *162*, 1444–1447. [CrossRef] [PubMed]
34. Dworkin, R.H.; Turk, D.C.; Wyrwich, K.W.; Beaton, D.; Cleeland, C.S.; Farrar, J.T.; Haythornthwaite, J.A.; Jensen, M.P.; Kerns, R.D.; Ader, D.N.; et al. Interpreting the clinical importance of treatment outcomes in chronic pain clinical trials: Immpact recommendations. *J. Pain* **2008**, *9*, 105–121. [CrossRef] [PubMed]
35. Moyer, C.A.; Rounds, J.; Hannum, J.W. A meta-analysis of massage therapy research. *Psychol. Bull.* **2004**, *130*, 3–18. [CrossRef]
36. Sherman, K.J.; Cook, A.J.; Wellman, R.D.; Hawkes, R.J.; Kahn, J.R.; Deyo, R.A.; Cherkin, D.C. Five-week outcomes from a dosing trial of therapeutic massage for chronic neck pain. *Ann. Fam. Med.* **2014**, *12*, 112–120. [CrossRef] [PubMed]
37. Hoppe, F. *Hamburger Schmerz-Adjektiv-Liste (HSAL)*; Beltz: Weinheim, Germany, 1991.
38. Lehrl, S.; Cziske, R.; Blaha, L. *Schmerzmessung Durch die Mehr Dimensionale Schmerzskala—MSS*; Vless GmbH: Munich, Germany, 1980.
39. Laux, L.; Glanzmann, P.; Schaffner, P.; Spielberger, C.D. *Das State-Trait-Angstinventar. Theoretische Grundlagen und Handanweisung*; State Trait Anxiety Inventory. Theoretical Foundations and Manual; Beltz: Weinheim, Germany, 1981.
40. Hautzinger, M.; Keller, F.; Kühner, C. *BDI-II Beck-Depressions-Inventar Revision*, 2nd ed.; Pearson Assessment: Frankfurt, Germany, 2009.
41. Beck, A.T.; Steer, R.A.; Brown, G.K. Manual for the beck depression inventory-II. San Antonio. *TX Psychol. Corp.* **1996**, *1*, 82.
42. Hiroe, T.; Kojima, M.; Yamamoto, I.; Nojima, S.; Kinoshita, Y.; Hashimoto, N.; Watanabe, N.; Maeda, T.; Furukawa, T.A. Gradations of clinical severity and sensitivity to change assessed with the Beck Depression Inventory-II in Japanese patients with depression. *Psychiatry Res.* **2005**, *135*, 229–235. [CrossRef]
43. Fairbank, J.C.; Couper, J.; Davies, J.B.; O'Brien, J.P. The Oswestry low back pain disability questionnaire. *Physiotherapy* **1980**, *66*, 271–273.
44. Mannion, A.F.; Junge, A.; Fairbank, J.C.T.; Dvořák, J.; Grob, D. Development of a German version of the Oswestry Disability Index. Part 1: Cross-cultural adaptation, reliability, and validity. *Eur. Spine J.* **2005**, *15*, 55–65. [CrossRef]
45. Mannion, A.F.; Junge, A.; Grob, D.; Dvořák, J.; Fairbank, J.C.T. Development of a German version of the Oswestry Disability Index. Part 2: Sensitivity to change after spinal surgery. *Eur. Spine J.* **2005**, *15*, 66–73. [CrossRef]
46. Van Hooff, M.L.; Spruit, M.; Fairbank, J.C.T.; van Limbeek, J.; Wilco, J.C.H. The Oswestry Disability Index (version 2.1 a): Validation of a Dutch language version. *Spine* **2015**, *40*, 83–90. [CrossRef]
47. Fairbank, J.C.T.; Pynsent, P.B. The Oswestry Disability Index. *Spine* **2000**, *25*, 2940–2953. [CrossRef] [PubMed]
48. Tal-Akabi, A.; Oesch, P. Behinderung bei rückenbeschwerden: Oswestry Disability questionnaire—Deutsche version (ODI-D.). In *Assessments in der Rehabilitation*, 2nd ed.; Oesch, P., Hilfiker, R., Keller, S., Kool, J., Luomajoki, H., Schädler, S., Tal-Akabi, A., Verra, M., Leu, C.W., Eds.; Verlag Hans Huber: Bern, Switzerland, 2011; Volume 2, pp. 296–300.
49. Dworkin, R.H.; Turk, D.C.; Farrar, J.T.; Haythornthwaite, J.A.; Jensen, M.P.; Katz, N.P.; Kerns, R.D.; Stucki, G.; Allen, R.R.; Bellamy, N.; et al. Core outcome measures for chronic pain clinical trials: IMMPACT recommendations. *Pain* **2005**, *113*, 9–19. [CrossRef] [PubMed]
50. Boonstra, A.M.; Preuper, H.R.S.; Reneman, M.F.; Posthumus, J.B.; Stewart, R.E. Reliability and validity of the visual analogue scale for disability in patients with chronic musculoskeletal pain. *Int. J. Rehabil. Res.* **2008**, *31*, 165–169. [CrossRef]
51. Cherkin, D.C.; Sherman, K.J.; Kahn, J.; Wellman, M.R.; Cook, A.J.; Johnson, M.E.; Erro, R.J.; Delaney, M.K.; Deyo, R.A. A comparison of the effects of 2 types of massage and usual care on chronic low back pain. *Ann. Intern. Med.* **2011**, *155*. [CrossRef]
52. Walach, H.; Güthlin, C.; König, M. Efficacy of massage therapy in chronic pain: A pragmatic randomized trial. *J. Altern. Complement. Med.* **2003**, *9*, 837–846. [CrossRef]

53. Hamre, H.J.; Witt, C.M.; Glockmann, A.; Ziegler, R.; Willich, S.N.; Kiene, H. Rhythmical massage therapy in chronic disease: A 4-year prospective cohort study. *J. Altern. Complement. Med.* **2007**, *13*, 635–642. [CrossRef] [PubMed]
54. Lloyd, D.M.; McGlone, F.P.; Yosipovitch, G. Somatosensory pleasure circuit: From skin to brain and back. *Exp. Dermatol.* **2015**, *24*, 321–324. [CrossRef] [PubMed]
55. Krahé, C.; Drabek, M.M.; Paloyelis, Y.; Fotopoulou, A. Affective touch and attachment style modulate pain: A laser-evoked potentials study. *Philos. Trans. R. Soc. B Biol. Sci.* **2016**, *371*, 20160009. [CrossRef]
56. Liljencrantz, J.; Olausson, H. Tactile C fibers and their contributions to pleasant sensations and to tactile allodynia. *Front. Behav. Neurosci.* **2014**, *8*, 37. [CrossRef]
57. Kaplan, C. An Examination of Brain Network Organization and the Analgesic Mechanisms of a Non-Pharmacological Treatment in Chronic Centralized Pain. Ph.D. Thesis, University of Michigan, Ann Arbor, MI, USA, 2018.
58. Boehme, R.; van Ettinger-Veenstra, H.; Olausson, H.; Gerdle, B.; Nagi, S.S. Anhedonia to gentle touch in fibromyalgia: Normal sensory processing but abnormal evaluation. *Brain Sci.* **2020**, *10*, 306. [CrossRef] [PubMed]
59. Weiss, T. Fibromyalgie-ein chronisch-generalisierendes Sensitivierungssyndrom? *PiD Psychother. im Dialog* **2005**, *6*, 59–65. [CrossRef]
60. Craig, A.D. How do you feel–now? The anterior insula and human awareness. *Nat. Rev. Neurosci.* **2009**, *10*, 59–70. [CrossRef] [PubMed]
61. Devue, C.; Collette, F.; Balteau, E.; Degueldre, C.; Luxen, A.; Maquet, P.; Brédart, S. Here I am: The cortical correlates of visual self-recognition. *Brain Res.* **2007**, *1143*, 169–182. [CrossRef]
62. Damasio, A.R. *Descartes' Error: Emotion, Reason and the Human Brain*; Putnam: New York, NY, USA, 1994.
63. Paulus, M.P.; Stein, M.B. Interoception in anxiety and depression. *Brain Struct. Funct.* **2010**, *214*, 451–463. [CrossRef]
64. Pfeifer, A.-C.; Ditzen, B.; Neubauer, E.; Schiltenwolf, M. Wirkung von Oxytocin auf das menschliche Schmerzerleben Effect of oxytocin on human pain perception. *Schmerz* **2016**, *30*, 457–469. [CrossRef]
65. Lund, I.; Yu, L.C.; Uvnäs-Moberg, K.; Wang, J.; Yu, C.; Kurosawa, M.; Agren, G.; Rosen, A.; Lekman, M.; Lundeberg, T. Repeated massage-like stimulation induces long term effects on nociception: Contribution of oxytonergic mechanisms. *Eur. J. Neurosci.* **2005**, *22*, 1553–1554. [CrossRef]
66. Miranda-Cardenas, Y.; Rojas-Piloni, G.; Martínez-Lorenzana, G.; Rodríguez-Jiménez, J.; López-Hidalgo, M.; Freund-Mercier, M.J.; Condés-Lara, M. Oxytocin and electrical stimulation of the paraventricular hypothalamic nucleus produce antinociceptive effects that are reversed by an oxytocin antagonist. *Pain* **2006**, *122*, 182–189. [CrossRef]
67. DeLaTorre, S.; Rojas-Piloni, G.; Martinez-Lorenzana, G.J.; Villanueva, L.; Rodrigues-Jimenez, J.; Villanueva, L.; Condes-Lara, M. Paraventricular oxitocinergic hypothalamic prevention or interruption of long-term potentiation in dorsal horn nociceptive neurons: Electrophysiological and behavioral evidence. *Pain* **2009**, *144*, 320–328. [CrossRef] [PubMed]
68. Jo, Y.H.; Stoeckel, M.E.; Freund-Mercier, M.J.; Schlichter, R. Oxytocin modulates glutamatergic synaptic transmission between cultured neonatal spinal cord dorsal horn neurons. *J. Neurosci.* **1998**, *18*, 2377–2386. [CrossRef]
69. Sprott, H. Pathophysiologie der peripheren Schmerzentstehung–therapeutische Angriffspunkte. *Praxis* **2016**, *105*, 1267–1271. [CrossRef]
70. Schleip, R.; Jäger, H. *Lehrbuch Faszien: Grundlagen, Forschung, Behandlung*; Urban & Fischer: Munich, Germany, 2014; pp. 65–68.
71. Chiesa, A.; Serretti, A.; Jakobsen, J.C. Mindfulness: Top–down or bottom–up emotion regulation strategy? *Clin. Psychol. Rev.* **2013**, *33*, 82–96. [CrossRef] [PubMed]
72. Triscoli, C.; Croy, I.; Steudte-Schmiedgen, S.; Olausson, H.; Sailer, U. Heart rate variability is enhanced by long-lasting pleasant touch at CT-optimized velocity. *Biol. Psychol.* **2017**, *128*, 71–81. [CrossRef] [PubMed]

6

Depression, Olfaction and Quality of Life: A Mutual Relationship

Marion Rochet [1], Wissam El-Hage [1,2], Sami Richa [3], François Kazour [1,4] and Boriana Atanasova [1,*]

1 UMR 1253, iBrain, Université de Tours, Inserm, 37200 Tours, France; marion.rochet@etu.univ-tours.fr (M.R.); wissam.elhage@univ-tours.fr (W.E.-H.); francoiskazour@hotmail.com (F.K.)
2 CHRU de Tours, Clinique Psychiatrique Universitaire, 37044 Tours, France
3 Department of Psychiatry, Faculty of Medicine, Saint-Joseph University, P.O. Box 17-5208, 11-5076 Beirut, Lebanon; richasami@hotmail.com
4 Psychiatric Hospital of the Cross, 60096 Jal Eddib, Lebanon
* Correspondence: atanasova@univ-tours.fr;

Abstract: Olfactory dysfunction has been well studied in depression. Common brain areas are involved in depression and in the olfactory process, suggesting that olfactory impairments may constitute potential markers of this disorder. Olfactory markers of depression can be either state (present only in symptomatic phases) or trait (persistent after symptomatic remission) markers. This study presents the etiology of depression, the anatomical links between olfaction and depression, and a literature review of different olfactory markers of depression. Several studies have also shown that olfactory impairment affects the quality of life and that olfactory disorders can affect daily life and may be lead to depression. Thus, this study discusses the links between olfactory processing, depression, and quality of life. Finally, olfaction is an innovative research field that may constitute a new therapeutic tool for the treatment of depression.

Keywords: depression; olfaction; markers; quality of life; therapeutic tool

1. Introduction

Depression and olfactory dysfunction induce long-term impairments that affect individuals and have a major impact on subjects' social skills, relationships, wellbeing, and quality of life [1,2]. Major depression is one of the two most debilitating diseases according to the World Health Organization (2010). Depression affects 8 to 12% of the world's population [3]. In France, 9 million people experience at least one depressive episode during their lifetime (INPES, National Institute for Prevention and Health Education). Olfactory dysfunctions are present in 22% of individuals aged between 25 and 75 years old [4]. In these situations, the impact of this olfactory impairment on patients' life is often neglected. However, olfaction provides people with valuable input from the chemical environment around them. Smell can also impact different psychological aspects of the subject's life by forming positive and negative emotional memories related to smell. It can also affect the social abilities and the interpersonal relationships of the individual. When the olfactory input is distorted, disability and decreased quality of life are reported [5].

In the last two decades, several studies have investigated olfactory dysfunction in depression. Several reasons are behind the study of olfaction in depression. First, the rapid expansion of structural and functional imagery techniques that uncover overlapping brain areas involved in olfactory processing and depression. These regions are mainly the orbitofrontal cortex, the anterior and posterior cingulate cortices, the insula, the amygdala, the hippocampus, and the thalamus [6–8]. Second, olfactory stimuli are encoded and may activate emotional memory. This could be explained by the close anatomical links between the olfactory system and the brain circuits involved in memory [9] and emotion [10]. These two cognitive functions are frequently altered in depression [11]. Third, olfactory dysfunction may induce symptoms of depression, due to the impact of odors on emotions, mood, or behaviors [12]. Indeed, a recent systematic review has shown a reciprocity and a close association between olfactory impairment and depression [13]. Thus, depressed patients have lower olfactory performance than healthy controls, and patients with olfactory dysfunction have symptoms of depression that worsen with the severity of olfactory impairment. Fourth, bilateral olfactory bulbectomy in rodents induces changes in behavior, as well as in the endocrine, immune, and neurotransmitter systems. These changes are similar to those seen in patients with major depression [14,15]. These alterations are reversed by antidepressants, suggesting that the dysfunctions seen in depression could be related to alterations in the olfaction system. However, these findings cannot be replicated in humans. Nevertheless, studies showed that olfactory bulb volume differs significantly between depressed and non-depressed individuals and seems to be a promising marker for depression [16]. Fifth, stress, a triggering factor of depression in vulnerable subjects, induces behavior similar to some symptoms of depression, as well as decreased cell proliferation or neurogenesis, both in the hippocampus and in the olfactive bulbs [17]. Finally, it has been suggested in human [18–21] and animal studies [22–24] that olfaction can be used as a therapeutic tool for depression.

The exact relationship between depression and olfactory dysfunction is still unclear, even if both disorders coexist and affect quality of life, social and professional integration, as well as family balance [25]. Several reviews have studied olfactory perception in depression [26,27], the relationship between olfactory loss and quality of life [28,29], and between depression and quality of life [1]. In the present review, we overview the links between depression, olfaction, and quality of life of patients in order to understand the relationship between olfactory function and depression, and to determine if olfactory loss affects patients' quality of life. In addition, we discuss the possible use of olfactory stimulation as a promising therapeutic tool to potentiate the antidepressant effect of medication.

2. Depression

Depression is a multifactorial disease involving multiple etiologies, with the contribution of biological, genetic, and environmental factors [30].

From a biological perspective, depression is associated to a monoaminergic deficiency in the brain [31]. Indeed, the role of monoaminergic neurotransmitters (noradrenaline, serotonin, and dopamine) has been demonstrated in the control of mood and cognitive functions. Neurotransmitter-based drug treatments accelerate clinical improvement, but resistance to antidepressants implies the involvement of other etiologies. One hypothesis is the inhibition of hippocampal neurogenesis, since long-term use of antidepressants leads to an increase of adult hippocampal neurogenesis [32]. A decrease in hippocampal volume has been demonstrated in depression [33] at the earliest stages of the disease and was correlated with patients' cognitive impairment [34]. Brain abnormalities have also been observed in the orbitofrontal cortex, anterior cingulate cortex [35], and the amygdala [36]. It has been shown that amygdala volume is reduced in untreated depressed patients, but increases with treatment [37].

As for the genetic etiologies of depression, studies show contradicting results. A meta-analysis suggested that depression is a familial disorder and with an estimated heritability of 31 to 42% [38]. For instance, a functional polymorphism of the serotonin transporter gene would change the impact of stressful life events on depression [39]. However, another meta-analysis was not able to show any association between the serotonin transporter genotype and depression [40]; and a genome-wide association study could not clearly identify the involvement of several genes in depression [41].

Concerning the psychological perspective, Beck [42] proposed a model based on the fact that negative life events may trigger depressive episodes. Therefore, certain life experiences can modify the psychological functioning of the individual and induce emotional instability. Kendler et al. [43] proposed the kindling-sensitization hypothesis where negative life events that were initially unable to trigger a depressive episode later gained a capacity to trigger a recurring episode.

Pathophysiology of depression is complex and remains partially elucidated. According to the latest edition of the Diagnostic and Statistical Manual (DSM-5, [44]), a major depressive episode is diagnosed, when (i) five (or more) of the following symptoms are present during the same two-week period: depressed mood most of the day, markedly diminished interest or pleasure in all, or almost all, activities most of the day, nearly every day, significant weight loss when not dieting or weight gain, insomnia or hypersomnia, psychomotor agitation or retardation, fatigue or loss of energy, feelings of worthlessness or excessive or inappropriate guilt, diminished ability to think or concentrate and recurrent thoughts of death; and (ii) a change from previous functioning with at least one of the two major symptoms of depression: depressed mood or loss of interest or pleasure. These symptoms are associated with significant clinical distress or impairment in social, occupational, or other important areas of functioning. It was shown that depression alters aspects of information processing, including perception and attention, memory processes (e.g., preferential recall of negative information rather than positive one), and interpretation of ambiguous information [11]. Recent literature explored the presence of depression-associated sensorial biases, particularly at the olfactory level by investigating the state (disappearance of olfactory alterations in clinically improved patients) and the trait (persistent olfactory alterations after clinical improvement) olfactory markers of major depression [27,45–48].

3. Olfaction

3.1. Functioning of Olfactory Perception

The olfactory information (i.e., the chemical molecule), will first settle at the level of the olfactory receptors, within the olfactory epithelium. There are two ways for volatile chemical molecules to reach the olfactory epithelium. The first is the orthonasal pathway (so-called "direct" pathway) and takes place during inspiration through the nose. The second is the retronasal pathway (so-called "indirect" pathway) and takes place during mastication through the mouth. The binding of the molecule on specific olfactory neuroreceptors, triggers an action potential on these cells [49]. The information then reaches the olfactory bulb, located at the base of the frontal lobe [2]. The olfactory bulb sends projections via the lateral olfactory tract to different brain areas, such as the olfactory tubercle, the anterior olfactory nucleus, the piriform cortex, the lateral entorhinal cortex, or the ventral tenia tectae [50], allowing olfactory information to reach different brain levels (e.g., the thalamus, hypothalamus, or hippocampus). Indeed, the olfactory system is connected to the limbic system through the amygdala, the piriform cortex, the anterior cingulate cortex, the insula, and the orbitofrontal cortex [7]. These connections may explain how odors an induce mood changes [51] and impact cognitions and behaviors [52].

3.2. Evaluation of Olfactory Functions

Various olfactory tests are available for the evaluation of olfactory function. Psychophysical measures have been used to establish a link between measurable parameters (i.e., product concentration, chemical composition) and the qualitative (i.e., odor's identification, odor's naming) and quantitative (i.e., perception of odor's intensity) characteristics of the evoked stimulus. It is, thus, possible to evaluate parameters, such as the odor's intensity, familiarity, or hedonic level by using scales of measurements. The psychophysical tests provide a quantitative measure of sensory function by using the verbal response of the subject as an indicator of the olfactory perception. Generally, the psychophysical tests include investigation of odor detection threshold, odor discrimination, and identification. Standardized tests have been developed to evaluate these three olfactory functions. They were validated with several hundred healthy participants (men and women) of different ages. Doty et al. [53] has developed the University of Pennsylvania Smell Identification Test (UPSIT), an olfactory evaluation tool in the form of a scratch 'n sniff test. This test can measure individuals' odor identification ability. The Sniffin' Stick Test created by Hummel et al. [54] evaluates odor detection threshold, odor discrimination, and identification ability. This test is formed of several odorous pens (sticks). For the olfactory threshold test, stick triplets with increasing odor concentrations are presented to the subject. In every triplet, only one stick contains the odorant (2-phenyl ethyl alcohol). The subject is asked to identify in every triplet the pen that contains the odorant, the other two being without odor. The discrimination test is done with the following presentation of 16 odorous pen triplets. In this test, the subject has to detect if the pen with the odorant is different from the other two. Finally, during the odor identification test, 12 or 16 odorous pens are presented to the subject. Using a multiple forced-choice task, odors are identified from a list of four descriptors for each odor. A final score evaluates the overall olfactory capacity of the subject and determines whether the individual is normosmic, hyposmic, or anosmic.

Occasionally, devices called olfactometers are used to carry out the psychophysical measures while providing a better control of the delivery conditions of the odorant. It allows the delivery of a precise concentration of the odorant at the entrance of the nostrils via a controlled airflow. It is also possible with this device to have either unilateral or bilateral nostril stimulations. This tool seems to be more appropriate in situations where the control of odors' concentration is important, like in olfactory threshold measures.

The psychophysical tests described above are easy to administer, to transport, are not expensive, and provide a rapid time of analysis (between 5 and 40 min depending on the test). They are the most used in the clinical field. However, the psychophysical evaluation of the olfactory functions demands an active participation of the subject. To avoid this inconvenience neurophysiological techniques are used to measure the human electrophysiologic response to an odorant stimulus. They include odor event-related potentials (OERPs) and a summated potential recorded from the surface of the olfactory epithelium (the electro-olfactogram, EOG). Many other techniques have also been developed, including electroencephalographic testing, measurement of psychogalvanic skin response to olfactory stimuli, measurement of respiratory, cardiovascular, papillary, and oculomotor reflexes [55]. More recently, structural and functional imaging technologies (positron emission tomography, single photon emission tomography, and high-resolution structural magnetic resonance imaging) were developed in order to study the central pattern associated to the olfactory perception.

In summary, a number of techniques and tools are available to explore the olfactory function, each having its own advantages and disadvantages. It is important to note that all these methods (psychophysical, neurophysiological, and neuroimaging techniques) are complementary because they do not measure the same olfactory parameters, function, and process. Some authors described and compared the existing methods and techniques (see [55,56]).

The methods described above can be used to study olfactory function and to detect the presence of olfactory disorders. Olfactory disorders are divided into quantitative and qualitative disorders. Quantitative olfactory disorders are hyposmia, hyperosmia, or anosmia [50]. They are defined, respectively, as a decrease, an increase, or a complete loss of olfactory perception. Qualitative olfactory disorders are parosmia (bad perception of smell) and fantosmia (an olfactory hallucination, or perception of odors that are not present within the olfactory field) [57]. Two thirds of cases of anosmia and hyposmia are due to either an upper respiratory tract infection, a brain trauma, or to nasal pathologies that damage the olfactory neuroepithelium [58]. Moreover, it has been demonstrated that olfactory perception is altered in patients with neurodegenerative diseases. Indeed, olfactory disorders are seen in 85 to 90% of patients with Alzheimer and Parkinson diseases. However, these patients are rarely aware of their olfactory impairment.

4. What Is the Link between Olfaction and Depression?

4.1. Anatomical Link

Several brain areas play a role in olfactory perception and are involved in the etiology of depression. First, the olfactory bulb transmits olfactory information to other brain areas, like the amygdala, the hippocampus, and the anterior angular cortex [50]. It has been shown that bilateral olfactory bulbectomy in rodents causes changes to the immune and endocrine systems similar to those seen in depression [15]. Indeed, bilateral destruction of olfactory bulbs leads to alteration in serotonin and dopamine concentration [14]. Bilateral olfactory bulbectomy can also induce behavioral changes, such as a reduction in sexual behavior [59], an odd food-motivated behavior [60], a decrease in anxiety-like behavior [61], and an increase in depression-like behavior [15,62]. In addition, a study found a reduced volume of the olfactory bulb in depressed patients [63]. A study using a rat model of depression, with unpredictable chronic mild stress (UCMS), has observed a reduced amount of olfactory receptor neurons in olfactory epithelium [64]. These results may explain some of the impairment in olfactory sensitivity observed in depressed patients.

A recent study showed that in a murine model that mimics the hyperactivation of the HPA axis (and thus causes a phenotype of depression), olfactory function, and also adult neurogenesis at the subventricular zone and the dentate gyrus, were affected [48]. In this study, mice receiving chronic administration of corticosterone had deficits in their olfactory acuity, fine odor discrimination, and olfactory memory. In addition, cell proliferation in the subventricular zone and the dentate gyrus (two niches of adult neurogenesis), and the survival of new neurons in the dentate gyrus and olfactory bulbs, were decreased by corticosterone administration. Antidepressant treatment (fluoxetine) allowed a return to normal olfactory function and adult neurogenesis [48]. Therefore, the link between olfaction and depression can also be explained by the decrease in neurogenesis.

Other areas, such as the amygdala or hippocampus, also have a role in olfaction and depression. Indeed, the hippocampus is involved in odor storage tasks [65] and in depressive symptoms, such as deficits in autobiographical memory [66]. In addition, studies have shown decreases in hippocampal volume associated to depression [33]. It has been shown that the amygdala of healthy individuals is activated during the evaluation of intensity, hedonic aspect and memory of odor-related emotions [67]. The amygdala would be hyper-activated in depression [68].

The orbitofrontal cortex is also implicated in the link between olfaction and depression. It is involved in attention, emotional, and cognitive processes of depression. On one hand, the ventromedial part is involved in rumination, anxiety, and sensitivity to pain, and is hyper-activated in depressed patients. On the other hand, the dorsal part is involved in psychomotor retardation, apathy, attention disorders, and working memory, and hypoactive in depressed patients [69]. The role of this cortex is crucial in olfaction, but is still controversial in depression [70,71]. Some authors consider that an unpleasant stimulus activates the left part of this cortex and a pleasant stimulus activates the right side [71], but other authors have shown that the activation of the orbitofrontal cortex is not a function of positive or negative valence of odorants [72]. The orbitofrontal cortex is involved in the identification of odors and in olfactory memorization [71,73].

The cingulate cortex is involved in both olfactory function and depression. In depression, the volume of its anterior part is diminished [35,74]. This would be partly responsible for the increased recurrence of depressive episodes [75]. As for its role in olfaction, the activation of this brain area depends on the hedonic valence of the odor [76].

The insula participates in the evaluation of emotional states and more particularly of the bodily sensations during an emotional experience [77]. A study showed that the insular cortex contributes to odor quality coding by representing the taste-like aspects of food odors [78]. The insula has higher levels of activity in resting states, increasing the inability of depressed patients to disengage from externally-cued events, and leading to pathological self-focused mental ruminative behaviors [79].

Finally, the habenula is affected by olfactory bulb input and is involved in the regulation of psychomotor and psychosocial behaviors [57]. Its metabolic activity is increased in animal models of depression [80]. The role of the habenula is the transfer of olfactory information to other brain areas [81]. It is activated in response to emotionally-negative stimuli [82]. According to Oral et al. [83] habenula plays a decisive role in the link between olfactory disorders and depression since a bilateral bulbectomy induces a structural degeneration by apoptosis of the habenula, leading to the appearance of the main symptoms of depression. A summary of the brains areas involved in olfaction and depression is presented in Table 1.

4.2. Olfaction: A Marker of Depression?

Over the years, several studies have focused on the impact of depression on olfactory functions like detection thresholds, identification, and discrimination capabilities, and the assessment of hedonicity or intensity. The strong link between depression and olfaction has allowed researchers to espouse the hypothesis that a reduced olfactory capacity may be a marker of depression [45,84]. Two types of olfactory markers have been proposed: (i) the state olfactory markers where olfactory impairments disappear after antidepressant treatment; and (ii) the trait olfactory marker, where olfactory impairments persist after clinical remission.

Most studies have shown that the detection threshold of depressed subjects was increased compared to controls [27,63,85,86]. However, some authors reported an unchanged olfactory threshold [87–89]. Few studies investigated the olfactory threshold in remitted patients after antidepressant treatment and showed conflicting results. Gross-Isseroff et al. [90] have demonstrated an increase of olfactory odor sensitivity in remitted patients suggesting that this could be due to antidepressant treatment. Another study observed a significant negative correlation between olfactory sensitivity and depressive symptoms [91]. Pause et al. [86] reported remission of odor threshold impairment in depressed patients after antidepressant treatment. All these observations suggest that the reduced olfactory sensitivity may be a marker of depression. However, further studies are needed to confirm whether this olfactory function is restored by antidepressant treatment.

Some studies have shown that depression is associated with a lower olfactory identification capacity [92–94]. Two studies reported that depressed subjects had a lower identification capacity of the components of a complex odorant environment (binary iso-intense mixtures), during the major depressive episode [46,95]. Naudin et al. [46] also showed that the olfactory alteration persists after clinical improvement reflecting olfactory trait markers of depression. The majority of studies have demonstrated that olfactory identification capacities are not altered in depression [46,85,87–89,91,96–100]. In summary, odor identification function didn't seem to be altered in depression when standardized olfactory tests were used. Moreover, it has been proposed that an odor identification parameter could be used to differentiate between depressed patients and Alzheimer's disease (AD) patients since comparative studies showed that this function is altered in AD, but not in depression (for review, see [8]).

Concerning odor hedonic perception, only two studies have shown unchanged scores between depressed patients and healthy controls [89] before or after antidepressant treatment [92]. For the majority of the investigations, this parameter is influenced by depressive state [46,47,85,86,95,101]. Atanasova et al. [95] showed that depressed patients would perceive unpleasant odors as more unpleasant (negative olfactory alliesthesia), while pleasant odorants would be perceived as less pleasant (olfactory anhedonia) in comparison to controls. Naudin et al. [46] reported that this hedonic olfactory bias concerns a highly emotional odorant and that it vanishes after antidepressant treatment. Therefore, it is considered as an olfactory state marker of depression. In contrast to these observations, other studies revealed that depressed patients over-evaluate the hedonic perception of odors [85,86]. Lombion-Pouthier et al. [85] suggested that this over-evaluation could be due to modifications in the orbitofrontal cortex observed in depression (this structure is also applied in hedonic perception of odor).

Several studies investigated changes in olfactory intensity rating in depression [85,86,92,95,102,103]. Only one showed that depressed patients perceived pleasant stimuli as less intense and unpleasant stimuli as more intense than controls [95]. However, the majority of the studies did not find any associations between that hedonic value of odors and changes in the perception of odor intensity.

As for the perception of familiarity, studies show contradictory results. Some authors could not find any change in familiarity ratings associated with depression [47,102,103], whereas others found lower familiarity ratings in depressed patients compared to controls [46]. Future studies are needed to clarify this aspect of olfaction. The edibility perception of odors has not been studied in depression. However, knowing that eating disorders are frequently observed in depression, this parameter should be a subject for future investigation.

Studies show that odor discrimination abilities are not different in depressed patients compared to controls [63,84,92,95]. These same studies found similar results with respect to odor intensity assessment capabilities. A summary of the studies exploring the deficits in the different olfactory functions in depressed patients and in clinically-improved patients are presented in Table 2.

Table 1. Brain areas involved in the processing of olfaction and depression.

Brain Areas	Olfaction		Depression	
	Observations	References	Observations	References
Olfactory bulb	• Transmission of olfactory information to other brain areas	Brand, 2001 [50]	• A bulbectomy causes changes (molecular and behavioral) similar to those of depression • Reduced volume observed in depression	Song and Leonard, 2005 [15] Negoias et al. 2010 [63]
Amygdala	• Activation during the evaluation of intensity, hedonic aspect and emotional memory related to odors	Pouliot and Jones-Gotman, 2008 [67]	• Hyperactivated in depression	Drevets, 2003 [68]
Hippocampus	• Role in odor storage tasks	Kesner et al. 2002 [65]	• Deficit in autobiographical memory • Reduced volume observed in depression	Lemogne et al. 2006 [66] Campbell et al. 2004 [33]
Orbitofrontal cortex	• Controversial data: left part activated by unpleasant stimulus and right part activated by pleasant stimulus vs. activation not dependent of hedonic valence • Identification of odors and memorization	Grabenhorst et al. 2011 [72] Zald and Pardo, 1997 [71] Zald et al. 2002 [73]	• Ventromedian part (hyperactivated) involved in rumination anxiety and sensitivity to pain and dorsal part (hypoactivated) psychomotor retardation, apathy, attention disorders, and working memory	Rogers et al. 2004 [69]
Cingulate cortex	• Activation dependent of hedonic valence of the odor	Fulbright et al. 1998 [76]	• Reduced volume of anterior part: partly responsible for the increased recurrence of depressive episodes	Phillips et al. 2003 [74] van Tol et al. 2010 [35] Bhagwagar et al. 2008 [75]
Insula	• Odor quality coding	Veldhuizen et al. 2010 [78]	• Increased of activity during states of rest can be involved in inabilitiy to disengage from external events and lead to rumination	Sliz and Hayley, 2012 [79]
Habenula	• Transfer olfactory information to other brain areas • Activated in response to emotionally-negative stimuli	Da Costa et al. 1997 [81] Hikosaka et al. 2008 [82]	• Metabolic activity increased	Shumake et al. 2003 [80]

Table 2. Summary of publications on olfactory function in depression.

Study	Number of Patients Female (f)/Male (m)	Mean Age ± Standard Deviation	Measures and Tools	Conclusions
Swiecicki et al. (2009) [89]	D: 46 (f) C: 30 (f)	D: 38.2 ± 1.6 C: 35.4 ± 2.1	One testing session Sniffin' Stick Test: • Odor threshold • Odor identification • Odor characterization: pleasant/unpleasant/neutral	• Intact odor threshold • Intact identification abilities • Intact odor hedonicity
Scinska et al. (2008) [88]	D: 25 (17/7) C: 60 (38/22)	D: 67.2 ± 1.2 C: 66.7 ± 0.9	One testing session Sniffin' Stick Test: • Odor threshold (n-butanol) • Odor identification	• Intact odor threshold • Intact identification abilities
Postolache et al. (1999) [87]	D: 24 C: 24	D: 42.8 ± 9.7 C: 42.1 ± 11.8	One testing session • Odor threshold: single stair-case procedure (PEA) • Identification: L-UPSIT and R-UPSIT	• Intact odor threshold • Intact identification abilities
Negoias et al. (2010) [63]	D: 21 (17/4) C: 21 (15/6)	D: 36.9 ± 10.1 C: 39.6 ± 11.4	One testing session Sniffin' Stick test: • Odor threshold (PEA) • Odor discrimination • Odor identification	• Modified odor threshold • Intact odor discrimination ability • Intact odor identification ability
Lombion-Pouthier et al. (2006) [85]	D: 49 (35/14) C: 58 (36/22)	D: 43.4 ± 17.5 C: 38.4 ± 13.9	One testing session Olfactory test (Ezus) • Odor sensibility • Detection/evaluation abilities (16 odors) • Odor Identification • Intensity rating • Hedonic rating	• Modified odor threshold • Intact detection/evaluation abilities • Intact identification abilities • Intact odor intensity • Modified odor hedonicity
Pause et al. (2001) [86]	D: 24 (15/9) C: 25 (15/9)	D: 48.4 ± 13.2 C: 44.2 ± 12.6	Two testing sessions (S1 and S2) • Odor threshold (PEA and eugenol) • Subjective odors rating (intensity and hedonicity, 10 odors)	• Modified odor threshold (S1) • Modified odor hedonicity (S1) and intact odor intensity (S1/S2)

Table 2. *Cont.*

Study	Number of Patients Female (f)/Male (m)	Mean Age ± Standard Deviation	Measures and Tools	Conclusions
Pentzek et al. (2007) [99]	C: 20 (15/5) C: 30 (24/6)	D: 73.4 ± 5.6 C: 77.1 ± 6.8	One testing session Sniffin' Stick Test • Odor identification	• Intact identification abilities
McCaffrey et al. (2000) [98]	D: 20 (11/9) A: 20 (13/7)	D: 67.55 ± 7.29 A: 74.15 ± 7.86	One testing session • Pocket Smell Test	• Intact identification abilities
Solomon et al. (1998) [100]	D: 20 (13/7) A: 20 (12/8)	D: 69.4 ± 7.7 A: 74.5 ± 7.7	One testing session • Pocket Smell test	• Intact identification abilities
Kopala et al. (1994) [97]	D: 21 (13/8) C: 77 (47/30)	D: 37.0 ± 9.6 C: 32.5 ± 11.1	One testing session UPSIT • Odor identification	• Intact identification abilities
Amsterdam et al. (1987) [96]	D: 51 (34/17) C: 51 (34/17)	D: 43 ± 13 (f); 49 ± 14 (m) C: age-matched	One testing session UPSIT • Odor identification	• Intact identification abilities
Naudin et al. (2012) [46]	D: 20 (12/6) C: 54 (36/18)	D: 50.1 ± 13.3 C: 49.5 ± 12.5	Two testing sessions (during acute phase of depression and after 6 weeks of antidepressant treatment) • Eight odors (four pleasant, two unpleasant, two neutral) • Hedonic rating • Familiarity rating • Identification of single odors • Odor intensity discrimination • Odor identification abilities in binary mixture (one pleasant/one unpleasant)	• Modified odor hedonicity (S1) and improvement in (S2) • Modified odor familiarity (S1, S2 for vanillin) • Intact identification abilities of single odors (S1, S2) • Modified odor intensity discrimination (S1, S2) • Modified identification abilities in binary mixture) (S1, S2)
Zucco and Bollini (2011) [94]	Mild D: 12 (6/6) Severe D: 12 (6/6) C: 12 (6/6)	Mild D: 41.3 ± 6.4 Severe D: 41.9 ± 6.2 C: 39.8 ± 7.1	One testing session • Odor identification • Odor recognition memory (10 targets odors/30 distractors odors)	• Modified odor identification abilities • Modified odor recognition memory

Table 2. *Cont.*

Study	Number of Patients Female (f)/Male (m)	Mean Age ± Standard Deviation	Measures and Tools	Conclusions
Atanasova et al. (2010) [95]	D: 30 (12/18) C: 30 (12/18)	D: 34.6 ± 11.1 C: 33.4 ± 9.9	One testing session • Two odors: vanillin/butyric acid • Intensity rating • Odor intensity discrimination • Odor identification in binary mixture • Hedonics rating (single/binary mixture) • Odor discrimination	• Modified odor intensity • Modified odor intensity discrimination • Modified identification abilities in binary mixture • Modified odor hedonicity • Intact odor discrimination ability for unpleasant odor and modified for pleasant odor
Clepce et al. (2010) [92]	D: 37 (21/16) C: 37 (21/16)	D: 48.3 ± 11.9 (m); 47.5 ± 11.3 (f) C: age-matched	Two testing sessions (during acute phase of depression and six months after the 1st phase) Sniffin' Stick Test: • Odor identification • Hedonics and intensity rating	• Modified odor identification abilities (S1) • Intact odor hedonicity and intensity (S1, S2)
Pollatos et al. (2007) [91]	D: 48 (34/14)	28.2 ± 5.8	One testing session Sniffin' Stick test: • Odor threshold • Odor discrimination	• Modified odor threshold • Intact odor quality discrimination
Croy et al. (2014) [27]	D: 27 (f) C: 28 (f)	D: 38.5 ± 10.6 C: 353 ± 10.3	Two testing sessions (before and after therapy) Sniffin' Stick test: • Odor threshold • Odor discrimination • Odor identification	• Intact odor threshold (S1, S2) • Modified odor discrimination (S1, S2) • Intact odor identification (S1, S2)
Atanasova et al. (2012) [101]	D: 30 (12/18) C: 30 (12/18)	D: 36.6 ± 11.1 C: 33.4 ± 9.9	One testing session • Odor: vanillin/butyric acid • Hedonicity	• Modified odor hedonicity

Table 2. *Cont.*

Study	Number of Patients Female (f)/Male (m)	Mean Age ± Standard Deviation	Measures and Tools	Conclusions
Naudin et al. (2014) [47]	D: 22 (16/6) C: 41 (24/17)	D: 33,2 ± 11.2 C: 34 ± 11	Two testing sessions (one during acute phase of depression and 100 days ± 64 after the 1st phase) • Eight odors • Hedonicity, Familiarity and emotion' intensity rating	• Modified odor hedonicity (S1; restore in S2), intact odor familiarity (S1, S2) and modified intensity of emotion (S1)
Naudin et al. (2014) [102]	D: 20 (15/5) A: 20 (14/6) C: 24 (17/9)	D: 64.9 ± 11.2 A: 73.0 ± 11.2 C: 67.0 ± 12.7	One testing session (in elderly) • Eight odors: four familiar and four unfamiliar • Odor recognition memory • Pleasantness, intensity, familiarity	• Modified odor recognition memory for D and A • Intact odors pleasantness, intensity and familiarity perception for D and A
Gross-Isseroff et al. (1994) [90]	D: 9 (8/1) C: 9 (8/1)	D: 49 ± 4.6 C: 49.1 ± 4.8	Three testing sessions (1st: acute phase of depression; 2nd: three weeks after the 1st and 3rd: sox weeks after the 1st) • Odors threshold (androsteron and isoamylacetate)	• Intact odor threshold (1st and 2nd sessions) and modified odor threshold (3rd session)
Serby et al. (1990) [93]	D: 9 (m) C: 9 (m)	D: 50–59 years old C: age-matched	One testing phase • UPSIT (identification abilities) • Odor threshold (geraniol)	• Modified odor identification abilities • Intact odor threshold
Thomas et al. (2002) [103]	D: 16 C: 16	*i.i.*	• Odor threshold • Intensity and familiarity ratings	• Intact odor threshold • Intact intensity and familiarity ratings abilities
Postolache et al. (2002) [104]	SAD: 14 (7/7) C: 16 (9/7)	SAD: 42.3 ± 11.5 C: 39.0 ± 10.0	One testing session • Odor threshold	• Intact odor threshold
Oren et al. (1995) [105]	SAD: 21 (16/9) C: 21 (16/9)	SAD: 38 ± 9 C: 38 ± 9	One testing session • Odor identification	• Intact odor identification abilities
Kamath et al. (2017) [106]	BPI: 43 (28/15) BPII: 48 (29/19) D: 134 (97/34) Anxiety: 48 (36/12) C: 72 (30/42)	BPI: 43.66 ± 15.6 BPII: 44.85 ± 15.6 D: 30.31 ± 14.87 Anxiety: 48.78 ± 17.12 C: 50.50 ± 18.09	One testing session • UPSIT (identification abilities) • Sniffin' Stick Test: Discrimination abilities and odor threshold	• Modified odor identification abilities (BPI, D) • Intact discrimination abilities and odor threshold

A: Alzheimer patients; C: control group; D: depressed patients; SAD: seasonal affective disorder; *i.i.*: incomplete information; BP: bipolar depression; PEA: phenyl ethyl alcohol; UPSIT: University of Pennsylvania Smell Identification Test, S1: testing session during acute phase of depression, S2: testing session during remission and/or after therapy.

Olfactory impairments were also described in other psychiatric, disorders like schizophrenia [107], bipolar disorder [108], or posttraumatic stress disorder [109]. However, there are very few studies comparing olfactory dysfunction in depression and other affective disorders. When assessing olfactory thresholds and identification abilities, Swiecicki et al. [89] could not find any difference between patients with unipolar and bipolar depression. However, a recent study [106], showed that impairment in odor identification may be seen in mood disorders (major depressive and bipolar I disorder), with a more pronounced impairment associated to psychotic depression features. On the other hand, global olfactory dysfunction observed in schizophrenia may not be a feature of other neuropsychiatric conditions [106]. Olfactory markers of differentiation were also described in depression and Alzheimer's disease [8]. Future investigations are needed in order to investigate potential markers of differentiation between other neuropsychiatric disorders.

5. Quality of Life: Definition and Evaluation

The World Health Organization, defined the quality of life as "the perception of an individual of his place in existence, in the context of the culture and the system of values in which he lives, in relation to its objectives, expectations, norms and concerns. It is a very broad concept influenced in a complex way by the physical health of the subject, his psychological state, his level of independence, his social relations as well as his relation to the essential elements of its environment". Questionnaires have been created to assess the quality of life, like the Questionnaire of Olfactory Disorders [25]. This questionnaire was developed to assess the impact of olfactory disorders in daily life and is composed of 52 statements divided into three areas: (1) "negative statement", which provides information on the degree of suffering of the respondent; (2) "positive statement", that gives information on the way respondents cope with their olfactory disorders; and (3) "socially desired". This third area allows the evaluator to assess the credibility of participants' responses. Indeed, it helps knowing if the participant is trying to give a certain impression or socially desirable answers.

Other questionnaires used to assess quality of life include the "Short Form 36 Health Survey", "The General Well Being Schedule" [110], "The 90-item symptom checklist" [111], and "The Nottingham Health Profile" [112]. In these different questionnaires, several areas, like general health, vitality, depression, anxiety, sleep, and pain are evaluated. However, sensory functions, like taste and olfaction, are not evaluated. A study by MacDowell et al. [113] compared the reliability, validity, and duration needed for several of these instruments. They concluded that most of these tools perform adequately for survey research purposes.

This is a non-exhaustive list of standardized questionnaires used to assess quality of life, but researchers may prefer to use other non-standardized questionnaires targeting specific fields of research (olfactory disorders, etc.). For example, some studies used a self-report where participants had to write their feeling about their loss of olfaction [5,114].

6. Impact of Olfactory Disorders on Quality of Life

It is interesting to focus on the impact of olfactory loss (partial or total, reversible or not) on the diet in general. Individuals with olfactory disorders report having a more complicated alimentation because of the important link between smell and taste. Patients with olfactory disorders (69%, n = 239) had lower ratings of food since the beginning of their disorder [115]. This lower rating leads to a decrease in appetite in 56% (n = 278) [114], 32% (n = 72) [116] and 27% of subjects (n = 50) [117]. All the subjects included in these studies had olfactory disorders and the results were obtained through self-reporting questionnaires and the Multi-Clinic Smell and Taste Questionnaire [118].

Individuals sometimes develop coping strategies: they can increase the taste by adding salt, sugar, or spices [5,28]. Moreover, 3 to 20% of individuals with olfactory disorders report eating more than before, while from 20 to 36% report eating less [115]. The presence of olfactory dysfunction causes difficulty in maintaining a healthy balanced diet. Individuals with olfactory disorders also have difficulties cooking food because they have difficulties to detect burning food. They may burn or stale food because of their olfactory impairment [5,114,119,120]. They also have difficulties to detect gas leaks or smoke odors [120].

In addition, patients are no longer able to detect their own body odor (sweating, bad breath) [114] and report problems of hygiene. This can lead in some cases to excessive showers in order to have a higher self-confidence. For some individuals, this is the most negative effect of olfactory loss [116,117]. Between 1/4 and 1/3 of patients with olfactory disorders report having social difficulties related to hygiene problems [117,121]. Indeed, an individual with olfactory disorders is socially vulnerable if he is not able to smell his body odor or odors of others. This places him in an uncomfortable situation and increases the risk of social isolation.

Olfactory disturbance interferes with professional life in 3 to 8% of cases [116,117]. Temmel et al. [114] reported that 8% of participants with olfactory disorders had problems in their professional lives. The impact of an olfactory disorder on professional life depends on the type profession: people who work in oenology, in gastronomy, in the perfume industry, or even nurses or firefighters, can have major impairments in their professional lives [28]. A loss of smell can also be problematic in this kind of situation and add major concerns for the future professional. All of this can lead to anxiety, mood disturbances, and depression [58]. Olfactory disorders that cause food disturbance (whether cooking or eating) can also constitute factors that affect mood and lead to anhedonia [28].

Several studies have shown the impact of olfaction on social and family relations [122,123] such as the mother-child bond [124] and men-women relationships (i.e., in reproduction, avoidance of consanguinity, selection of partner) [125,126]. For example, olfaction is involved in the detection of fear signals. In a study by Ackerl et al. [122], women watched a terrifying movie while wearing axillary pads. A neutral film was presented the next day as control. Other women then had to smell and categorize the axillary pads obtained after the presentation of the terrifying film and those obtained after the presentation of the neutral film. As a result, women were able to distinguish between the pads of fear and those of non-fear. These results assume the existence of an odor of fear, present in perspiration and detectable by other individuals. Such behaviors may be also affected by olfactory disorders, but further studies still need to be done in this area.

7. Olfaction: A New Therapeutic Tool?

7.1. Animal Model and Odorants

Studies in animals have shown effects of odors on the emotional state. Komiya et al. [24] have demonstrated the anti-stress effects of lemon oil vapor on mice during behavioral tests (elevated plus maze and forced swim tests). The mechanism hypothesis is that lemon essential oil vapor affects the response to dopaminergic activity by modulating serotoninergic activity and/or GABA-benzodiazepines receptor complex.

In another study, Xu et al. [23] showed the effect of vanillin on the depressive-like behavior of non-bulbectomized and bulbectomized groups of rats. This was a comparative study of the effects of vanillin on depressive-like behavior rats induces by two ways: chronic unpredictable mild stress (CUMS) and olfactory bulbectomy. Results showed a significant decrease of depressive-like behavior for the CUMS group exposed to vanillin and the CUMS group exposed to fluoxetine. No changes were observed for the bulbectomy group exposed to vanillin. These results suggest that vanillin may have an effect on the symptoms of depression if the olfactory pathway is intact [23]. A study on Mongolian gerbil (which has more neuroendocrine similarity with humans than mice and rats) highlighted the anxiolytic effect of lavender odor. The authors showed that after chronic exposure to this odor, the anxiolytic effects were almost similar to those obtained after exposure to diazepam [22], but the mechanisms were not completely elucidated. Another study on rats demonstrated the antidepressant effect of lemon odor during behavioral tests (forced swim test and open field test) [127]. Lemon odor significantly reduced the depressive-like behavior. Further studies on the effects of odors on affective states in animal models are needed in order to understand the underlying mechanisms of these effects.

However, it is important to note that the cited studies have used bulbectomy to develop an animal model of depression. Their validity was, however criticized (for review, see [128]). Therefore, it is important to be careful before applying the findings obtained in animal models onto human subjects.

7.2. Use of Odors in Humans

Some studies have highlighted the sedative [129] and the anxiolytic effects [130,131] of odors in humans. Lehrner et al. [129] showed that participants exposed to the ambient odors of orange essential oils had lower levels of anxiety compared to control participants. The same authors extended their observations by using lavender odor [131]. The objective of this last study was to compare the effect of odor to the effect of music in the waiting room of a dental office. The results showed that the lavender odor had a more pronounced anxiolytic effect compared to music and control conditions. Indeed, studies showed that lavender acts post-synaptically and modulates the activity of cyclic adenosine monophosphate (cAMP). A reduction in cyclic adenosine monophosphate activity is associated with sedation [132].

Studies in humans have highlighted the interest of using odors as therapeutic tool. In a study by Hummel et al. [21], participants with olfactory loss (various origins: post-infectious, post-traumatic or idiopathic) followed a 12-week olfactory training program. At the end of this training, measurements of olfactory function were performed and it appeared that repeated daily olfactory stimulation improved the olfactory function of participants.

Haehner et al. [19] has proposed olfactory training in patients with Parkinson's disease. They used the same protocol as Hummel et al. [21]. The results of the study showed that olfactory training produced an increased olfactory sensitivity for the four odors used during the training, but also an overall increase of the olfactory function, whereas no anti-Parkinsonian treatment allowed this type of result.

Finally, a recent study highlighted the effects of olfactory training on symptoms of depression [20]. In this study, the subjects followed an olfactory training over a period of five months or had to perform Sudoku daily for the control group. The odors used were the same as in Hummel's study presented previously [21]. The results showed a significant decrease in the depression score (obtained with the Beck Depression Inventory) for the group who followed the five-month olfactory training compared to the group who performed Sudoku daily.

The mechanisms of action of odors' effects on depression are not known yet. However, several hypotheses were developed: the volatile odorant compound could act as a pharmacological agent and enter the bloodstream. In such a situation, its effects will be dependent on the concentration of the compound [133]. Studies are still needed to understand the mechanisms of action of odors on behavior in animals or humans.

8. Conclusions

We have shown here the links between the olfactory system, depression, and quality of life. Different brain areas are involved in both depression and olfaction, and patients with depression regularly suffer from an impaired sense of smell. Further studies are needed to confirm that only olfactory threshold and hedonic perception are altered in depression while the odor identification capabilities are preserved. In the future, it is important to study the olfactory perception of depressed patients in a more natural environment reflecting everyday life and using more complex sensory (olfactory and gustatory) stimuli. These investigations could explain the role of olfactory impairment in the eating disorders frequently observed in depression.

In this review, we have also demonstrated that the presence of olfactory disorders can lead to a decrease in the quality of life of patients in several areas: food, social life, and work. Previous studies have demonstrated that other perceptual deficits affecting gustation [134], vision [135], or audition [136] may lead to depression by decreasing quality of life. There are no comparative studies investigating the importance of different perceptual sensory deficits on depressed patients' quality of life. However, it is known that all senses participate in some sensory experiences like food intake. Such sensory experience will involve vision, audition, and kinesthesis, as well as the chemosensory modalities of olfaction, gustation, and chemesthesis that underlies flavor perception. However, sensory deficits are only partially assessed in some of the questionnaires evaluating the quality of life. Future improvement of the existing questionnaires are needed to create the tools suitable to the real problems of the clinical populations with olfactory deficits. Moreover, current clinical practice does not take into account olfactory impairments in depressed patients; olfactory deficits are not described in depression clinical criteria defined in DSM-5 [44]. The present review confirms the presence of sensory impairments and, specifically, the olfactory ones in the clinical spectrum of depression patients, and suggests that simple and inexpensive tools could be used to improve olfactory deficits. Furthermore, the current literature provides emerging evidence that olfactory stimulation (olfactory training) may be a promising tool for future therapeutic prospects. As suggested by Hummel et al. [21], it would be interesting to study the effects of this stimulation over time in order to know if the changes observed during olfactory training persist in time or not. Finally, studying the precise mechanisms of action of olfactory training is a must, in order to develop better olfactory training methods and to deepen knowledge about the olfactory system, depression, and how they affect quality of life.

Author Contributions: M.R., B.A., W.E.-H., F.K. and S.R. wrote the paper.

References

1. Sivertsen, H.; Bjørkløf, G.H.; Engedal, K.; Selbæk, G.; Helvik, A.-S. Depression and Quality of Life in Older Persons: A Review. *Dement. Geriatr. Cogn. Disord.* **2015**, *40*, 311–339. [CrossRef] [PubMed]
2. Doty, R. The Olfactory System and Its Disorders. *Semin. Neurol.* **2009**, *29*, 74–81. [CrossRef] [PubMed]
3. Andrade, L.; Caraveo-Anduaga, J.J.; Berglund, P.; Bijl, R.V.; De Graaf, R.; Vollebergh, W.; Dragomirecka, E.; Kohn, R.; Keller, M.; Kessler, R.C.; et al. The epidemiology of major depressive episodes: Results from the International Consortium of Psychiatric Epidemiology (ICPE) Surveys. *Int. J. Methods Psychiatr. Res.* **2003**, *12*, 3–21. [CrossRef] [PubMed]
4. Vennemann, M.M.; Hummel, T.; Berger, K. The association between smoking and smell and taste impairment in the general population. *J. Neurol.* **2008**, *255*, 1121–1126. [CrossRef] [PubMed]
5. Miwa, T.; Furukawa, M.; Tsukatani, T.; Costanzo, R.M.; DiNardo, L.J.; Reiter, E.R. Impact of olfactory impairment on quality of life and disability. *Arch. Otolaryngol. Head Neck Surg.* **2001**, *127*, 497–503. [CrossRef] [PubMed]
6. Höflich, A.; Baldinger, P.; Savli, M.; Lanzenberger, R.; Kasper, S. Imaging treatment effects in depression. *Rev. Neurosci.* **2012**, *23*, 227–252. [CrossRef] [PubMed]
7. Soudry, Y.; Lemogne, C.; Malinvaud, D.; Consoli, S.-M.; Bonfils, P. Olfactory system and emotion: Common substrates. *Eur. Ann. Otorhinolaryngol. Head Neck Dis.* **2011**, *128*, 18–23. [CrossRef] [PubMed]
8. Naudin, M.; Atanasova, B. Olfactory markers of depression and Alzheimer's disease. *Neurosci. Biobehav. Rev.* **2014**, *45*, 262–270. [CrossRef] [PubMed]
9. Savic, I.; Gulyas, B.; Larsson, M.; Roland, P. Olfactory functions are mediated by parallel and hierarchical processing. *Neuron* **2000**, *26*, 735–745. [CrossRef]
10. Anderson, A.K.; Christoff, K.; Stappen, I.; Panitz, D.; Ghahremani, D.G.; Glover, G.; Gabrieli, J.D.E.; Sobel, N. Dissociated neural representations of intensity and valence in human olfaction. *Nat. Neurosci.* **2003**, *6*, 196–202. [CrossRef] [PubMed]
11. Kircanski, K.; Joormann, J.; Gotlib, I.H. Cognitive aspects of depression: Cognitive aspects of depression. *Wiley Interdiscip. Rev. Cogn. Sci.* **2012**, *3*, 301–313. [CrossRef] [PubMed]
12. Seo, H.-S.; Roidl, E.; Müller, F.; Negoias, S. Odors enhance visual attention to congruent objects. *Appetite* **2010**, *54*, 544–549. [CrossRef] [PubMed]

13. Kohli, P.; Soler, Z.M.; Nguyen, S.A.; Muus, J.S.; Schlosser, R.J. The Association between Olfaction and Depression: A Systematic Review. *Chem. Senses* **2016**, *41*, 479–486. [CrossRef] [PubMed]
14. Masini, C.V.; Holmes, P.V.; Freeman, K.G.; Maki, A.C.; Edwards, G.L. Dopamine overflow is increased in olfactory bulbectomized rats: An in vivo microdialysis study. *Physiol. Behav.* **2004**, *81*, 111–119. [CrossRef] [PubMed]
15. Song, C.; Leonard, B.E. The olfactory bulbectomised rat as a model of depression. *Neurosci. Biobehav. Rev.* **2005**, *29*, 627–647. [CrossRef] [PubMed]
16. Rottstaedt, F.; Weidner, K.; Strauß, T.; Schellong, J.; Kitzler, H.; Wolff-Stephan, S.; Hummel, T.; Croy, I. Size matters—The olfactory bulb as a marker for depression. *J. Affect. Disord.* **2018**, *229*, 193–198. [CrossRef] [PubMed]
17. Mineur, Y.S.; Belzung, C.; Crusio, W.E. Functional implications of decreases in neurogenesis following chronic mild stress in mice. *Neuroscience* **2007**, *150*, 251–259. [CrossRef] [PubMed]
18. Croy, I.; Hummel, T. Olfaction as a marker for depression. *J. Neurol.* **2017**, *264*, 631–638. [CrossRef] [PubMed]
19. Haehner, A.; Tosch, C.; Wolz, M.; Klingelhoefer, L.; Fauser, M.; Storch, A.; Reichmann, H.; Hummel, T. Olfactory Training in Patients with Parkinson's Disease. *PLoS ONE* **2013**, *8*, e61680. [CrossRef] [PubMed]
20. Wegener, B.-A.; Croy, I.; Hähner, A.; Hummel, T. Olfactory training with older people: Olfactory training. *Int. J. Geriatr. Psychiatry* **2018**, *33*, 212–220. [CrossRef]
21. Hummel, T.; Rissom, K.; Reden, J.; Hähner, A.; Weidenbecher, M.; Hüttenbrink, K.-B. Effects of olfactory training in patients with olfactory loss. *Laryngoscope* **2009**, *119*, 496–499. [CrossRef] [PubMed]
22. Bradley, B.F.; Starkey, N.J.; Brown, S.L.; Lea, R.W. Anxiolytic effects of *Lavandula angustifolia* odour on the Mongolian gerbil elevated plus maze. *J. Ethnopharmacol.* **2007**, *111*, 517–525. [CrossRef] [PubMed]
23. Xu, J.; Xu, H.; Liu, Y.; He, H.; Li, G. Vanillin-induced amelioration of depression-like behaviors in rats by modulating monoamine neurotransmitters in the brain. *Psychiatry Res.* **2015**, *225*, 509–514. [CrossRef] [PubMed]
24. Komiya, M.; Takeuchi, T.; Harada, E. Lemon oil vapor causes an anti-stress effect via modulating the 5-HT and DA activities in mice. *Behav. Brain Res.* **2006**, *172*, 240–249. [CrossRef] [PubMed]
25. Frasnelli, J.; Hummel, T. Olfactory dysfunction and daily life. *Eur. Arch. Otorhinolaryngol.* **2005**, *262*, 231–235. [CrossRef] [PubMed]
26. Taalman, H.; Wallace, C.; Milev, R. Olfactory Functioning and Depression: A Systematic Review. *Front. Psychiatry* **2017**, *8*. [CrossRef] [PubMed]
27. Croy, I.; Symmank, A.; Schellong, J.; Hummel, C.; Gerber, J.; Joraschky, P.; Hummel, T. Olfaction as a marker for depression in humans. *J. Affect. Disord.* **2014**, *160*, 80–86. [CrossRef] [PubMed]
28. Croy, I.; Nordin, S.; Hummel, T. Olfactory Disorders and Quality of Life—An Updated Review. *Chem. Senses* **2014**, *39*, 185–194. [CrossRef] [PubMed]
29. Hummel, T.; Nordin, S. Olfactory disorders and their consequences for quality of life. *Acta Otolaryngol. (Stockh.)* **2005**, *125*, 116–121. [CrossRef]
30. El Hage, W.; Powell, J.F.; Surguladze, S.A. Vulnerability to depression: What is the role of stress genes in gene x environment interaction? *Psychol. Med.* **2009**, *39*, 1407–1411. [CrossRef] [PubMed]
31. Willner, P.; Scheel-Krüger, J.; Belzung, C. The neurobiology of depression and antidepressant action. *Neurosci. Biobehav. Rev.* **2013**, *37*, 2331–2371. [CrossRef] [PubMed]
32. Malberg, J.E.; Eisch, A.J.; Nestler, E.J.; Duman, R.S. Chronic antidepressant treatment increases neurogenesis in adult rat hippocampus. *J. Neurosci. Off. J. Soc. Neurosci.* **2000**, *20*, 9104–9110. [CrossRef]
33. Campbell, S.; Marriott, M.; Nahmias, C.; MacQueen, G.M. Lower hippocampal volume in patients suffering from depression: A meta-analysis. *Am. J. Psychiatry* **2004**, *161*, 598–607. [CrossRef] [PubMed]
34. Hickie, I.; Naismith, S.; Ward, P.B.; Turner, K.; Scott, E.; Mitchell, P.; Wilhelm, K.; Parker, G. Reduced hippocampal volumes and memory loss in patients with early- and late-onset depression. *Br. J. Psychiatry J. Ment. Sci.* **2005**, *186*, 197–202. [CrossRef] [PubMed]
35. Van Tol, M.-J.; van der Wee, N.J.A.; van den Heuvel, O.A.; Nielen, M.M.A.; Demenescu, L.R.; Aleman, A.; Renken, R.; van Buchem, M.A.; Zitman, F.G.; Veltman, D.J. Regional brain volume in depression and anxiety disorders. *Arch. Gen. Psychiatry* **2010**, *67*, 1002–1011. [CrossRef] [PubMed]
36. Kronenberg, G.; Tebartz van Elst, L.; Regen, F.; Deuschle, M.; Heuser, I.; Colla, M. Reduced amygdala volume in newly admitted psychiatric in-patients with unipolar major depression. *J. Psychiatr. Res.* **2009**, *43*, 1112–1117. [CrossRef] [PubMed]

37. Hamilton, J.P.; Siemer, M.; Gotlib, I.H. Amygdala volume in major depressive disorder: A meta-analysis of magnetic resonance imaging studies. *Mol. Psychiatry* **2008**, *13*, 993–1000. [CrossRef] [PubMed]

38. Sullivan, P.F.; Neale, M.C.; Kendler, K.S. Genetic epidemiology of major depression: Review and meta-analysis. *Am. J. Psychiatry* **2000**, *157*, 1552–1562. [CrossRef] [PubMed]

39. Caspi, A.; Sugden, K.; Moffitt, T.E.; Taylor, A.; Craig, I.W.; Harrington, H.; McClay, J.; Mill, J.; Martin, J.; Braithwaite, A.; et al. Influence of life stress on depression: Moderation by a polymorphism in the 5-HTT gene. *Science* **2003**, *301*, 386–389. [CrossRef] [PubMed]

40. Risch, N.; Herrell, R.; Lehner, T.; Liang, K.-Y.; Eaves, L.; Hoh, J.; Griem, A.; Kovacs, M.; Ott, J.; Merikangas, K.R. Interaction between the serotonin transporter gene (5-HTTLPR), stressful life events, and risk of depression: A meta-analysis. *JAMA* **2009**, *301*, 2462–2471. [CrossRef] [PubMed]

41. Hek, K.; Demirkan, A.; Lahti, J.; Terracciano, A.; Teumer, A.; Cornelis, M.C.; Amin, N.; Bakshis, E.; Baumert, J.; Ding, J.; et al. A genome-wide association study of depressive symptoms. *Biol. Psychiatry* **2013**, *73*, 667–678. [CrossRef] [PubMed]

42. Beck, A.T. *Cognitive Therapy and the Emotional Disorders*; Meridian: New York, NY, USA, 1976; ISBN 978-1-101-65988-5.

43. Kendler, K.S.; Thornton, L.M.; Gardner, C.O. Stressful life events and previous episodes in the etiology of major depression in women: An evaluation of the "kindling" hypothesis. *Am. J. Psychiatry* **2000**, *157*, 1243–1251. [CrossRef] [PubMed]

44. American Psychiatric Association. *Diagnostic and Statistical Manual of Mental Disorders (DSM-5®)*; American Psychiatric Publishing: Washington, UK, 2013.

45. Atanasova, B.; Graux, J.; El Hage, W.; Hommet, C.; Camus, V.; Belzung, C. Olfaction: A potential cognitive marker of psychiatric disorders. *Neurosci. Biobehav. Rev.* **2008**, *32*, 1315–1325. [CrossRef] [PubMed]

46. Naudin, M.; El-Hage, W.; Gomes, M.; Gaillard, P.; Belzung, C.; Atanasova, B. State and trait olfactory markers of major depression. *PLoS ONE* **2012**, *7*, e46938. [CrossRef] [PubMed]

47. Naudin, M.; Carl, T.; Surguladze, S.; Guillen, C.; Gaillard, P.; Belzung, C.; El-Hage, W.; Atanasova, B. Perceptive Biases in Major Depressive Episode. *PLoS ONE* **2014**, *9*. [CrossRef] [PubMed]

48. Siopi, E.; Denizet, M.; Gabellec, M.-M.; de Chaumont, F.; Olivo-Marin, J.-C.; Guilloux, J.-P.; Lledo, P.-M.; Lazarini, F. Anxiety- and Depression-Like States Lead to Pronounced Olfactory Deficits and Impaired Adult Neurogenesis in Mice. *J. Neurosci. Off. J. Soc. Neurosci.* **2016**, *36*, 518–531. [CrossRef] [PubMed]

49. Pevsner, J.; Snyder, S.H. Odorant-binding protein: Odorant transport function in the vertebrate nasal epithelium. *Chem. Senses* **1990**, *15*, 217–222. [CrossRef]

50. Brand, G. *L'olfaction: De la Molécule au Comportement*; SOLAL Editeurs: Marseille, France, 2001; ISBN 978-2-914513-12-8.

51. Delplanque, S.; Coppin, G.; Sander, D. Odor and Emotion. In *Springer Handbook of Odor*; Buettner, A., Ed.; Springer International Publishing: Cham, Switzerland, 2017; pp. 101–102. ISBN 978-3-319-26930-6.

52. Parma, V.; Bulgheroni, M.; Tirindelli, R.; Castiello, U. Facilitation of action planning in children with autism: The contribution of the maternal body odor. *Brain Cogn.* **2014**, *88*, 73–82. [CrossRef] [PubMed]

53. Doty, R.L.; Shaman, P.; Dann, M. Development of the University of Pennsylvania Smell Identification Test: A standardized microencapsulated test of olfactory function. *Physiol. Behav.* **1984**, *32*, 489–502. [CrossRef]

54. Hummel, T.; Sekinger, B.; Wolf, S.R.; Pauli, E.; Kobal, G. "Sniffin" sticks': Olfactory performance assessed by the combined testing of odor identification, odor discrimination and olfactory threshold. *Chem. Senses* **1997**, *22*, 39–52. [CrossRef] [PubMed]

55. Doty, R.; Kobal, G. Current trends in the measurement of olfactory function. In *Handbook of Olfaction and Gustation*; John Wiley & Sons: New York, NY, USA, 1995; pp. 191–225.

56. Atanasova, B.; Hernandez, N.; van Nieuwenhuijzen, P.; Belzung, C. Psychophysical, neurophysiological and neurobiological investigation of the olfactory process in humans: Olfactory impairment in some neuropsychiatric disorders. In *The Biology of Odors: Sources, Olfaction and Response*; Nova Science Publishers Incorp: Hauppauge, NY, USA, 2011; pp. 1–67.

57. Brand, G.; Schaal, B. L'olfaction dans les troubles dépressifs: Intérêts et perspectives. *L'Encéphale* **2016**. [CrossRef] [PubMed]

58. Deems, D.A.; Doty, R.L.; Settle, R.G.; Moore-Gillon, V.; Shaman, P.; Mester, A.F.; Kimmelman, C.P.; Brightman, V.J.; Snow, J.B. Smell and taste disorders, a study of 750 patients from the University of Pennsylvania Smell and Taste Center. *Arch. Otolaryngol. Head Neck Surg.* **1991**, *117*, 519–528. [CrossRef] [PubMed]
59. Larsson, K. Impaired mating performances in male rats after anosmia induced peripherally or centrally. *Brain. Behav. Evol.* **1971**, *4*, 463–471. [CrossRef] [PubMed]
60. Kelly, J.P.; Leonard, B.E. Effects of chronic desipramine on waiting behaviour for a food reward in olfactory bulbectomized rats. *J. Psychopharmacol. (Oxf.)* **1996**, *10*, 153–156. [CrossRef] [PubMed]
61. Song, C.; Earley, B.; Leonard, B.E. The effects of central administration of neuropeptide Y on behavior, neurotransmitter, and immune functions in the olfactory bulbectomized rat model of depression. *Brain. Behav. Immun.* **1996**, *10*, 1–16. [CrossRef] [PubMed]
62. Kelly, J.P.; Wrynn, A.S.; Leonard, B.E. The olfactory bulbectomized rat as a model of depression: An update. *Pharmacol. Ther.* **1997**, *74*, 299–316. [CrossRef]
63. Negoias, S.; Croy, I.; Gerber, J.; Puschmann, S.; Petrowski, K.; Joraschky, P.; Hummel, T. Reduced olfactory bulb volume and olfactory sensitivity in patients with acute major depression. *Neuroscience* **2010**, *169*, 415–421. [CrossRef] [PubMed]
64. Li, Q.; Yang, D.; Wang, J.; Liu, L.; Feng, G.; Li, J.; Liao, J.; Wei, Y.; Li, Z. Reduced amount of olfactory receptor neurons in the rat model of depression. *Neurosci. Lett.* **2015**, *603*, 48–54. [CrossRef] [PubMed]
65. Kesner, R.P.; Gilbert, P.E.; Barua, L.A. The role of the hippocampus in memory for the temporal order of a sequence of odors. *Behav. Neurosci.* **2002**, *116*, 286–290. [CrossRef] [PubMed]
66. Lemogne, C.; Piolino, P.; Friszer, S.; Claret, A.; Girault, N.; Jouvent, R.; Allilaire, J.-F.; Fossati, P. Episodic autobiographical memory in depression: Specificity, autonoetic consciousness, and self-perspective. *Conscious. Cogn.* **2006**, *15*, 258–268. [CrossRef] [PubMed]
67. Pouliot, S.; Jones-Gotman, M. Medial temporal-lobe damage and memory for emotionally arousing odors. *Neuropsychologia* **2008**, *46*, 1124–1134. [CrossRef] [PubMed]
68. Drevets, W.C. Neuroimaging abnormalities in the amygdala in mood disorders. *Ann. N. Y. Acad. Sci.* **2003**, *985*, 420–444. [CrossRef] [PubMed]
69. Rogers, M.A.; Kasai, K.; Koji, M.; Fukuda, R.; Iwanami, A.; Nakagome, K.; Fukuda, M.; Kato, N. Executive and prefrontal dysfunction in unipolar depression: A review of neuropsychological and imaging evidence. *Neurosci. Res.* **2004**, *50*, 1–11. [CrossRef] [PubMed]
70. Grabenhorst, F.; Rolls, E.T.; Margot, C. A hedonically complex odor mixture produces an attentional capture effect in the brain. *NeuroImage* **2011**, *55*, 832–843. [CrossRef] [PubMed]
71. Zald, D.H.; Pardo, J.V. Emotion, olfaction, and the human amygdala: Amygdala activation during aversive olfactory stimulation. *Proc. Natl. Acad. Sci. USA* **1997**, *94*, 4119–4124. [CrossRef] [PubMed]
72. Grabenhorst, F.; Rolls, E.T.; Margot, C.; da Silva, M.A.A.P.; Velazco, M.I. How pleasant and unpleasant stimuli combine in different brain regions: Odor mixtures. *J. Neurosci. Off. J. Soc. Neurosci.* **2007**, *27*, 13532–13540. [CrossRef] [PubMed]
73. Zald, D.H.; Mattson, D.L.; Pardo, J.V. Brain activity in ventromedial prefrontal cortex correlates with individual differences in negative affect. *Proc. Natl. Acad. Sci. USA* **2002**, *99*, 2450–2454. [CrossRef] [PubMed]
74. Phillips, M.L.; Drevets, W.C.; Rauch, S.L.; Lane, R. Neurobiology of emotion perception II: Implications for major psychiatric disorders. *Biol. Psychiatry* **2003**, *54*, 515–528. [CrossRef]
75. Bhagwagar, Z.; Wylezinska, M.; Jezzard, P.; Evans, J.; Boorman, E.; Matthews, P.M.; Cowen, P.J. Low GABA concentrations in occipital cortex and anterior cingulate cortex in medication-free, recovered depressed patients. *Int. J. Neuropsychopharmacol.* **2008**, *11*, 255–260. [CrossRef] [PubMed]
76. Fulbright, R.K.; Skudlarski, P.; Lacadie, C.M.; Warrenburg, S.; Bowers, A.A.; Gore, J.C.; Wexler, B.E. Functional MR imaging of regional brain responses to pleasant and unpleasant odors. *AJNR Am. J. Neuroradiol.* **1998**, *19*, 1721–1726. [PubMed]
77. Paulus, M.P.; Stein, M.B. An insular view of anxiety. *Biol. Psychiatry* **2006**, *60*, 383–387. [CrossRef] [PubMed]
78. Veldhuizen, M.G.; Nachtigal, D.; Teulings, L.; Gitelman, D.R.; Small, D.M. The Insular Taste Cortex Contributes to Odor Quality Coding. *Front. Hum. Neurosci.* **2010**, *4*. [CrossRef] [PubMed]
79. Sliz, D.; Hayley, S. Major Depressive Disorder and Alterations in Insular Cortical Activity: A Review of Current Functional Magnetic Imaging Research. *Front. Hum. Neurosci.* **2012**, *6*. [CrossRef] [PubMed]

80. Shumake, J.; Edwards, E.; Gonzalez-Lima, F. Opposite metabolic changes in the habenula and ventral tegmental area of a genetic model of helpless behavior. *Brain Res.* **2003**, *963*, 274–281. [CrossRef]
81. Da Costa, A.P.; Broad, K.D.; Kendrick, K.M. Olfactory memory and maternal behaviour-induced changes in c-fos and zif/268 mRNA expression in the sheep brain. *Brain Res. Mol. Brain Res.* **1997**, *46*, 63–76. [CrossRef]
82. Hikosaka, O.; Sesack, S.R.; Lecourtier, L.; Shepard, P.D. Habenula—Crossroad between the Basal Ganglia and the Limbic System. *J. Neurosci. Off. J. Soc. Neurosci.* **2008**, *28*, 11825–11829. [CrossRef] [PubMed]
83. Oral, E.; Aydin, M.D.; Aydin, N.; Ozcan, H.; Hacimuftuoglu, A.; Sipal, S.; Demirci, E. How olfaction disorders can cause depression? The role of habenular degeneration. *Neuroscience* **2013**, *240*, 63–69. [CrossRef] [PubMed]
84. Pause, B.M.; Raack, N.; Sojka, B.; Göder, R.; Aldenhoff, J.B.; Ferstl, R. Convergent and divergent effects of odors and emotions in depression. *Psychophysiology* **2003**, *40*, 209–225. [CrossRef] [PubMed]
85. Lombion-Pouthier, S.; Vandel, P.; Nezelof, S.; Haffen, E.; Millot, J.-L. Odor perception in patients with mood disorders. *J. Affect. Disord.* **2006**, *90*, 187–191. [CrossRef] [PubMed]
86. Pause, B.M.; Miranda, A.; Göder, R.; Aldenhoff, J.B.; Ferstl, R. Reduced olfactory performance in patients with major depression. *J. Psychiatr. Res.* **2001**, *35*, 271–277. [CrossRef]
87. Postolache, T.T.; Doty, R.L.; Wehr, T.A.; Jimma, L.A.; Han, L.; Turner, E.H.; Matthews, J.R.; Neumeister, A.; No, C.; Kroger, H.; et al. Monorhinal odor identification and depression scores in patients with seasonal affective disorder. *J. Affect. Disord.* **1999**, *56*, 27–35. [CrossRef]
88. Scinska, A.; Wrobel, E.; Korkosz, A.; Zatorski, P.; Sienkiewicz-Jarosz, H.; Lojkowska, W.; Swiecicki, L.; Kukwa, W. Depressive symptoms and olfactory function in older adults. *Psychiatry Clin. Neurosci.* **2008**, *62*, 450–456. [CrossRef] [PubMed]
89. Swiecicki, L.; Zatorski, P.; Bzinkowska, D.; Sienkiewicz-Jarosz, H.; Szyndler, J.; Scinska, A. Gustatory and olfactory function in patients with unipolar and bipolar depression. *Prog. Neuropsychopharmacol. Biol. Psychiatry* **2009**, *33*, 827–834. [CrossRef] [PubMed]
90. Gross-Isseroff, R.; Luca-Haimovici, K.; Sasson, Y.; Kindler, S.; Kotler, M.; Zohar, J. Olfactory sensitivity in major depressive disorder and obsessive compulsive disorder. *Biol. Psychiatry* **1994**, *35*, 798–802. [CrossRef]
91. Pollatos, O.; Albrecht, J.; Kopietz, R.; Linn, J.; Schoepf, V.; Kleemann, A.M.; Schreder, T.; Schandry, R.; Wiesmann, M. Reduced olfactory sensitivity in subjects with depressive symptoms. *J. Affect. Disord.* **2007**, *102*, 101–108. [CrossRef] [PubMed]
92. Clepce, M.; Gossler, A.; Reich, K.; Kornhuber, J.; Thuerauf, N. The relation between depression, anhedonia and olfactory hedonic estimates—A pilot study in major depression. *Neurosci. Lett.* **2010**, *471*, 139–143. [CrossRef] [PubMed]
93. Serby, M.; Larson, P.; Kalkstein, D. Olfactory sense in psychoses. *Biol. Psychiatry* **1990**, *28*, 830. [CrossRef]
94. Zucco, G.M.; Bollini, F. Odour recognition memory and odour identification in patients with mild and severe major depressive disorders. *Psychiatry Res.* **2011**, *190*, 217–220. [CrossRef] [PubMed]
95. Atanasova, B.; El-Hage, W.; Chabanet, C.; Gaillard, P.; Belzung, C.; Camus, V. Olfactory anhedonia and negative olfactory alliesthesia in depressed patients. *Psychiatry Res.* **2010**, *176*, 190–196. [CrossRef] [PubMed]
96. Amsterdam, J.D.; Settle, R.G.; Doty, R.L.; Abelman, E.; Winokur, A. Taste and smell perception in depression. *Biol. Psychiatry* **1987**, *22*, 1481–1485. [CrossRef]
97. Kopala, L.C.; Good, K.P.; Honer, W.G. Olfactory hallucinations and olfactory identification ability in patients with schizophrenia and other psychiatric disorders. *Schizophr. Res.* **1994**, *12*, 205–211. [CrossRef]
98. McCaffrey, R.J.; Duff, K.; Solomon, G.S. Olfactory dysfunction discriminates probable Alzheimer's dementia from major depression: A cross-validation and extension. *J. Neuropsychiatry Clin. Neurosci.* **2000**, *12*, 29–33. [CrossRef] [PubMed]
99. Pentzek, M.; Grass-Kapanke, B.; Ihl, R. Odor identification in Alzheimer's disease and depression. *Aging Clin. Exp. Res.* **2007**, *19*, 255–258. [CrossRef] [PubMed]
100. Solomon, G.S.; Petrie, W.M.; Hart, J.R.; Brackin, J.; Henry, B. Olfactory Dysfunction Discriminates Alzheimer's Dementia from Major Depression. *J. Neuropsychiatry Clin. Neurosci.* **1998**, *10*, 64–67. [CrossRef] [PubMed]
101. Atanasova, B.; Gaillard, P.; Minier, F.; Belzung, C.; El-Hage, W. Hedonic Olfactory Perception in Depression: Relationship between Self-Evaluation and Autonomic Response. *Psychology* **2012**, *3*, 959–965. [CrossRef]
102. Naudin, M.; Mondon, K.; El-Hage, W.; Desmidt, T.; Jaafari, N.; Belzung, C.; Gaillard, P.; Hommet, C.; Atanasova, B. Long-term odor recognition memory in unipolar major depression and Alzheimer's disease. *Psychiatry Res.* **2014**, *220*, 861–866. [CrossRef] [PubMed]

103. Thomas, H.J.; Fries, W.; Distel, H. Evaluation of olfactory stimuli by depressed patients. *Nervenarzt* **2002**, *73*, 71–77. [CrossRef] [PubMed]
104. Postolache, T.T.; Wehr, T.A.; Doty, R.L.; Sher, L.; Turner, E.H.; Bartko, J.J.; Rosenthal, N.E. Patients with Seasonal Affective Disorder Have Lower Odor Detection Thresholds Than Control Subjects. *Arch. Gen. Psychiatry* **2002**, *59*, 1119–1122. [CrossRef] [PubMed]
105. Oren, D.A.; Schwartz, P.J.; Turner, E.H.; Rosenthal, N.E. Olfactory function in winter seasonal affective disorder. *Am. J. Psychiatry* **1995**, *152*, 1531–1532. [PubMed]
106. Kamath, V.; Paksarian, D.; Cui, L.; Moberg, P.J.; Turetsky, B.I.; Merikangas, K.R. Olfactory processing in bipolar disorder, major depression, and anxiety. *Bipolar Disord.* **2018**. [CrossRef] [PubMed]
107. Striebel, K.M.; Beyerstein, B.; Remick, R.A.; Kopala, L.; Honer, W.G. Olfactory identification and psychosis. *Biol. Psychiatry* **1999**, *45*, 1419–1425. [CrossRef]
108. Krüger, S.; Frasnelli, J.; Bräunig, P.; Hummel, T. Increased olfactory sensitivity in euthymic patients with bipolar disorder with event-related episodes compared with patients with bipolar disorder without such episodes. *J. Psychiatry Neurosci.* **2006**, *31*, 263–270. [PubMed]
109. Vasterling, J.J.; Brailey, K.; Sutker, P.B. Olfactory identification in combat-related posttraumatic stress disorder. *J. Trauma. Stress* **2000**, *13*, 241–253. [CrossRef] [PubMed]
110. McDowell, I. *Measuring Health*; Oxford University Press: Oxford, UK, 2006; ISBN 978-0-19-516567-8.
111. Derogatis, L.R.; Unger, R. Symptom Checklist-90-Revised. In *The Corsini Encyclopedia of Psychology*; Weiner, I.B., Craighead, W.E., Eds.; John Wiley & Sons, Inc.: Hoboken, NJ, USA, 2010; ISBN 978-0-470-47921-6.
112. Wiklund, I.; Romanus, B.; Hunt, S.M. Self-assessed disability in patients with arthrosis of the hip joint. Reliability of the Swedish version of the Nottingham Health Profile. *Int. Disabil. Stud.* **1988**, *10*, 159–163. [CrossRef] [PubMed]
113. McDowell, I. Measures of self-perceived well-being. *J. Psychosom. Res.* **2010**, *69*, 69–79. [CrossRef] [PubMed]
114. Temmel, A.F.P.; Quint, C.; Schickinger-Fischer, B.; Klimek, L.; Stoller, E.; Hummel, T. Characteristics of olfactory disorders in relation to major causes of olfactory loss. *Arch. Otolaryngol. Head Neck Surg.* **2002**, *128*, 635–641. [CrossRef] [PubMed]
115. Ferris, A.M.; Duffy, V.B. Effect of olfactory deficits on nutritional status. Does age predict persons at risk? *Ann. N. Y. Acad. Sci.* **1989**, *561*, 113–123. [CrossRef] [PubMed]
116. Blomqvist, E.H.; Brämerson, A.; Stjärne, P.; Nordin, S. Consequences of olfactory loss and adopted coping strategies. *Rhinology* **2004**, *42*, 189–194. [PubMed]
117. Nordin, S.; Hedén Blomqvist, E.; Olsson, P.; Stjärne, P.; Ehnhage, A.; NAF2S2 Study Group. Effects of smell loss on daily life and adopted coping strategies in patients with nasal polyposis with asthma. *Acta Otolaryngol. (Stockh.)* **2011**, *131*, 826–832. [CrossRef] [PubMed]
118. Nordin, S.; Brämerson, A.; Murphy, C.; Bende, M. A Scandinavian adaptation of the Multi-Clinic Smell and Taste Questionnaire: Evaluation of questions about olfaction. *Acta Otolaryngol. (Stockh.)* **2003**, *123*, 536–542. [CrossRef]
119. Croy, I.; Negoias, S.; Novakova, L.; Landis, B.N.; Hummel, T. Learning about the functions of the olfactory system from people without a sense of smell. *PLoS ONE* **2012**, *7*, e33365. [CrossRef] [PubMed]
120. Santos, D.V.; Reiter, E.R.; DiNardo, L.J.; Costanzo, R.M. Hazardous events associated with impaired olfactory function. *Arch. Otolaryngol. Head Neck Surg.* **2004**, *130*, 317–319. [CrossRef] [PubMed]
121. Brämerson, A.; Johansson, L.; Ek, L.; Nordin, S.; Bende, M. Prevalence of olfactory dysfunction: The skövde population-based study. *Laryngoscope* **2004**, *114*, 733–737. [CrossRef] [PubMed]
122. Ackerl, K.; Atzmueller, M.; Grammer, K. The scent of fear. *Neuro Endocrinol. Lett.* **2002**, *23*, 79–84. [PubMed]
123. Prehn-Kristensen, A.; Wiesner, C.; Bergmann, T.O.; Wolff, S.; Jansen, O.; Mehdorn, H.M.; Ferstl, R.; Pause, B.M. Induction of empathy by the smell of anxiety. *PLoS ONE* **2009**, *4*, e5987. [CrossRef] [PubMed]
124. Schaal, B.; Montagner, H.; Hertling, E.; Bolzoni, D.; Moyse, A.; Quichon, R. Les stimulations olfactives dans les relations entre l'enfant et la mère. *Reprod. Nutr. Dév.* **1980**, *20*, 843–858. [CrossRef] [PubMed]
125. Gelstein, S.; Yeshurun, Y.; Rozenkrantz, L.; Shushan, S.; Frumin, I.; Roth, Y.; Sobel, N. Human tears contain a chemosignal. *Science* **2011**, *331*, 226–230. [CrossRef] [PubMed]
126. Stevenson, R.J. An initial evaluation of the functions of human olfaction. *Chem. Senses* **2010**, *35*, 3–20. [CrossRef] [PubMed]
127. Komori, T.; Fujiwara, R.; Tanida, M.; Nomura, J. Potential antidepressant effects of lemon odor in rats. *Eur. Neuropsychopharmacol. J. Eur. Coll. Neuropsychopharmacol.* **1995**, *5*, 477–480. [CrossRef]

128. Harkin, A.; Kelly, J.P.; Leonard, B.E. A review of the relevance and validity of olfactory bulbectomy as a model of depression. *Clin. Neurosci. Res.* **2003**, *3*, 253–262. [CrossRef]
129. Lehrner, J.; Eckersberger, C.; Walla, P.; Pötsch, G.; Deecke, L. Ambient odor of orange in a dental office reduces anxiety and improves mood in female patients. *Physiol. Behav.* **2000**, *71*, 83–86. [CrossRef]
130. Diego, M.A.; Jones, N.A.; Field, T.; Hernandez-Reif, M.; Schanberg, S.; Kuhn, C.; McAdam, V.; Galamaga, R.; Galamaga, M. Aromatherapy positively affects mood, EEG patterns of alertness and math computations. *Int. J. Neurosci.* **1998**, *96*, 217–224. [CrossRef] [PubMed]
131. Lehrner, J.; Marwinski, G.; Lehr, S.; Johren, P.; Deecke, L. Ambient odors of orange and lavender reduce anxiety and improve mood in a dental office. *Physiol. Behav.* **2005**, *86*, 92–95. [CrossRef] [PubMed]
132. Lis-Balchin, M.; Hart, S. Studies on the mode of action of the essential oil of Lavender (*Lavandula angustifolia* P. Miller). *Phytother. Res.* **1999**, *13*, 540–542. [CrossRef]
133. Herz, R.S. Aromatherapy facts and fictions: A scientific analysis of olfactory effects on mood, physiology and behavior. *Int. J. Neurosci.* **2009**, *119*, 263–290. [CrossRef] [PubMed]
134. Maheswaran, T.; Abikshyeet, P.; Sitra, G.; Gokulanathan, S.; Vaithiyanadane, V.; Jeelani, S. Gustatory dysfunction. *J. Pharm. Bioallied Sci.* **2014**, *6*, S30–S33. [CrossRef] [PubMed]
135. Ribeiro, M.V.M. R.; Hasten-Reiter Júnior, H.N.; Ribeiro, E.A.N.; Jucá, M.J.; Barbosa, F.T.; Sousa-Rodrigues, C.F. de Association between visual impairment and depression in the elderly: A systematic review. *Arq. Bras. Oftalmol.* **2015**, *78*, 197–201. [CrossRef] [PubMed]
136. Mosaku, K.; Akinpelu, V.; Ogunniyi, G. Psychopathology among a sample of hearing impaired adolescents. *Asian J. Psychiatry* **2015**, *18*, 53–56. [CrossRef] [PubMed]

7

Can Anhedonia Be Considered a Suicide Risk Factor?

Luca Bonanni [1], Flavia Gualtieri [1], David Lester [2], Giulia Falcone [1], Adele Nardella [1], Andrea Fiorillo [3] and Maurizio Pompili [4,*]

1 Psychiatry Residency Training Program, Faculty of Medicine and Psychology, Sapienza University of Rome, 00189 Rome, Italy
2 Psychology Program, Stockton University, Galloway, NJ 08205, USA
3 Department of Psychiatry, University of Campania Luigi Vanvitelli, 80138 Naples, Italy
4 Department of Neurosciences, Mental Health and Sensory Organs, Suicide Prevention Center, Sant'Andrea Hospital, Sapienza University of Rome, 00189 Rome, Italy
* Correspondence: maurizio.pompili@uniroma1.it;

Abstract: *Background and Objectives*: At present, data collected from the literature about suicide and anhedonia are controversial. Some studies have shown that low levels of anhedonia are associated with serious suicide attempts and death by suicide, while other studies have shown that high levels of anhedonia are associated with suicide. *Materials and Methods*: For this review, we searched PubMed, Medline, and ScienceDirect for clinical studies published from 1 January 1990 to 31 December 2018 with the following search terms used in the title or in the abstract: "anhedonia AND suicid*." We obtained a total of 155 articles; 133 items were excluded using specific exclusion criteria, the remaining 22 articles included were divided into six groups based on the psychiatric diagnosis: mood disorders, schizophrenia spectrum disorders, post-traumatic stress disorder (PTSD), other diagnoses, attempted suicides, and others (healthy subjects). *Results*: The results of this review reveal inconsistencies. Some studies reported that high anhedonia scores were associated with suicidal behavior (regardless of the diagnosis), while other studies found that low anhedonia scores were associated with suicidal behavior, and a few studies reported no association. The most consistent association between anhedonia and suicidal behavior was found for affective disorders (7 of 7 studies reported a significant positive association) and for PTSD (3 of 3 studies reported a positive association). In the two studies of patients with schizophrenia, one found no association, and one found a negative association. For patients who attempted suicide (undiagnosed), one study found a positive association, one a positive association only for depressed attempters, and one a negative association. *Conclusions*: We found the most consistent positive association for patients with affective disorders and PTSD, indicating that the assessment of anhedonia may be useful in the evaluation of suicidal risk.

Keywords: anhedonia; PTSD; suicide; suicide risk; suicidal behavior

---

1. Introduction

Suicide is a severe public health problem with more than one million deaths reported each year worldwide [1] and with nearly 20 times more people attempting suicide each year [2]. Moreover, suicide ranks among the ten major causes of death worldwide and is a leading cause of death among youth and young adults in many countries [3–6]. Given the prevalence of suicidal ideation and behaviors and the associated medical expenses, it is important to know what factors lead to both suicidal thoughts and suicide attempts in order to identify reliably those transitioning from suicidal ideation to fatal suicidal behaviors [7]. Developing this ability will inform suicide risk assessment methods and early intervention tools.

The MATRICS consensus conference on negative symptoms, convened under the auspices of the National Institutes of Mental Health (NIMH) in 2005, suggested that there are five general categories of negative symptoms: avolition, anhedonia, asociality, affective blunting, and alogia. The most common negative symptoms are avolition and anhedonia, and one of the most persistent negative symptoms is anhedonia, that is not experiencing pleasure or having the ability to obtain pleasure from activities or interpersonal relationships. In DSM-5, anhedonia is defined as "Lack of enjoyment from, engagement in, or energy for life's experiences; deficits in the capacity to feel pleasure and take an interest in things." Anhedonia is present in both patients with schizophrenia and patients with depression. It is estimated that half of schizophrenia patients experience anhedonia, although estimates of its prevalence vary greatly. Anhedonia and social isolation predict schizophrenia in high-risk populations [8].

Lately, there has been a growing interest in anhedonia with the evidence suggesting that this symptom may be a unique predictor of psychopathology [9], including suicidality [10–12]. For example, a study of 40 patients with depression and 20 controls showed that individuals who had suicidal ideation and previous suicidal attempts were less likely to respond to rewarding stimuli on a task designed to assess the presence of anhedonia [12].

The results of the research, however, are inconsistent. Some research has shown that low levels of anhedonia are associated with serious suicide attempts and death by suicide [13,14], while other research has shown that high levels of anhedonia are associated with suicide [15–18]. A study conducted by Winer et al. [19] showed that anhedonia is associated with suicidal ideation but not with previous suicide attempts. Regarding the observed relationship between anhedonia and suicidal behavior, Nock and Kazdin [10] suggested that anhedonia is experienced as an intolerable state leading to suicidal behavior to escape a current stressor. Other research shows that those who think of suicide feel less pleasure and are focused on efforts to avoid psychological pain [12], and a reduction in psychological pain has been observed when individuals engage in suicidal behavior [20]. Some studies have suggested that anhedonia is a modifiable clinical factor associated with suicidal ideation, independently of depressive symptoms [21].

As mentioned above, several studies have shown that anhedonia is related to an increased risk of suicide, while others have claimed the opposite. This discrepancy can be understood using the following considerations [22]. First, anhedonia can be considered either as a trait or as a state. When anhedonia is a state, presenting and persisting as a symptom of a specific psychiatric disorder and, particularly, depression, it may be a risk factor for suicide. When it is considered as a trait, with long-term stability and not associated with depression, it may not act as a risk factor for suicide or it may be associated with a low risk of suicide [23]. Also significant is the difference between consummatory and anticipatory anhedonia [24], although this is rarely taken into consideration. A deficit in consummatory pleasure can characterize endogenomorphic depression, a subtype of depression associated with a higher risk of suicide [25]. Moreover, there is not just one but several types of suicide risk: suicidal ideation, suicide attempt (recent or not), and completed suicide. In addition, there is a great deal of difference in the methodology used in studies proposing to demonstrate a correlation between anhedonia and suicide risk which should be kept in mind. In fact, these studies do not have homogeneity in the types of sample chosen (differentiating for example by age, gender, etc.,) as well as a control of the confounding variables (such as outpatients or inpatients) and a control for depression level (that is, the effect of the anhedonia independently of depression) [22].

Although some medications, such as lithium [26,27] and clozapine [27,28], as well as psychotherapy, have shown effectiveness in managing suicidal behavior, the rates of suicidal ideation, suicide attempts, and completed suicides have not substantially decreased in recent years [29]. Hence, it will be useful to know in more detail the risk factors for suicide, such as anhedonia, in order to create alternative suicide prevention tactics, and the present review of the literature tries to understand the association between suicidal behaviors and anhedonia.

2. Materials and Methods

For this review, we searched PubMed, Medline, and ScienceDirect for clinical studies published from 1 January 1990 to 31 December 2018 with the following search terms used in the title or in the abstract: "anhedonia AND suicid*". Initially, two reviewers screened the abstracts of studies identified for eligibility with 100% agreement, and then another reviewer assessed the included studies. All three reviewers discussed any disagreements identified and reached an agreement before proceeding. We obtained a total of 155 articles of which 133 articles were excluded using the following exclusion criteria: reviews or meta-analyses (21), case reports (2), letters/opinions (1), non-psychiatric studies (6) or unfocused (98), and studies conducted on adolescents (5). The 22 articles included in this review were divided into six groups based on the psychiatric diagnosis: mood disorders, schizophrenia spectrum disorders, post-traumatic stress disorder, other diagnoses (such as anxiety disorders), attempted suicide, and others (that is, without a psychiatric diagnosis). Details of the trials included (study design, sample size, criteria, objectives, evaluation tools, outcomes) were extracted and are reported in Table 1.

Table 1. Summary of reports on suicide behavior and anhedonia.

Mood Disorder						
Reference	**Study Design**	**Sample**	**Criteria**	**Objectives**	**Methods**	**Results**
Zielinski et al. 2017	Prospective longitudinal study	187 participants	Participants (mean age = 34.41) with a history of non-suicidal self-injury or previous suicide attempts	To verify if modifications in depressive symptoms and anhedonia can be considered as predictive factors of suicide and self-harm behavior	- DASS-21 © to assess depressive symptoms - SLIPS [¥] to evaluate anhedonia - SBQ-R [↓] to assess several dimensions of suicidal risk - OSI[€] to evaluate self -harm behavior	Anhedonia scores were higher in those with prior suicide attempts than in those with a history of non-suicidal self-injury. Depressive symptoms predicted suicidal behavior directly and also via mediation through anhedonia
Ballard et al. 2017	Retrospective longitudinal study	100 participants	Patients (18–65 years) affected by treatment-resistant major depressive disorder (n = 65) or bipolar disorder without psychotic features (n = 35) recruited from several clinical trials of ketamine	To evaluate the relationship between the decrease of suicidal ideation after ketamine administration and the reduction of anhedonia	- BDI [*]-II and the SHAPS [#] to assess anhedonia - SSI5 [Ø] to assess suicidal ideation	At baseline, anhedonia scores were associated with suicidal ideation. After administration of ketamine, both suicidal ideation and anhedonia declined. The change in anhedonia accounted for an additional 13% of the variance for changes in suicidal thoughts beyond the effects of depressive symptoms
Ballard et al. 2016	Prospective study from the STEP-BD study (4360 patients)	530 participants	Subjects who attempted or died by suicide (n = 103) vs. controls (n = 427)	To individualize which clinical dimensions (suicidal ideation, loss of interest, anxiety, psychomotor agitation, high-risk behavior) increase before suicidal conduct	- Clinical Monitoring Form (CMF) for clinic evaluation	Patients with suicidal behavior had an elevation of all symptoms, including loss of interest. Suicidal ideation and loss of interest were highly intense in the months before the suicidal behavior and can be considered a risk factor for suicidal behavior in bipolar patients
Xie et al. 2014	Cross-sectional study	60 participants	Participants (18–60 years) included patients affected by major depressive disorder (n = 40) vs. control subjects without psychiatric disorder (n = 20). Based on BSS scores, psychiatric patients were divided into two subgroups: high suicidal ideation (HSI) group and low suicidal ideation (LSI) group	To analyze the association between anhedonia, pain avoidance motivation, and suicidal ideation	- BDI [*]-II to assess depressive symptoms - BSS [$] for suicidal ideation - PAS [%] and TDPPS [¢] to evaluatephysical and mental pain - MID [~] and AID [§]	In AID task, the HSI had longer response times (RTs) under the reward condition than those under the punishment condition ($p = 0.002$); the LSI group and control groups had shorter RTs under the reward condition than those under the neutral condition ($p < 0.001$ and $p = 0.008$, respectively); the LSI group had shorter RTs under the reward condition than under the punishment condition ($p = 0.003$). Pain arousal ($p < 0.01$) and BSS scores were significantly negatively correlated with differences in RTs between neutral and reward conditions and positively correlated with differences in RTs between neutral and punishment conditions. The AID was the best task for detection of hedonic approach to experiences and of pain avoidance so that a reduced motivation to experience anhedonia and an increased one to avoid pain can be considered reliable predictors of suicidal behavior
Spijker et al. 2010	Prospective epidemiologic survey	586 participants	Data were extracted from the Netherlands Mental Health Survey and Incidence Study (NEMESIS). Participants were adults (18–64 years) with a depressive spectrum disorder (≥2 depressive symptoms—according to Composite International Diagnostic Interview—CIDI)	To individuate determinants of suicidality (suicidal ideation and suicide attempts) and compare these two factors	- One item of the CIDI to evaluate suicidal ideation and suicide attempts	Suicidal ideation was influenced by different clinical features: longer duration of depression—13 months—($p = 0.01$), anhedonia ($p = 0.05$), feeling worthless ($p = 0.03$), comorbid anxiety ($p < 0.01$), previous suicidal ideation ($p < 0.001$), and use of professional care ($p = 0.05$). Anxiety, suicidal ideation, previous suicide attempts, and living alone were significantly related with suicide attempts (respectively $p = 0.01$; $p = 0.05$; $p < 0.01$; $p = 0.02$)

Table 1. *Cont.*

Reference	Study Design	Sample	Criteria	Objectives	Methods	Results
Oei et al. 1990	Cross-sectional study	46 participants	Patients (18–65 years) with depressive symptoms (according to DSM-III) were recruited from Department of Psychiatry of the University Hospital in Utrecht (The Netherlands)	To evaluate the relationship between anhedonia, suicidal behavior, and dexamethasone non suppression	- HDRS [ß] and MADRS [†] for depression - BSS [$] for suicidal ideation - CPAS [°] to assess anhedonia - STAI [%] for anxiety -Dexamethasone (DEX) Suppression	The combination of anhedonia ($p < 0.001$), suicidal ideation ($p < 0.05$), and DEX-non-suppression ($p < 0.05$) identified a subgroup of patients affected by depressive disorder who presented three positive symptoms
Fawcett et al. 1990	Prospective study	954 participants	954 subjects (mean age = 38.1) affected by major affective disorder (according to Research Diagnostic Criteria)	To identify clinical factors related to suicidal risk	- Schedules for affective disorders and schizophrenia (SADS)	3% of the subjects committed suicide; 41% of the patients died during the first year of follow-up. Suicide was associated with anhedonia ($p = 0.005$) in the 12-month follow-up
				Schizophrenic Spectrum Disorder		
Reference	**Study Design**	**Sample**	**Criteria**	**Objectives**	**Methods**	**Results**
Jahn et al. 2016	Prospective study	162 participants	Patients (mean age = 46.84) affected by schizophrenia or schizoaffective disorder (according to DSM-IV)	To examine the role of social functioning on suicidal ideation	- BPRS [↔] (24-item expanded version) to assess symptoms - RFS [Σ] and Social Closeness Scale from MPQ - SC [◦] for social role functioning - CAINS [Ł] to assess negative symptoms	Motivation and pleasure-related negative symptoms influenced the relationship between social role functioning and suicidal ideation ($p < 0.001$). A low level of suicidal ideation was associated with better social role functioning in patients who had low motivation and pleasure-related negative symptoms
Loas et al. 2009	Prospective study	150 participants	150 in- or outpatients affected by chronic schizophrenia were included from April 1991 to July 1995 and followed-up for 14 years	To compare clinical symptoms (positive and negative) of schizophrenic patients who died by suicide vs. patients who died by other causes	- BPRS [↔] - CPAS [°] to assess anhedonia - BDI [*]-II - PANSS [⊙]	Patients who died from suicide had a shorter duration of illness, and a higher level of education vs. patients died from other causes ($p = 0.02$). Negative symptoms and deficit syndrome can be considered as protective factors in schizophrenia.Anhedonia was associated with a higher risk of suicide in schizophrenia ($p = 0.19$)
				Post-Traumatic Stress Disorder		
Reference	**Study Design**	**Sample**	**Criteria**	**Objectives**	**Methods**	**Results**
Spitzer et al. 2018	Cross-sectional study	373 participants	Psychology undergraduates students (mean age = 19.9) enrolled in a public university in the southeastern United States who satisfied criterion A of PTSD (DSM-5)	To analyze the association between PTSD dimensionality (based on the six-factor anhedonia model) and acquired capability for suicide (including fearlessness of pain involved in dying and fearlessness about death)	- FOP [⋇] and FAD [∞] - DSM-5 to assess the diagnosis of PTSD - BDI [*]-II	Anhedonia cluster symptoms of PTSD was significantly related to the fearlessness of pain involved in dying ($p = 0.04$) and also fearlessness about death ($p = 0.03$)
Guina et al. 2017	Cross-sectional self-report survey	480 participants	Adults outpatients recruited at a military medical center with previous trauma	To investigate the relationships between suicide attempts and PTSD, trauma types, demographics, use of substance and benzodiazepine prescriptions	- Diagnostic and Statistical Manual of Mental Disorders -5(DSM-5) to assess the diagnosis of PTSD and to evaluate suicide attempts, previous traumatic events and abuse of alcohol or drugs	Suicide attempts were significantly associated with severity of PTSD symptom ($p < 0.0001$), childhood physical abuse ($p = 0.0002$), violent death of a loved one ($p = 0.0037$), childhood neglect ($p = 0.0099$), childhood sexual abuse ($p = 0.0246$), substance and alcohol problems (respectively $p = 0.0189$ and $p = 0.0128$), and benzodiazepine prescriptions ($p = 0.0006$)
Chen et al. 2017	Survey	36,309 participants	Participants (≥18 years) were recruited in 2012–2013. A sample of 23,936 subjects (2457 veterans and 21,479 non-veterans) had a history of at least a traumatic event	To evaluate the clinical dimension of PTSD and its relationship with suicide attempts	- Lifetime suicide attempts-AUDADIS -5 [•] to assess the diagnosis of PTSD	PTSD can be considered as a risk factor for suicide attempts and anhedonia. Anhedonia was recognized as a latent factor of PTSD and had a statistically significant effect on suicide attempts ($p < 0.05$)

Table 1. *Cont.*

Reference	Study Design	Sample	Criteria	Objectives	Methods	Results
Other Diagnoses						
Reference	**Study Design**	**Sample**	**Criteria**	**Objectives**	**Methods**	**Results**
Hawes et al. 2018	Prospective study	395 participants	Participants (≥18 years) recruited from three adult psychiatric outpatient centers in New York City between January 2016 and March 2017	To explore the different effects of chronic vs. acute anhedonia on suicidal ideation and lifetime suicide attempts	- SHAPS [#] to assess anhedonia; - BDI [*]-II to assess depression; - [%] STAI to assess anxiety; - [$] BSS and [§] C-SSRS to assess severity of suicidal ideation and history of suicide attempts;	Recent changes in the capacity to experience pleasure is better for predicting near-term suicidal ideation than is chronic anhedonia. The acutely anhedonic group reported greater severity of suicidal ideation in the past-week ($p = 0.02$) and past-month ($p = 0.04$)
Loas et al. 2016	Cross-sectional study	122 participants	122 adult patients (mean age = 44.64) recruited between 2010 and 2013 in the Psychiatric Unit of the CHU of Amiens. Subjects had a diagnosis of mood disorder ($n = 37$) or anxiety disorder ($n = 85$) according to ICD-10. Forty-one patients were admitted for a suicide attempt	To explore the association between anhedonia, alexithymia, impulsivity, suicidal ideation, recent suicide attempt, C-Reactive Protein (CRP) and serum lipid profile	- TAS-20 [¤] for alexithymia - BIS-10 [¬] for impulsivity - Subscales of the Temporal Experience Pleasure Scale for trait anhedonia - BDI [*]-II for anhedonia, depression and suicidal ideation - Blood samples for CRP and serum lipid profile (between 7:00 and 8:00 a.m. after at least 12 h of fast)	Anhedonia was related to low total cholesterol level ($p = 0.043$) and low triglycerides level ($p = 0.077$). There was an association between a low level of HDL cholesterol and high suicidal ideation ($p = 0.015$). Patients who committed suicide presented a higher level of CRP vs. patients without suicidal behavior ($p = 0.033$)
Winer et al.2014	Prospective cohort study	1529 participants	Adult inpatients (mean age: 35.55 years) of a private, not-for-profit Psychiatric structure in the southern United States recruited between April 2008 and August 2011. Participants were affected by: depressive disorder (53.0%); bipolar disorder (16.06%); anxiety disorder (4.86%)	To investigate the association between suicidality and anhedonia	- BDI [*]-II (Anhedonia, depression symptoms and suicidal ideation were assessed at admission and discharge)	Anhedonia was associated with suicidality at baseline ($p = 0.001$) and at the end of hospitalization ($p = 0.001$). Change in anhedonia from baseline to termination predicted a change in suicidality
Attempted Suicides						
Reference	**Study Design**	**Sample**	**Criteria**	**Objectives**	**Methods**	**Results**
Yaseen et al. 2016	Cross-sectional analysis	135 participants	Attempted suicides or high-risk patients admitted to an emergency room at Mount Sinai Beth Israel Hospital (New York)	To explore the association of anhedonia with suicidal ideation in attempted suicides and high-risk patients	- C-SSRS [§] to assess suicidal behavior - Items 4 and 12 of BDI [*]-II to assess anhedonia	Prior suicidal ideation was significantly associated with anhedonia, anxiety, and feelings of entrapment. Entrapment and anhedonia were independently associated also with the severity of suicidal ideation
Loas 2007	Follow-up study	106 participants	Attempted suicides admitted to the Hospital Nord d'Amiens	To predict suicide in a sample of attempted suicides	- PAS [%] to assess anhedonia	Patients who died from suicide in 6.5-year follow-up had lower anhedonia scores than those who did not die
Loas et al. 2000	Cross-sectional study	207 participants	Depressed patients ($n = 73$) and not-depressed patients ($n = 30$) admitted to the Centre Hospitalier Universitaire (CHU) Nord d'Amiens after a suicide attempt from September 1993 to August 1996 vs. 104 control subjects	To assess the effect of anhedonia on suicide and parasuicide in patients with depressive disorder and in healthy subjects	- CPAS [°] to assess anhedonia - BDI [*]-II to evaluate depression	Level of anhedonia was higher in depressed attempters vs. not-depressed attempters ($p < 0.001$) and vs. controls ($p < 0.001$). There was no difference in PAS score between healthy subjects and non-depressed attempters ($p = 0.05$)

Table 1. *Cont.*

Reference	Study Design	Sample	Criteria	Objectives	Methods	Results
Others						
Daghigh et al. 2018	Cross-sectional study	404 participants	Students of Kashan University (center of Persia)	To replicate in an Iranian sample finding of the association between anhedonia, suicide ideation and suicide attempts	- SLIPS ¥ for anhedonia - CES-D ҁ for depression - SBQ-R for suicidal behavior	Anhedonia was associated with suicidal risk ($p = 0.030$), independent of other symptoms of depression, and with suicide attempts ($p = 0.000$)
Loas et al. 2018	Cross-sectional study	557 participants	Participants were physicians	To explore the relationship between suicidality and anhedonia in a general population	- An abridged version of BDI *-13	Anhedonia was associated with both suicidal ideation ($p = 0.001$) and suicide attempts ($p = 0.001$). Anhedonia influenced the relationship between suicidal ideation and perceived burdensomeness ($p = 0.001$) and thwarted belongingness ($p = 0.001$). Suicide attempts were mediated only by thwarted belongingness. "Dissatisfaction" and "work inhibition" (two different component of anhedonia) can influence respectively suicidal ideation (lifetime- $p = 0.003$; recent- $p = 0.001$) and suicide attempts ($p = 0.001$)
Winer et al. 2016	Cross-sectional study	1122 participants	Undergraduate students (18–36 years) of a public university in the Southern United States	To assess the relationship between anhedonia, suicidal ideation, and suicide attempt	- SLIPS ¥ for anhedonia - CES-Dҁ for depression - SBQ-R ↓ for suicidal behavior	Suicidal ideation was influenced by anhedonia ($p < 0.05$). Anhedonia was not associated with suicide attempts ($p = 0.33$). Other depressive symptoms presented a correlation with suicide attempts ($p < 0.001$)
Loas et al. 1995	Cross-sectional study	224 participants	Healthy adult subjects of the Picardie (region of France) were included	To investigate the association between anhedonia, depression, and suicidal risk	- CPAS ° to assess anhedonia - BDI *-II to evaluate depression	There was no association between anhedonia and depression or anhedonia and suicidal ideation (p = ns)

§ AID: Affective Incentive Delay; • AUDADIS-5: The Alcohol Use Disorder and Associated Disabilities Interview Schedule; * BDI: Beck Depression Inventory; ˥ BIS-10: Barratt impulsivity scale; ↔ BPRS: Brief Psychiatric Rating Scale; $ BSS: Beck Scale for Suicide Ideation; Ł CAINS: Clinical Assessment Interview for Negative Symptoms; ҁ CES-D: Center of Epidemiological Studies Depression Scale; ᶾ C-SSRS: Columbia Suicide Severity Rating Scale; ° CPAS: Chapman Physical Anhedonia Scale; © DASS: Depression Anxiety Stress Scale; ∞ FAD: Fearlessness About Death; ↑ FDI-24: Future Disposition Inventory-24; ⋇ FOP: Scales for Fearlessness of Pain Involved in Dying; ß HDRS: Hamilton Rating Scale for depression; † MADRS: Montgomery–Asberg Depression Rating Scale; ~ MID: Monetary Incentive Delay; ^ MPQ-SC: Multidimensional Personality Questionnaire; € OSI: Ottawa Self-Injury Inventory-Clinical; ʘ PANSS: Positive and Negative Syndrome Scale; % PAS: Psychache Scale; Σ RFS: Role Functioning Scale; ↓ SBQ-R: Suicide Behaviors Questionnaire-Revised; # SHAPS: Snaith–Hamilton Pleasure Scale; ¥ SLIPS: Specific Loss of Interest and Pleasure Scale; Ø SSI5: Scale for Suicide Ideation; ‰ STAI: State-Trait-Anxiety Inventory; Ω TAS-20: 20-item Toronto Alexithymia Scale; ¢ TDPPS: Three-Dimensional Psychological Pain Scale.

3. Results

3.1. *Affective Disorders*

In a retrospective longitudinal study, Ballard et al. [21] studied 100 treatment-resistant patients with major depressive disorder ($n = 65$) or bipolar disorder ($n = 35$) using data from several clinical trials of ketamine to evaluate whether anhedonia can be considered a clinical correlate of suicidal thoughts. At baseline, anhedonia measured both by the Snaith–Hamilton Pleasure Scale (SHAPS) scale and the anhedonia subscale of the Beck Depression Inventory (BDI) was associated with suicidal ideation. A reduction in suicidal thoughts 230 min after the administration of ketamine was associated with a reduction in anhedonia, independently of a reduction in depressive symptoms. The change in anhedonia accounted for an additional 13% of the variance for changes in suicidal thoughts beyond the effects of depressive symptoms.

In a prospective longitudinal study of 187 adult patients with suicidal and/or non-suicidal self-injury history, Zielinsky and colleagues [30] found that anhedonia scores were higher in those with prior suicide attempts than in those with a history of non-suicidal self-injury. Depressive symptoms predicted suicidal behavior directly and also via mediation through anhedonia.

Ballard and colleagues [31] carried out a prospective study in order to identify which clinical dimensions (suicidal ideation, loss of interest, anxiety, psychomotor agitation, high-risk behavior) increase before suicidal behavior. Data were collected from the Systematic Treatment Enhancement Program for Bipolar Disorder (STEP-BD) study. All the patients included were affected by bipolar disorders. Ballard et al. compared the participants who attempted suicide or completed suicide ($n = 103$) with patients without suicidal behavior ($n = 427$). The results indicated that patients with suicidal behavior had an elevation of all symptoms, including loss of interest. Moreover, suicidal ideation and loss of interest were highly intense in the months before the suicidal behavior so that they could be considered to be a risk factor for suicidal behavior in bipolar patients.

In a cross-sectional study [12], Xie et al. explored the contribution of anhedonia and avoidance of pain as central factors in influencing the suicidal mind in a cohort of 40 depressed outpatients and 20 healthy control subjects. In the Affective Incentive Delay (AID) task, the High Suicidal Ideation (HIS) group had longer response times (RTs) under the reward condition than under the punishment condition, while the Low Suicidal Ideation (LSI) group and control groups had shorter RTs under the reward condition than under the neutral condition. The LSI group had also shorter RTs under the reward condition than under the punishment condition. Moreover, pain arousal and scores on the Beck Scale for Suicide Ideation (BSS) were negatively associated with differences in RTs between neutral and reward conditions, while pain avoidance and BSS scores were positively associated with differences in RTs between neutral and punishment conditions. Xie et al. concluded that the AID task was the best task for the detection of a hedonic approach to experience and of pain avoidance so that a reduced motivation to experience pleasure and an increased motivation to avoid pain could be considered reliable predictors of suicidal behavior.

In order to explore determinants of suicidal ideation and suicide attempts, Spijker and colleagues [32] carried out a prospective epidemiologic survey in the 2009 Netherlands Mental Health Survey and Incidence Study. They studied 586 adults with ≥ 2 depressive symptoms (according to the Composite International Diagnostic Interview-CIDI). The results indicated that the rates of suicidal ideation and suicide attempts in the observed population were, respectively, 16.6% and 3.2%. Several clinical factors seemed to be related to an increased risk of suicide: longer duration (13 months) of depression ($p = 0.01$), anhedonia ($p = 0.005$), feeling useless ($p = 0.03$), anxiety ($p < 0.01$), previous suicidal ideation ($p < 0.001$), and access to professional care ($p = 0.05$).

Oei and colleagues [34] conducted a cross-sectional study on 46 patients with depressive symptoms recruited from the Department of Psychiatry at the University Hospital in Utrecht (Netherlands). Using several measures of both suicidal ideation and anhedonia, they found that anhedonia scores were positively associated with suicidal ideation scores. Of the anhedonic patients, 71% had suicidal ideation.

Fawcett and colleagues [16] investigated the possible role of anhedonia in suicidal behavior as a time-related predictor of suicide in major affective disorder, together with other clinical features. In this prospective study of 954 patients affected by major affective disorder, among the nine clinical features studied, the following were correlated with the risk of dying by suicide within 13 months from baseline: anhedonia, panic attacks, severe anxiety, diminished concentration, moderate alcohol abuse, and global insomnia. Long-term suicides (after 13 months from the baseline) were associated with hopelessness and prior suicidal ideation.

3.2. *Schizophrenic Spectrum Disorders*

Jahn and colleagues [35] studied 162 patients affected by schizophrenia or schizoaffective disorder and found that motivation and pleasure scores as rated by the Clinical Assessment Interview for negative symptoms (CAINS) were not directly associated with recent suicidal ideation. However, motivation and pleasure-related scores moderated the relationship between social role functioning and suicide ideation.

Loas and colleagues [18] investigated the protective nature of negative symptoms by comparing positive and negative symptoms in schizophrenic patients who died by suicide with non-suicidal schizophrenic patients in a prospective study of 150 patients with chronic schizophrenia. They found out that negative symptoms and the deficit syndrome [defined as a subgroup of schizophrenic patients with at least two enduring, primary or idiopathic, negative symptoms (e.g., poverty of speech, restricted affect, diminished emotional range, interests, sense of purpose or social drive) as assessed by the Positive and Negative Syndrome Scale (PANSS) and the subscale of the Brief Psychiatric Rating Scale (BPRS)] were associated with a lower risk of suicide in these patients. The incidence of the deficit syndrome in the suicides (0%) was lower than the incidence in non-suicidal patients (23.5%).

3.3. *Post-Traumatic Stress Disorder (PTSD)*

Spitzer and colleagues [36] conducted a cross-sectional study in a sample of 373 trauma-exposed psychology undergraduate students to examine the relationship between acquired capability for suicide (ACS) and DSM–5 PTSD symptom clusters. Whereas most PTSD symptom clusters had a negative association with ACS, the anhedonia cluster was positively related to both facets of ACS: fearlessness of the pain involved in dying (FOP) and fearlessness about death (FAD). The relationship between anhedonia and ACS may explain the decreased fear of death and the higher levels of pain tolerance that contribute to lethal suicidal behavior in PTSD patients.

Guina and colleagues [37] studied 480 adults from military medical centers with previous trauma. The PTSD symptoms most strongly associated with suicide attempts were anhedonia, negative beliefs, and recklessness. Suicide attempts were also significantly associated with worse total PTSD symptom severity, childhood physical abuse, the violent death of a loved one, childhood neglect, childhood sexual abuse, substance, alcohol problem, and benzodiazepine prescriptions.

Chen and colleagues [38] analyzed the data from 36,309 U.S. adults (≥18 years) from the National Epidemiologic Survey on Alcohol and Related Conditions-III and found that both PTSD and anhedonia were associated with attempting suicide.

3.4. *Other Diagnoses*

Hawes et al. [50] explored the different effects of chronic vs. acute anhedonia on suicidal ideation and lifetime suicide attempt history in a prospective study of 395 adult psychiatric outpatient centers in New York City between January 2016 and March 2017. They found out that recent changes in the capacity to experience pleasure was more powerful in predicting near-term suicidal ideation than was chronic anhedonia.

Winer et al. [11] investigated the association between suicidal ideation and anhedonia in a prospective cohort study of 1529 adult psychiatric inpatients with various diagnoses from DSM-IV using the Beck Depression Inventory II. Anhedonia was associated with suicidal ideation at baseline and at the termination of the study. Changes in anhedonia from baseline to termination predicted a change in suicidal ideation, and anhedonia was a predictor of suicidal ideation regardless of cognitive/affective symptoms of depression.

Loas and colleagues [40] studied 122 psychiatric patients hospitalized in the psychiatric unit of the CHU of Amiens between 2010 and 2013. They found that suicidal ideation as measured by the Beck Depression Inventory was associated with anticipatory anhedonia as measured by the Physical Anhedonia Scale (PAS) (but not PAS consummatory anhedonia) and with anhedonia as measured by the BDI, but not with scores on the Temporal Experience of Pleasure Scale (TEPS).

3.5. *Attempted Suicides*

Yaseen and colleagues [39] conducted a cross-sectional study to evaluate the relationship between suicidal behavior and anhedonia, anxiety, feelings of being trapped, and frightened attachment in 135 adults admitted to the Emergency Room of the Mount Sinai Beth Israel Hospital (New York) for a suicide attempt or with high suicidal risk. All participants reported suicidal ideation in the past month. Suicidal behavior was assessed with the Columbia Suicide-Severity Rating Scale (C-SSRS). The results showed that prior suicidal ideation was significantly associated with anhedonia, anxiety, and feelings of entrapment. Entrapment and anhedonia were independently associated also with the severity of suicidal ideation.

Loas and colleagues [33] examined the correlation between anhedonia and suicide risk in a cross-sectional study of 106 attempted suicides (30 non-depressed and 73 depressed) and 104 normal controls. The participants were evaluated using the PAS and BDI. Depressed attempters were significantly more anhedonic than controls and non-depressed attempters, while no statistically significant difference on the PAS score emerged between healthy subjects and non-depressed attempters.

Loas [13] followed-up for 6.5 years 106 patients who attempted suicide and who were admitted to the Hospital Nord d'Amiens (between September 1993 and August 1996). During the follow-up period, 6.7% of the patients died by suicide. The patients who completed suicide had a significantly lower score on the PAS as compared to the non-suicide group. Thus, this prospective cohort study indicated that a low level of anhedonia was associated with death from suicide.

3.6. *Others*

In a cross-sectional study, Daghigh et al. [51] tried to replicate findings of the association between anhedonia, suicide ideation ad suicide attempts [19] in an Iranian sample of 404 students at Kashan University (in the center of Iran). In addition to the surprising finding that the Iranian students were more anhedonic than were the American students (more than double), the authors reported that anhedonia was associated with suicidal risk, independently of other symptoms of depression, and also with suicide attempts.

Loas and colleagues [41] found that anhedonia was related to both suicidal ideation and suicide attempts in a population of 557 physicians. Anhedonia mediated the relationship between suicidal ideation and perceived burdensomeness and thwarted belongingness, variables relevant to Joiner's Interpersonal Theory of Suicide [44]. Two different features of anhedonia (lack of satisfaction and loss of energy) were associated with suicidal behavior. Lack of satisfaction had an impact on suicidal ideation, while loss of energy had an impact on suicide attempts.

In a cross-sectional study, Winer and colleagues [19] studied a population of 1122 undergraduate students at a public university in the southern United States and found that anhedonia was associated with suicidal ideation, but not with suicide attempts.

A cross-sectional study by Loas [42] investigated the association between anhedonia, depression, and suicidal behavior in 224 healthy patients (using the PAS and the BDI) and found that anhedonia scores were not associated with depression scores or current suicidal ideation.

4. Discussion

The present review of the literature suggested that findings on anhedonia and suicidal behavior are inconsistent, and it is difficult to propose a theoretical framework that could explain all the research findings. Some studies in this review reported a positive association between the presence of anhedonia and suicidal behavior (high anhedonia scores were associated with suicidal behavior), regardless of the diagnosis of the patients. Other studies found a negative association (low anhedonia scores were associated with suicidal behavior), and a few studies reported no association. The included studies, organized by type of disorder, are summarized in Table 1.

The role of psychiatric diagnosis in the association of anhedonia with suicidal behavior appears to be important. The most consistent association was found for patients with affective disorders (7 of 7 studies reported a significant positive association) and for patients with PTSD (3 of 3 studies reported a positive association). For the two studies of patients with schizophrenia, one found no association (Jahn et al. [35]) and the other found a negative association (Loas et al. [18]). For patients who had attempted suicide (and who were undiagnosed), one study found a positive association [39], one a positive association but only for depressed attempters [33], and one found a negative association [13].

The results are also made complex by the type of suicidal risk studied. Winer et al. [19] reported a positive association between anhedonia and suicidal ideation but not for anhedonia and attempted suicide. A meta-analysis by Ducasse and colleagues [45] confirmed that anhedonia scores are higher among patients with than without current suicidal ideation. That meta-analysis evaluated the results of 15 case-control studies, which included 7347 participants (mean age = 30 yrs.) and compared the results for subjects with current suicidal ideation ($n = 657$) vs. subjects without current suicidal ideation ($n = 6690$). Patients affected by different psychiatric disorders (depression; schizophrenia; personality disorders; substance abuse disorder) and subjects without psychiatric diagnosis were included. The results demonstrated that the group with current suicidal ideation presented higher level of anhedonia vs. the group without suicidal ideation ($p < 0.001$; CI = 0.37–0.79). Moreover, the subgroup analysis conducted for a group of patients with homogenous depression scale scores showed that the association between anhedonia and suicidal ideation was not influenced by depression. Those results suggested that people with suicidal ideation had higher level of anhedonia, independently of the presence of depression. For completed suicides, Ballard et al. [31] reported a positive association, whereas Loas et al. [13] reported a negative association. The results may also be made complex by the high incidence of anhedonia in psychiatric patients, as high as 50% as reported in a study from Silverstone [43].

Why is there an association between suicide and anhedonia? The tendency to avoid emotions experienced as unpleasant can be a maladaptive coping strategy [46], and suicidal ideation could also be an avoidance strategy [47,48]. However, avoiding experiences leads to the attenuation of pleasant emotions and the exacerbation of unpleasant ones [49]. The association between current suicidal ideation and anhedonia may also be related to the interaction between the social component of anhedonia (loss of interest in people) and thwarted belongingness, as described by Joiner's Interpersonal Theory of Suicide [44].

This review had several limitations. The studies differed in sample size, study design, and methodology. There were several different measures of anhedonia used in the various studies, and not all of them may be reliable, valid, and equivalent measures. Furthermore, some of the studies did not accurately diagnose the patients, and we have seen in the present review that psychiatric diagnosis may affect the results of the research. Finally, we respected the choice of some authors to use the generic term of "suicidality" [12,32,39,41] to indicate different aspects of the issue, even if we believe that it could be a source of misunderstanding. A more specific term, such as "suicidal risk," is preferable.

5. Conclusions

The relationship between anhedonia and suicidal behavior is complex. The majority of studies included in our review reported a positive correlation between anhedonia and suicidal risk. The most consistent positive association was found for patients with affective disorders and for patients with PTSD. The positive association was most consistent for suicidal ideation, but less consistent for attempted suicide and completed suicide. However, our review suggests that the assessment of anhedonia may be useful in the evaluation of suicidal risk in depressed patients.

Author Contributions: The main contributions of the individual authors are illustrated as follows: conceptualization, M.P. and L.B.; methodology, L.B.; validation, D.L., L.B. and A.F.; formal analysis, D.L.; investigation, L.B. and F.G.; resources, G.F.; data curation, L.B.; writing—original draft preparation, L.B. and F.G.; writing—review and editing, D.L.; visualization, A.N.; supervision, M.P.; project administration, L.B.

References

1. World Health Organization. *Preventing Suicide: A Global Imperative*; WHO Press: Geneva, Switzerland, 2014; ISBN 978-924-156-477-9.
2. Jimenez-Trevino, L.; Saiz, P.A.; Corcoran, P.; Garcia-Portilla, M.P.; Buron, P.; Garrido, M.; Bobes, J. The incidence of hospital-treated attempted suicide in Oviedo, Spain. *Crisis* **2012**, *33*, 46–53. [CrossRef] [PubMed]
3. Pompili, M.; Gonda, X.; Serafini, G.; Innamorati, M.; Sher, L.; Amore, M.; Rihmer, Z.; Girardi, P. Epidemiology of suicide in bipolar disorders: A systematic review of the literature. *Bipolar Disord.* **2013**, *15*, 457–490. [CrossRef] [PubMed]
4. Associate Minister of Health. *The New Zealand Suicide Prevention Strategy 2006–2016*; Ministry of Health: Wellington, New Zealand, 2006; ISBN 047-829-995-8.
5. White, J. *Suicide-Related Research in Canada: A Descriptive Overview*; A Background Paper Prepared for the Workshop on Suicide-Related Research; Centre for Suicide Prevention and Centre for Research and Intervention on Suicide and Euthanasia: Montreal, QC, Canada, 2003.
6. World Health Organization. Depression/Suicide. 2002. Available online: http://www.int/health_topics/suicide/en/ (accessed on 12 February 2019).
7. Klonsky, E.D.; May, A.M. Differentiating suicide attempters from suicide ideators: A critical frontier for suicidology research. *Suicide Life Threat. Behav.* **2014**, *44*, 1–5. [CrossRef] [PubMed]
8. Sadock, B.J.; Sadock, V.A.; Ruiz, P. *Kaplan & Sadock's Comprehensive Textbook of Psychiatry*, 10th ed.; Lippincott Williams & Wilkins (LWW): Philadelphia, PA, USA, 2017; ISBN 978-145-110-047-1.
9. Winer, E.S.; Veilleux, J.C.; Ginger, E.J. Development and validation of the specific loss of interest and pleasure scale (SLIPS). *J. Affect. Disord.* **2014**, *152*, 193–201. [CrossRef] [PubMed]
10. Nock, M.K.; Kazdin, A.E. Examination of affective, cognitive, and behavioral factors and suicide-related outcomes in children and young adolescents. *J. Clin. Child Adolesc. Psychol.* **2002**, *31*, 48–58. [CrossRef] [PubMed]
11. Winer, E.S.; Nadorff, M.R.; Ellis, T.E.; Allen, J.G.; Herrera, S.; Salem, T. Anhedonia predicts suicidal ideation in a large psychiatric inpatient sample. *Psychiatry Res.* **2014**, *218*, 124–128. [CrossRef] [PubMed]
12. Xie, W.; Li, H.; Luo, X.; Fu, R.; Ying, X.; Wang, N.; Shi, C. Anhedonia and pain avoidance in the suicidal mind: Behavioral evidence for motivational manifestations of suicidal ideation in patients with major depressive disorder. *J. Clin. Psychol.* **2014**, *70*, 681–692. [CrossRef]
13. Loas, G. Anhedonia and suicide: A 6.5-yr follow-up study of patients hospitalised for a suicide attempt. *Psychol. Rep.* **2007**, *100*, 183–190. [CrossRef]
14. Watson, C.G.; Kucala, T. Anhedonia and death. *Psychol. Rep.* **1978**, *43*, 1120–1122. [CrossRef]
15. Fawcett, J.; Clark, D.C.; Busch, K. Assessing and treating the patient at risk for suicide. *Psychiatr. Ann.* **1993**, *23*, 244–255. [CrossRef]
16. Fawcett, J.; Scheftner, W.A.; Fogg, L.; Clark, D.C.; Young, M.A.; Hedeker, D.; Gibbons, R. Time-related predictors of suicide in major affective disorder. *Am. J. Psychiatry* **1990**, *147*, 1189–1194. [CrossRef] [PubMed]
17. Hall, R.C.; Platt, D.E.; Hall, R.C.W. Suicide risk assessment: A review of risk factors for suicide in 100 patients who made severe suicide attempts. Evaluation of suicide risk in a time of managed care. *Psychosomatics* **1999**, *40*, 18–27. [CrossRef]

18. Loas, G.; Azi, A.; Noisette, C.; Legrand, A.; Yon, V. Fourteen-year prospective follow-up study of positive and negative symptoms in chronic schizophrenic patients dying from suicide compared to other causes of death. *Psychopathology* **2009**, *42*, 185–189. [CrossRef] [PubMed]
19. Winer, E.S.; Drapeau, C.W.; Veilleux, J.C.; Nadorff, M.R. The Association between Anhedonia, Suicidal Ideation, and Suicide Attempts in a Large Student Sample. *Arch. Suicide Res.* **2016**, *20*, 265–272. [CrossRef] [PubMed]
20. Reisch, T.; Seifritz, E.; Esposito, F.; Wiest, R.; Valach, L.; Michel, K. An fMRI study on mental pain and suicidal behavior. *J. Affect. Disord.* **2010**, *126*, 321–325. [CrossRef] [PubMed]
21. Ballard, E.D.; Wills, K.; Lally, N.; Richards, E.M.; Luckenbaugh, D.A.; Walls, T.; Zarate, C.A., Jr. Anhedonia as a clinical correlate of suicidal thoughts in clinical ketamine trials. *J. Affect. Disord.* **2017**, *218*, 195–200. [CrossRef] [PubMed]
22. Loas, G. Anhedonia and Risk of Suicide: An Overview. In *Anhedonia: A Comprehensive Handbook Volume II: 247 Neuropsychiatric and Physical Disorder*; Ritsner, M.S., Ed.; Springer Science + Business Media: Dordrecht, The Netherlands, 2014.
23. Fawcett, J.; Busch, K.A.; Jacobs, D.; Kravitz, H.M.; Fogg, L. Suicide: A four-pathway clinical-biochemical model. *Ann. N. Y. Acad. Sci.* **1997**, *836*, 288–301. [CrossRef] [PubMed]
24. Gard, D.E.; Germans, M.G.; Kring, A.M.; John, O.P. Anticipatory and consummatory components of the experience of pleasure: a scale development study. *J. Res. Personal.* **2006**, *40*, 1086–1102. [CrossRef]
25. Klein, D.F. Depression and anhedonia. In *Anhedonia and Affect Deficit States*; Clark, D.C., Fawcett, J., Eds.; PMA Publishing Corporation: New York, NY, USA, 1987; pp. 1–14.
26. Cipriani, A.; Hawton, K.; Stockton, S.; Geddes, J.R. Lithium in the prevention of suicide in mood disorders: Updated systematic review and meta-analysis. *BMJ* **2013**, *27*, f3646. [CrossRef]
27. Zalsman, G.; Hawton, K.; Wasserman, D.; van Heeringen, K.; Arensman, E.; Sarchiapone, M.; Carli, V.; Höschl, C.; Barzilay, R.; Balazs, J.; et al. Suicide prevention strategies revisited: 10-year systematic review. *Lancet Psychiatry* **2016**, *3*, 646–659. [CrossRef]
28. Hennen, J.; Baldessarini, R.J. Suicidalriskduring treatment with clozapine: A meta-analysis. *Schizophr. Res.* **2005**, *73*, 139–145. [CrossRef]
29. Kessler, R.C.; Berglund, P.; Borges, G.; Nock, M.; Wang, P.S. Trends in suicide ideation, plans, gestures, and attempts in the United States, 1990–1992 to 2001–2003. *JAMA* **2005**, *293*, 2487–2495. [CrossRef]
30. Zielinski, M.J.; Veilleux, J.C.; Winer, E.S.; Nadorff, M.R. A short-term longitudinal examination of the relations between depression, anhedonia, and self-injurious thoughts and behaviors in adults with a history of self-injury. *Compr. Psychiatry* **2017**, *73*, 187–195. [CrossRef]
31. Ballard, E.D.; VandeVoort, J.L.; Luckenbaugh, D.A.; Machado-Vieira, R.; Tohen, M.; Zarate, C.A. Acute risk factors for suicide attempts and death: Prospective findings from the STEP-BD study. *Bipolar Disord.* **2016**, *18*, 363–372. [CrossRef]
32. Spijker, J.; de Graaf, R.; Ten Have, M.; Nolen, W.A.; Speckens, A. Predictors of suicidality in depressive spectrum disorders in the general population: Results of the Netherlands MentalHealth Survey and Incidence Study. *Soc. Psychiatry Psychiatr. Epidemiol.* **2010**, *45*, 513–521. [CrossRef]
33. Loas, G.; Perot, J.M.; Chignague, J.F.; Trespalacios, H.; Delahousse, J. Parasuicide, anhedonia, and depression. *Compr. Psychiatry* **2000**, *41*, 369–372. [CrossRef]
34. Oei, T.I.; Verhoeven, W.M.; Westenberg, H.G.; Zwart, F.M.; van Ree, J.M. Anhedonia, suicide ideation and dexamethasone nonsuppression in depressed patients. *J. Psychiatr. Res.* **1990**, *24*, 25–35. [CrossRef]
35. Jahn, D.R.; Bennett, M.E.; Park, S.G.; Gur, R.E.; Horan, W.P.; Kring, A.M.; Blanchard, J.J. The interactive effects of negative symptoms and social role functioning on suicide ideation in individuals with schizophrenia. *Schizophr. Res.* **2016**, *170*, 271–277. [CrossRef]
36. Spitzer, E.G.; Zuromski, K.L.; Davis, M.T.; Witte, T.K.; Weathers, F. Posttraumatic Stress Disorder Symptom Clusters and Acquired Capability for Suicide: A Reexamination Using DSM-5 Criteria. *Suicide Life Threat. Behav.* **2018**, *48*, 105–115. [CrossRef]
37. Guina, J.; Nahhas, R.W.; Mata, N.; Farnsworth, S. Which Posttraumatic Stress Disorder Symptoms, Trauma Types, and Substances Correlate with Suicide Attempts in Trauma Survivors? *Prim. Care Companion CNS Disord.* **2017**, *19*. [CrossRef]

38. Chen, C.M.; Yoon, Y.H.; Harford, T.C.; Grant, B.F. Dimensionality of DSM-5 posttraumatic stress disorder and its association with suicide attempts: Results from the National Epidemiologic Survey on Alcohol and Related Conditions-III. *Soc. Psychiatry Psychiatr. Epidemiol.* **2017**, *52*, 715–725. [CrossRef] [PubMed]
39. Yaseen, Z.S.; Galynker, I.I.; Briggs, J.; Freed, R.D.; Gabbay, V. Functional domains as correlates of suicidality among psychiatric inpatients. *J. Affect. Disord.* **2016**, *203*, 77–83. [CrossRef] [PubMed]
40. Loas, G.; Dalleau, E.; Lecointe, H.; Yon, V. Relationships between anhedonia, alexithymia, impulsivity, suicidal ideation, recent suicide attempt, C-reactive protein and serum lipid levels among 122 inpatients with mood or anxious disorders. *Psychiatry Res.* **2016**, *246*, 296–302. [CrossRef] [PubMed]
41. Loas, G.; Lefebvre, G.; Rotsaert, M.; Englert, Y. Relationships between anhedonia, suicidal ideation and suicide attempts in a large sample of physicians. *PLoS ONE* **2018**, *13*, e0193619. [CrossRef] [PubMed]
42. Loas, G.; Fremaux, D.; Gayant, C.; Boyer, P. Anhedonia, depression, and suicidal ideation. *Percept. Mot. Ski.* **1995**, *80*, 978. [CrossRef] [PubMed]
43. Silverstone, P. Is anhedonia a good measure of depression? *Acta Psychiatr. Scand.* **1991**, *83*, 249–250. [CrossRef] [PubMed]
44. Van Orden, K.A.; Witte, T.K.; Cukrowicz, K.C.; Braithwaite, S.; Selby, E.A.; Joiner, T.E., Jr. The interpersonal theory of suicide. *Psychol. Rev.* **2010**, *117*, 575–600. [CrossRef] [PubMed]
45. Ducasse, D.; Loas, G.; Dassa, D.; Gramaglia, C.; Zeppegno, P.; Guillaume, S.; Olié, E.; Courtet, P. Anhedonia is associated with suicidal ideation independently of depression: A meta-analysis. *Depress. Anxiety* **2018**, *35*, 382–392. [CrossRef]
46. Hayes, S.C.; Wilson, K.G.; Gifford, E.V.; Follette, V.M.; Strosahl, K. Experimental avoidance and behavioral disorders: A functional dimensional approach to diagnosis and treatment. *J. Consult. Clin. Psychol.* **1996**, *64*, 1152–1168. [CrossRef]
47. Harris, R. *Passez à l'ACT: Pratique de la Thérapie D'acceptation et D'engagement*, 2nd ed.; De Boeck Supérieur: Louvain-la-Neuve, Belgium, 2017; ISBN 978-280-730-849-7.
48. Shneidman, E.S. Suicide as psychache. *J. Nerv. Ment. Dis.* **1993**, *181*, 145–147. [CrossRef]
49. Machell, K.A.; Goodman, F.R.; Kashdan, T.B. Experiential avoidance and well-being: A daily diary analysis. *Cogn. Emot.* **2015**, *29*, 351–359. [CrossRef] [PubMed]
50. Hawes, M.; Galynker, I.; Barzilay, S.; Yaseen, Z.S. Anhedonia and suicidal thoughts and behaviors in psychiatric outpatients: The role of acuity. *Depress. Anxiety* **2018**, *35*, 1218–1227. [CrossRef] [PubMed]
51. Daghigh, A.; Daghigh, V.; Niazi, M.; Nadorff, M.R. The association between anhedonia, suicide ideation, and suicide attempts: A replication in a Persian student sample. *Suicide Life Threat. Behav.* **2018**, *49*, 678–683. [CrossRef] [PubMed]

8

Transcranial Direct Current Stimulation (tDCS): A Promising Treatment for Major Depressive Disorder?

Djamila Bennabi * and Emmanuel Haffen

Department of Clinical Psychiatry, CIC-1431 INSERM, CHU de Besançon, EA Neurosciences, University Bourgogne Franche-Comte, FondaMental Foundation, 94000 Creteil, France; emmanuel.haffen@univ-fcomte.fr

* Correspondence: djamila.bennabi@univ-fcomte.fr;

Abstract: Background: Transcranial direct current stimulation (tDCS) opens new perspectives in the treatment of major depressive disorder (MDD), because of its ability to modulate cortical excitability and induce long-lasting effects. The aim of this review is to summarize the current status of knowledge regarding tDCS application in MDD. **Methods:** In this review, we searched for articles published in PubMed/MEDLINE from the earliest available date to February 2018 that explored clinical and cognitive effects of tDCS in MDD. **Results:** Despite differences in design and stimulation parameters, the examined studies indicated beneficial effects of tDCS for MDD. These preliminary results, the non-invasiveness of tDCS, and its good tolerability support the need for further research on this technique. **Conclusions**: tDCS constitutes a promising therapeutic alternative for patients with MDD, but its place in the therapeutic armamentarium remains to be determined.

Keywords: transcranial direct current stimulation; depression; cognition

---

1. Introduction

Major depressive disorder (MDD) is a widespread psychiatric disease characterized by a high risk of morbidity and mortality and a high level of comorbidity with several psychiatric and non-psychiatric disorders [1]. Epidemiological surveys have repeatedly indicated a high lifetime prevalence of this illness, amounting to 6.7% of the population worldwide [2]. The costs of MDD to society, in terms of personal and familial suffering and health care consumption, are high [3,4]. Despite the progress in pharmacopoeia and in psychological therapies, clinicians involved in the management of MDD are regularly faced with clinical situations marked by treatment resistance. About 30% of depressed patients fail to experience significant clinical benefits from currently available treatments [5,6], leading to a chronically deteriorating course of the illness. Consequences of the illness and limitations of the usual pharmacological and psychological strategies highlight the necessity to develop alternative therapeutic options.

Brain stimulation therapies have emerged as relevant alternative strategies, on the basis of emerging knowledge about specific brain areas involved in psychiatric diseases. Among these techniques, transcranial direct current stimulation (tDCS) appears to hold particular promise because of its cost, ease of use, and favorable tolerability profile [7]. tDCS was used from the 1960s to generate modifications of cortical excitability in preclinical studies and as a therapeutic tool for MDD. More recently, this technique has gained renewed interest as a practical tool for the modulation of cortical excitability and the treatment of psychiatric disorders [7,8]. tDCS relies on the application of a weak direct current of 1–2 mA directly to the scalp through electrodes to induce regional changes in cortical excitability that can last up to a few hours after stimulation [9]. Sustainable effects seem to be mediated by bidirectional modifications of postsynaptic connections similar to long-term potentiation and depression, occurring through NMDA-dependent mechanisms [10,11]. Because of the implication of pathological alterations of neuroplasticity in psychiatric disorders, tDCS appears to be a promising therapeutic alternative to modify such pathological plasticity [12]. Beneficial effects of tDCS have been reported in the treatment of psychiatric (mainly depression and schizophrenia) and neurological diseases, as well as in the rehabilitation of cognitive, motor, and sensory functions after a stroke [8,13].

In this review, we summarize data obtained from trials with the aim of assessing the effectiveness of tDCS as a putative treatment option for MDD.

1.1. Method

To identify studies reporting the effects of tDCS on depression and cognition in MDD, two authors (E.H. and D.B.) searched the Pub-med database following PRISMA recommendations [14]. The identification of articles was based on the following keywords: "depression", "transcranial direct current stimulation".

Inclusion criteria for this review were: (a) publication in English; (b) inclusion of depressed patients treated with tDCS; (c) meta-analysis, randomized controlled studies (RCTs) and open-label trials; (d) assessment of depressive symptoms and/or cognition. Working independently and in duplicate, the two reviewers examined all titles and abstracts, obtained full texts of potentially relevant papers, and read the papers to determine whether they met the inclusion criteria. Of the 381 initial references, 67 papers were retained. We excluded seven studies exploring the effects of tDCS in healthy subjects, one review, and one protocol. Thus, we obtained data from 58 articles that met our eligibility criteria.

1.2. Technical and Safety Aspects of Transcranial Direct Current Stimulation

During tDCS sessions, a constant direct current of low intensity (generally 1–2 mA) is passed across the brain via electrodes wrapped in an electrode gel or saline-soaked sponge pockets. [8]. Wide variations in the amount of current delivered can be observed according to the stimulation parameters applied (i.e., position and size of the electrodes, current intensity, duration, frequency, and number of sessions). In the majority of protocols, the currents ranged from 0.5 to 2 mA and were delivered for 5–30 min via electrodes of 25–35 cm, generating current densities of 0.28–0.8 mA/cm^2. The placement of the electrodes is typically based on the 10–20 electrode placement system to locate the area of interest. More recent studies suggest the use of an initial magnetic resonance imaging (MRI) scan to refine the position of the electrode, taking into account the inter-individual variability [15]. From a neurobiological standpoint, tDCS is considered a technique of neuromodulation, given that it does not directly induce action potentials, unlike transcranial magnetic stimulation. The polarity of the stimulation determines the type of effect; anodal stimulation induces a depolarization of the neuronal membranes and an increase of the spontaneous neuronal firing rate, whereas cathodal stimulation leads to neuronal hyperpolarization and inhibition [16,17]. Depending on the duration and intensity of the stimulation, it has been shown that the modulation of electrophysiological properties is directly measurable in healthy volunteers and could last up to 90 min after stopping the stimulation [9].

tDCS may induce mild to moderate side effects, including light itching beneath the electrodes, mild headache, tingling, burning sensations, and discomfort. Skin irritation and lesions under the electrodes have also been reported, as well as some cases of mood switching [18,19].

1.3. Effects of tDCS on Symptoms

The rationale for using tDCS in this indication is based on historical observations of hypometabolism of the left dorsolateral prefrontal cortex (dlPFC) associated with right prefrontal hyperfunction in MDD and dysfunction of brain plasticity, characterized by an alteration of long-term potentiation and depression [20,21]. In the majority of the protocols, the currents used were 1 or 2 mA and were applied for 30 min via two large conductive electrodes (32–35 cm^2) soaked with a saline solution. The anode was typically placed over the left dlPFC, and the cathode over the contralateral supraorbital area, corresponding to F3 and FP2 according to the international 10–20 EEG system [22]. Transcranial direct current stimulation was proposed either alone or as an add-on treatment to psychotropic medication or cognitive training programs.

Following the seminal work of Fregni et al. [23] which produced positive results on the efficacy of five sessions of anodal tDCS applied over the left dlPFC (1 mA, 10 min) in ten patients with MDD, a series of controlled and open-label studies have been published. Subsequently, two RCTs conducted by Boggio et al. [24,25] have replicated these results. The authors observed an average reduction of 40.4% in the Hamilton Depression Rating Scale (HDRS) score after anodal tDCS (2 mA, 20 min) versus 10.4% after placebo stimulation in 40 patients with mild to moderate MDD. In 2010, Loo et al. [26] showed no superior antidepressant efficacy of ten sessions of tDCS (1 mA, 20 min) versus placebo in 40 patients with MDD. However, in a second study, these authors demonstrated a greater decrease in the Hamilton Depression Rating Scale (HDRS scores in 64 unipolar and bipolar depressed patients after 15 sessions of anodal tDCS of the left dlPFC (2 mA, 20 min) (28.4%) versus placebo (15.9%) [27]. Rigonatti et al. [28] compared the effect of fluoxetine and ten tDCS sessions (2 mA, 20 min) in 42 depressed patients, and noted a similar improvement in depressive symptoms following brain stimulation and pharmacological treatment, with an earlier antidepressant action in the tDCS group. In the field of treatment-resistant depression, three RCTs were conducted and did not show any significant difference between active stimulation and placebo [29–31]. Regarding post-stroke depression, Valiengo et al. [32] studied the effects after active versus sham stimulation in 45 patients and reported a higher response rate with active stimulation (37.5% and 20.8%, respectively) and higher remission rates (4.1% and 0%, respectively).

In this context, in 2013, a larger study was conducted involving 120 unipolar depressed patients, which compared tDCS versus a pharmacological treatment (sertraline) and versus tDCS plus sertraline. The results showed a greater reduction in Montgomery–Asberg Depression Rating Scale scores in patients receiving the combined intervention (tDCS + sertraline) versus those receiving sertraline alone (mean difference 8.5 points), tDCS alone (mean difference 5.9 points), or placebo (mean difference 11.5 points) [33]. More recently, these authors published the results of a non-inferiority trial involving 245 depressed patients and compared active tDCS (2 mA, 30 min) versus a pharmacological treatment (escitalopram) and versus placebo. They concluded that escitalopram was significantly superior to tDCS [34]. Moreover, a large-scale RCT involving 84 unipolar and 36 bipolar depressed patients reported comparable effects of active (2.5 mA, 30 min, 20 sessions over four weeks) and sham tDCS applied over the left dlPFC, suggesting that the low level of stimulation delivered in sham conditions may have been biologically active [35].

Studies evaluating the effectiveness of tDCS in a maintenance therapy for relapse prevention have shown that the reduction in treatment frequency from two to one week or a high level of pre-treatment resistance was associated with a greater rate of relapse [36,37].

Several meta-analyses pooling available data about the antidepressant efficacy of tDCS have yielded contradictory results. Kalu et al. [38] showed a higher efficacy of active tDCS versus placebo, as evidenced by a greater reduction in severity scores on depression scales. Berlim et al. [39] did not find any significant difference between active tDCS and placebo in response rates (23.3% versus 12.4%, respectively, p = 0.11) and remission (12.2% versus 5.4%, respectively, p = 0.22). Shiozawa et al. [40] included seven controlled trials in their meta-analysis and showed a superiority of active tDCS over placebo in terms of clinical response and remission, which was confirmed by Meron et al. [41] in a meta-analysis of 10 RCTs. In a meta-analysis of individual data from 289 patients, Brunoni et al. [42] demonstrated the superiority of active tDCS compared to placebo in terms of alleviation of depressive symptoms, with a response rate of 33.3% versus 19 %, respectively, and a remission rate of 23.1 versus 12.7%, respectively. The level of response was correlated with various parameters, namely, the number of sessions and the amount of energy delivered, but was inversely associated with the level of antidepressant resistance. Other variables, such as the severity of the current depressive episode, the presence of bipolar disorder, female gender, or treatment with sertraline, as well as pre-treatment motor retardation or better verbal fluency, were also identified as potential predictors of a positive response [42–45]. From a neurobiological point of view, 5-HTTLPR polymorphism has shown a predictive property, while brain-derived neurotrophic factor, cytokine levels, neurotrophins 3 and 4, nerve growth factor, and glial cell line-derived neurotropic factor have failed to predict the clinical response [46–49].

1.4. *Effects of tDCS on Cognition*

Current evidence suggests that tDCS may have an impact on some cognitive functions in healthy volunteers, such as working memory, attentional performance, procedural learning, and emotional information processing [50]. In MDD, although most studies reported an improvement in at least some cognitive functions, suggesting a potential pro-cognitive role of tDCS, no firm conclusions could be drawn. To date, the improvement of attention and working memory has been reported after 1 [27,51,52], 5 [53], and 10 [25] anodal tDCS sessions applied over the left DLPFC. Positive results have also been observed in other cognitive domains, such as cognitive control [54,55], processing speed [56], or emotion recognition [57]. Bifrontal tDCS has been shown to promote more accurate and faster responses to the n-back task, exploring working memory, and to prevent procedural learning during the probabilistic classification learning task in depressive states [51]. Moreover, a few clinical cases of improvement in cognitive performances after treatment with tDCS have been reported in the context of treatment-resistant depression or post-traumatic depression [29,58]. However, several RCTs applying a set of standardized cognitive tests did not record tDCS-related changes with offline stimulations, suggesting that repeated sessions have no cumulative effects [26,31,59]. Beyond the variability in the stimulations parameters (i.e., site of stimulation or use of off- or online sessions) and the impact of inter- and intraindividual differences, in most of the studies it is difficult to differentiate the "pure" effects of cognitive improvement of tDCS from a "collateral" effect relied on a cognitive improvement due to the alleviation of depression [60].

1.5. *Parameters Influencing Clinical Outcomes*

Multiple factors are likely to modulate the therapeutic effects of tDCS. Among them, the stimulation parameters and clinical characteristics of the population are key contributors to the variability of its effects [60–62]. With regard to MDD, there is a dearth of clinical trials exploring the impact of the stimulation parameters on clinical outcomes. Typically, bifrontal montages (F3–F8 and F3–F4 montages) targeting the left dlPFC are used in MDD. However, a computational modelling study suggested that other montages, using a fronto-extracephalic or fronto-occipital approach, could result in greater stimulation of brain regions of critical interest, such as the anterior cingulate cortex, which may be advantageous for treating MDD [63]. In fact, two open-label trials observed improvement in depressive symptoms following tDCS sessions applied over the fronto-occipital or -temporal regions [64,65] in a total of 18 patients and 20 sessions. Moreover, combined with sertraline, tDCS applied for 20 or 30 min was found to be effective for the treatment of mild and moderate depression, and the effect of the stimulation for 30 min was more pronounced than that of the 20 min stimulation [66]. Meta-analyses have noted that increasing the number of sessions or the intensity of the stimulation (1 versus 2 mA) does not improve tDCS effects on depressive symptoms [38,39]. In addition, the delay between sessions could have an impact on tDCS effects [67]. For example, Alonzo et al. [68] reported that daily tDCS induced a greater increase in cortical excitability than second daily stimulation of the motor cortex. Another, often overlooked, point is the influence of patient characteristics. Two open-label trials reported that depression severity was positively related to clinical improvement [69,70]. Evidence from three RCTs indicated that dlPFC tDCS had lesser efficacy in treatment-resistant depressed patients [29,31]. Finally, a meta-analysis of data from seven RCTs showed the superiority of active tDCS versus placebo in bipolar depression in terms of reduction in severity scores on depression scales from the first week of treatment [71]. Besides the features of the ongoing episode, the effects of interindividual variables, such as anatomical differences, genetic factors, personality, comorbidities, cognitive strategy, lifestyle, and baseline neuronal activation state, need to be explored [50]. Likewise, the age at which the stimulation is delivered might be a key determinant of the physiological and behavioral outcomes of tDCS. In children and adolescents, specific effects of tDCS on cortical excitability have been demonstrated [72,73]. In this population, the choice of the stimulation parameters, especially the dose selection, requires special attention [74].

It should also be emphasized that the final effects of tDCS depend on the concomitant use of pharmacotherapy with other interventions, such as cognitive therapy. A synergistic therapeutic action was observed with the combination of tDCS and sertraline in MDD patients in a large-scale RCT which compared the efficacy of tDCS, sertraline, and a combination of both [33]. Conversely, benzodiazepines were reported to reduce tDCS effects [75]. Concerning the effects of adjunctive tDCS and cognitive control therapy, Segrave et al. [76] showed that active tDCS coupled with weekly cognitive behavioral therapy (CBT) potentiated the treatment response, while Brunoni et al. [77] failed to demonstrate the superiority of combined cognitive control training (CCT) and active tDCS intervention versus CCT and sham tDCS. In resistant depression, one open study reported an improvement in depressive symptoms after 18 sessions of tDCS over six weeks, administered during Cognitive Emotional Training [78]. More recently, Mayur et al. failed to demonstrate differences in terms of speed of response or cognitive performance after the use of tDCS in combination with electroconvulsive therapy (ECT) versus ECT alone [79].

2. Conclusions

tDCS is a promising therapeutic strategy that offers the opportunity for non-invasive modulation of cortical excitability and plasticity in psychiatric disorders. With regard to MDD, the majority of meta-analyses have found that tDCS is superior to sham stimulation with an effect size (B coefficient = 0.35) comparable to that of repetitive transcranial magnetic stimulation (rTMS) and antidepressant medication in primary care [42]. This technique appears to be particularly indicated for patients with a mild-to-severe form of MDD who do not meet the criteria for resistant depression. In line with these data, a European expert group has recently proposed a Level B recommendation for its use in depressed patients, treated or not with antidepressants, without treatment resistance (minimum of 10 sessions (2 mA, 20–30 min) with the anode over the left dlPFC and the cathode over the right supra-orbital region) [7]. Questions still remain unanswered regarding the optimal stimulation parameters, the effect of tasks given during tDCS sessions, and the possible influence of add-on medications. Moreover, the clinical profile of depressed patients showing favorable responses to tDCS require clarification. Besides these critical questions, the promising preliminary results, the non-invasiveness of tDCS, and its good tolerability support the need for further research into this technique.

Author Contributions: Both authors contributed substantially to the preparation of the manuscript and approved the submitted version.

Acknowledgments: The authors received no specific funding for this work.

References

1. Rush, A.J.; Zimmerman, M.; Wisniewski, S.R.; Fava, M.; Hollon, S.D.; Warden, D.; Biggs, M.M.; Shores-Wilson, K.; Shelton, R.C.; Luther, J.F.; et al. Comorbid psychiatric disorders in depressed outpatients: Demographic and clinical features. *J. Affect. Disord.* **2005**, *87*, 43–55. [CrossRef] [PubMed]
2. Wittchen, H.U.; Jacobi, F.; Rehm, J.; Gustavsson, A.; Svensson, M.; Jönsson, B.; Olesen, J.; Allgulander, C.; Alonso, J.; Faravelli, C.; et al. The size and burden of mental disorders and other disorders of the brain in Europe 2010. *Eur. Neuropsychopharmacol.* **2011**, *21*, 655–679. [CrossRef] [PubMed]

3. Olesen, J.; Gustavsson, A.; Svensson, M.; Wittchen, H.-U.; Jönsson, B.; CDBE2010 Study Group. European Brain Council. The economic cost of brain disorders in Europe. *Eur. J. Neurol.* **2012**, *19*, 155–162. [CrossRef] [PubMed]
4. McCrone, P.; Rost, F.; Koeser, L.; Koutoufa, I.; Stephanou, S.; Knapp, M.; Goldberg, D.; Taylor, D.; Fonagy, P. The economic cost of treatment-resistant depression in patients referred to a specialist service. *J. Ment. Health* **2017**, 1–7. [CrossRef] [PubMed]
5. Rush, A.J.; Trivedi, M.H.; Wisniewski, S.R.; Nierenberg, A.A.; Stewart, J.W.; Warden, D.; Niederehe, G.; Thase, M.E.; Lavori, P.W.; Lebowitz, B.D.; et al. Acute and longer-term outcomes in depressed outpatients requiring one or several treatment steps: A STAR*D report. *Am. J. Psychiatry* **2006**, *163*, 1905–1917. [CrossRef] [PubMed]
6. Trivedi, M.H.; Rush, A.J.; Wisniewski, S.R.; Nierenberg, A.A.; Warden, D.; Ritz, L.; Norquist, G.; Howland, R.H.; Lebowitz, B.; McGrath, P.J.; et al. STAR*D study team evaluation of outcomes with citalopram for depression using measurement-based care in STAR*D: Implications for clinical practice. *Am. J. Psychiatry* **2006**, *163*, 28–40. [CrossRef] [PubMed]
7. Lefaucheur, J.-P.; Antal, A.; Ayache, S.S.; Benninger, D.H.; Brunelin, J.; Cogiamanian, F.; Cotelli, M.; De Ridder, D.; Ferrucci, R.; Langguth, B.; et al. Evidence-based guidelines on the therapeutic use of transcranial direct current stimulation (tDCS). *Clin. Neurophysiol.* **2017**, *128*, 56–92. [CrossRef] [PubMed]
8. Mondino, M.; Bennabi, D.; Poulet, E.; Galvao, F.; Brunelin, J.; Haffen, E. Can transcranial direct current stimulation (tDCS) alleviate symptoms and improve cognition in psychiatric disorders? *World J. Biol. Psychiatry* **2014**, *15*, 261–275. [CrossRef] [PubMed]
9. Nitsche, M.A.; Fricke, K.; Henschke, U.; Schlitterlau, A.; Liebetanz, D.; Lang, N.; Henning, S.; Tergau, F.; Paulus, W. Pharmacological modulation of cortical excitability shifts induced by transcranial direct current stimulation in humans. *J. Physiol.* **2003**, *553*, 293–301. [CrossRef] [PubMed]
10. Liebetanz, D.; Nitsche, M.A.; Tergau, F.; Paulus, W. Pharmacological approach to the mechanisms of transcranial DC-stimulation-induced after-effects of human motor cortex excitability. *Brain* **2002**, *125*, 2238–2247. [CrossRef] [PubMed]
11. Das, S.; Holland, P.; Frens, M.A.; Donchin, O. Impact of transcranial direct current stimulation (tDCS) on neuronal functions. *Front. Neurosci.* **2016**, *10*, 550. [CrossRef] [PubMed]
12. Kuo, M.-F.; Chen, P.-S.; Nitsche, M.A. The application of tDCS for the treatment of psychiatric diseases. *Int. Rev. Psychiatry* **2017**, *29*, 146–167. [CrossRef] [PubMed]
13. Kuo, M.-F.; Paulus, W.; Nitsche, M.A. Therapeutic effects of non-invasive Brain Stimul.ation with direct currents (tDCS) in neuropsychiatric diseases. *Neuroimage* **2014**, *85 Pt 3*, 948–960. [CrossRef] [PubMed]
14. Moher, D.; Liberati, A.; Tetzlaff, J.; Altman, D.G. PRISMA group preferred reporting items for systematic reviews and meta-analyses: The PRISMA statement. *J. Clin. Epidemiol.* **2009**, *62*, 1006–1012. [CrossRef] [PubMed]
15. Ko, J.H.; Tang, C.C.; Eidelberg, D. Brain Stimul.ation and functional imaging with fMRI and PET. *Handb. Clin. Neurol.* **2013**, *116*, 77–95. [CrossRef] [PubMed]
16. Nitsche, M.A.; Cohen, L.G.; Wassermann, E.M.; Priori, A.; Lang, N.; Antal, A.; Paulus, W.; Hummel, F.; Boggio, P.S.; Fregni, F.; et al. Transcranial direct current stimulation: State of the art 2008. *Brain Stimul.* **2008**, *1*, 206–223. [CrossRef] [PubMed]
17. Nitsche, M.A.; Doemkes, S.; Karaköse, T.; Antal, A.; Liebetanz, D.; Lang, N.; Tergau, F.; Paulus, W. Shaping the effects of transcranial direct current stimulation of the human motor cortex. *J. Neurophysiol.* **2007**, *97*, 3109–3117. [CrossRef] [PubMed]
18. Brunoni, A.R.; Moffa, A.H.; Sampaio-Júnior, B.; Gálvez, V.; Loo, C.K. Treatment-emergent mania/hypomania during antidepressant treatment with transcranial direct current stimulation (tDCS): A systematic review and meta-analysis. *Brain Stimul.* **2017**, *10*, 260–262. [CrossRef] [PubMed]
19. Bikson, M.; Grossman, P.; Thomas, C.; Zannou, A.L.; Jiang, J.; Adnan, T.; Mourdoukoutas, A.P.; Kronberg, G.; Truong, D.; Boggio, P.; et al. Safety of transcranial direct current stimulation: Evidence based update 2016. *Brain Stimul.* **2016**, *9*, 641–661. [CrossRef] [PubMed]
20. Cirillo, G.; Di Pino, G.; Capone, F.; Ranieri, F.; Florio, L.; Todisco, V.; Tedeschi, G.; Funke, K.; Di Lazzaro, V. Neurobiological after-effects of non-invasive Brain Stimul.ation. *Brain Stimul.* **2017**, *10*, 1–18. [CrossRef] [PubMed]

21. Brunoni, A.R.; Nitsche, M.A.; Bolognini, N.; Bikson, M.; Wagner, T.; Merabet, L.; Edwards, D.J.; Valero-Cabre, A.; Rotenberg, A.; Pascual-Leone, A.; et al. Clinical Research with Transcranial Direct Current Stimulation (Tdcs): Challenges and Future Directions. Available online: https://www.ncbi.nlm.nih.gov/pubmed/22037126 (accessed on 6 April 2018).
22. Dedoncker, J.; Brunoni, A.R.; Baeken, C.; Vanderhasselt, M.-A. A systematic review and meta-analysis of the effects of transcranial direct current stimulation (tDCS) over the dorsolateral prefrontal cortex in healthy and neuropsychiatric samples: Influence of stimulation parameters. *Brain Stimul.* **2016**, *9*, 501–517. [CrossRef] [PubMed]
23. Fregni, F.; Boggio, P.S.; Nitsche, M.A.; Marcolin, M.A.; Rigonatti, S.P.; Pascual-Leone, A. Treatment of major depression with transcranial direct current stimulation. *Bipolar Disord.* **2006**, *8*, 203–204. [CrossRef] [PubMed]
24. Boggio, P.S.; Rigonatti, S.P.; Ribeiro, R.B.; Myczkowski, M.L.; Nitsche, M.A.; Pascual-Leone, A.; Fregni, F. A randomized, double-blind clinical trial on the efficacy of cortical direct current stimulation for the treatment of major depression. *Int. J. Neuropsychopharmacol.* **2008**, *11*, 249–254. [CrossRef] [PubMed]
25. Boggio, P.S.; Bermpohl, F.; Vergara, A.O.; Muniz, A.L.C.R.; Nahas, F.H.; Leme, P.B.; Rigonatti, S.P.; Fregni, F. Go-no-go task performance improvement after anodal transcranial DC stimulation of the left dorsolateral prefrontal cortex in major depression. *J. Affect. Disord.* **2007**, *101*, 91–98. [CrossRef] [PubMed]
26. Loo, C.K.; Sachdev, P.; Martin, D.; Pigot, M.; Alonzo, A.; Malhi, G.S.; Lagopoulos, J.; Mitchell, P. A double-blind, sham-controlled trial of transcranial direct current stimulation for the treatment of depression. *Int. J. Neuropsychopharmacol.* **2010**, *13*, 61–69. [CrossRef] [PubMed]
27. Loo, C.K.; Alonzo, A.; Martin, D.; Mitchell, P.B.; Galvez, V.; Sachdev, P. Transcranial direct current stimulation for depression: 3-week, randomised, sham-controlled trial. *Br. J. Psychiatry* **2012**, *200*, 52–59. [CrossRef] [PubMed]
28. Rigonatti, S.P.; Boggio, P.S.; Myczkowski, M.L.; Otta, E.; Fiquer, J.T.; Ribeiro, R.B.; Nitsche, M.A.; Pascual-Leone, A.; Fregni, F. Transcranial direct stimulation and fluoxetine for the treatment of depression. *Eur. Psychiatry* **2008**, *23*, 74–76. [CrossRef] [PubMed]
29. Palm, U.; Schiller, C.; Fintescu, Z.; Obermeier, M.; Keeser, D.; Reisinger, E.; Pogarell, O.; Nitsche, M.A.; Möller, H.-J.; Padberg, F. Transcranial direct current stimulation in treatment resistant depression: A randomized double-blind, placebo-controlled study. *Brain Stimul.* **2012**, *5*, 242–251. [CrossRef] [PubMed]
30. Blumberger, D.M.; Tran, L.C.; Fitzgerald, P.B.; Hoy, K.E.; Daskalakis, Z.J. A randomized double-blind sham-controlled study of transcranial direct current stimulation for treatment-resistant major depression. *Front. Psychiatry* **2012**, *3*, 74. [CrossRef] [PubMed]
31. Bennabi, D.; Nicolier, M.; Monnin, J.; Tio, G.; Pazart, L.; Vandel, P.; Haffen, E. Pilot study of feasibility of the effect of treatment with tDCS in patients suffering from treatment-resistant depression treated with escitalopram. *Clin. Neurophysiol.* **2015**, *126*, 1185–1189. [CrossRef] [PubMed]
32. Valiengo, L.C.L.; Goulart, A.C.; de Oliveira, J.F.; Benseñor, I.M.; Lotufo, P.A.; Brunoni, A.R. Transcranial direct current stimulation for the treatment of post-stroke depression: Results from a randomised, sham-controlled, double-blinded trial. *J. Neurol. Neurosurg. Psychiatry* **2017**, *88*, 170–175. [CrossRef] [PubMed]
33. Brunoni, A.R.; Valiengo, L.; Baccaro, A.; Zanão, T.A.; de Oliveira, J.F.; Goulart, A.; Boggio, P.S.; Lotufo, P.A.; Benseñor, I.M.; Fregni, F. The sertraline vs. electrical current therapy for treating depression clinical study: Results from a factorial, randomized, controlled trial. *JAMA Psychiatry* **2013**, *70*, 383–391. [CrossRef] [PubMed]
34. Brunoni, A.R.; Sampaio-Junior, B.; Moffa, A.H.; Borrione, L.; Nogueira, B.S.; Aparício, L.V.M.; Veronezi, B.; Moreno, M.; Fernandes, R.A.; Tavares, D.; et al. The Escitalopram versus Electric Current Therapy for Treating Depression Clinical Study (ELECT-TDCS): Rationale and study design of a non-inferiority, triple-arm, placebo-controlled clinical trial. *Sao Paulo Med. J.* **2015**, *133*, 252–263. [CrossRef] [PubMed]
35. Loo, C.K.; Husain, M.M.; McDonald, W.M.; Aaronson, S.; O'Reardon, J.P.; Alonzo, A.; Weickert, C.S.; Martin, D.M.; McClintock, S.M.; Mohan, A.; et al. International Consortium of Research in tDCS (ICRT) International randomized-controlled trial of transcranial Direct Current Stimulation in depression. *Brain Stimul.* **2018**, *11*, 125–133. [CrossRef] [PubMed]
36. Martin, D.M.; Alonzo, A.; Ho, K.-A.; Player, M.; Mitchell, P.B.; Sachdev, P.; Loo, C.K. Continuation transcranial direct current stimulation for the prevention of relapse in major depression. *J. Affect. Disord.* **2013**, *144*, 274–278. [CrossRef] [PubMed]

37. Valiengo, L.; Benseñor, I.M.; Goulart, A.C.; de Oliveira, J.F.; Zanao, T.A.; Boggio, P.S.; Lotufo, P.A.; Fregni, F.; Brunoni, A.R. The sertraline versus electrical current therapy for treating depression clinical study (select-TDCS): Results of the crossover and follow-up phases. *Depress Anxiety* **2013**, *30*, 646–653. [CrossRef] [PubMed]
38. Kalu, U.G.; Sexton, C.E.; Loo, C.K.; Ebmeier, K.P. Transcranial direct current stimulation in the treatment of major depression: A meta-analysis. *Psychol. Med.* **2012**, *42*, 1791–1800. [CrossRef] [PubMed]
39. Berlim, M.T.; Van den Eynde, F.; Daskalakis, Z.J. Clinical utility of transcranial direct current stimulation (tDCS) for treating major depression: A systematic review and meta-analysis of randomized, double-blind and sham-controlled trials. *J. Psychiatr. Res.* **2013**, *47*, 1–7. [CrossRef] [PubMed]
40. Shiozawa, P.; Fregni, F.; Benseñor, I.M.; Lotufo, P.A.; Berlim, M.T.; Daskalakis, J.Z.; Cordeiro, Q.; Brunoni, A.R. Transcranial direct current stimulation for major depression: An updated systematic review and meta-analysis. *Int. J. Neuropsychopharmacol.* **2014**, *17*, 1443–1452. [CrossRef] [PubMed]
41. Meron, D.; Hedger, N.; Garner, M.; Baldwin, D.S. Transcranial direct current stimulation (tDCS) in the treatment of depression: Systematic review and meta-analysis of efficacy and tolerability. *Neurosci. Biobehav. Rev.* **2015**, *57*, 46–62. [CrossRef] [PubMed]
42. Brunoni, A.R.; Moffa, A.H.; Fregni, F.; Palm, U.; Padberg, F.; Blumberger, D.M.; Daskalakis, Z.J.; Bennabi, D.; Haffen, E.; Alonzo, A.; et al. Transcranial direct current stimulation for acute major depressive episodes: Meta-analysis of individual patient data. *Br. J. Psychiatry* **2016**, *208*, 522–531. [CrossRef] [PubMed]
43. Alonzo, A.; Chan, G.; Martin, D.; Mitchell, P.B.; Loo, C. Transcranial direct current stimulation (tDCS) for depression: Analysis of response using a three-factor structure of the Montgomery-Åsberg depression rating scale. *J. Affect. Disord.* **2013**, *150*, 91–95. [CrossRef] [PubMed]
44. D'Urso, G.; Dell'Osso, B.; Rossi, R.; Brunoni, A.R.; Bortolomasi, M.; Ferrucci, R.; Priori, A.; de Bartolomeis, A.; Altamura, A.C. Clinical predictors of acute response to transcranial direct current stimulation (tDCS) in major depression. *J. Affect. Disord.* **2017**, *219*, 25–30. [CrossRef] [PubMed]
45. Martin, D.M.; Yeung, K.; Loo, C.K. Pre-treatment letter fluency performance predicts antidepressant response to transcranial direct current stimulation. *J. Affect. Disord.* **2016**, *203*, 130–135. [CrossRef] [PubMed]
46. Brunoni, A.R.; Machado-Vieira, R.; Zarate, C.A.; Valiengo, L.; Vieira, E.L.; Benseñor, I.M.; Lotufo, P.A.; Gattaz, W.F.; Teixeira, A.L. Cytokines plasma levels during antidepressant treatment with sertraline and transcranial direct current stimulation (tDCS): Results from a factorial, randomized, controlled trial. *Psychopharmacology (Berl.)* **2014**, *231*, 1315–1323. [CrossRef] [PubMed]
47. Brunoni, A.R.; Machado-Vieira, R.; Zarate, C.A.; Vieira, E.L.M.; Valiengo, L.; Benseñor, I.M.; Lotufo, P.A.; Gattaz, W.F.; Teixeira, A.L. Assessment of non-BDNF neurotrophins and GDNF levels after depression treatment with sertraline and transcranial direct current stimulation in a factorial, randomized, sham-controlled trial (SELECT-TDCS): An exploratory analysis. *Prog. Neuropsychopharmacol. Biol. Psychiatry* **2015**, *56*, 91–96. [CrossRef] [PubMed]
48. Brunoni, A.R.; Machado-Vieira, R.; Zarate, C.A.; Vieira, E.L.M.; Vanderhasselt, M.-A.; Nitsche, M.A.; Valiengo, L.; Benseñor, I.M.; Lotufo, P.A.; Gattaz, W.F.; et al. BDNF plasma levels after antidepressant treatment with sertraline and transcranial direct current stimulation: Results from a factorial, randomized, sham-controlled trial. *Eur. Neuropsychopharmacol.* **2014**, *24*, 1144–1151. [CrossRef] [PubMed]
49. Brunoni, A.R.; Kemp, A.H.; Shiozawa, P.; Cordeiro, Q.; Valiengo, L.C.L.; Goulart, A.C.; Coprerski, B.; Lotufo, P.A.; Brunoni, D.; Perez, A.B.A.; et al. Impact of 5-HTTLPR and BDNF polymorphisms on response to sertraline versus transcranial direct current stimulation: Implications for the serotonergic system. *Eur. Neuropsychopharmacol.* **2013**, *23*, 1530–1540. [CrossRef] [PubMed]
50. Bennabi, D.; Pedron, S.; Haffen, E.; Monnin, J.; Peterschmitt, Y.; Van Waes, V. Transcranial direct current stimulation for memory enhancement: From clinical research to animal models. *Front. Syst. Neurosci.* **2014**, *8*, 159. [CrossRef] [PubMed]
51. Oliveira, J.F.; Zanão, T.A.; Valiengo, L.; Lotufo, P.A.; Benseñor, I.M.; Fregni, F.; Brunoni, A.R. Acute working memory improvement after tDCS in antidepressant-free patients with major depressive disorder. *Neurosci. Lett.* **2013**, *537*, 60–64. [CrossRef] [PubMed]
52. Moreno, M.L.; Vanderhasselt, M.-A.; Carvalho, A.F.; Moffa, A.H.; Lotufo, P.A.; Benseñor, I.M.; Brunoni, A.R. Effects of acute transcranial direct current stimulation in hot and cold working memory tasks in healthy and depressed subjects. *Neurosci. Lett.* **2015**, *591*, 126–131. [CrossRef] [PubMed]

53. Fregni, F.; Boggio, P.S.; Nitsche, M.A.; Rigonatti, S.P.; Pascual-Leone, A. Cognitive effects of repeated sessions of transcranial direct current stimulation in patients with depression. *Depress Anxiety* **2006**, *23*, 482–484. [CrossRef] [PubMed]
54. Wolkenstein, L.; Plewnia, C. Amelioration of cognitive control in depression by transcranial direct current stimulation. *Biol. Psychiatry* **2013**, *73*, 646–651. [CrossRef] [PubMed]
55. Salehinejad, M.A.; Ghanavai, E.; Rostami, R.; Nejati, V. Cognitive control dysfunction in emotion dysregulation and psychopathology of major depression (MD): Evidence from transcranial Brain Stimul.ation of the dorsolateral prefrontal cortex (DLPFC). *J. Affect. Disord.* **2017**, *210*, 241–248. [CrossRef] [PubMed]
56. Gögler, N.; Willacker, L.; Funk, J.; Strube, W.; Langgartner, S.; Napiórkowski, N.; Hasan, A.; Finke, K. Single-session transcranial direct current stimulation induces enduring enhancement of visual processing speed in patients with major depression. *Eur. Arch. Psychiatry Clin. Neurosci.* **2016**. [CrossRef] [PubMed]
57. Brennan, S.; McLoughlin, D.M.; O'Connell, R.; Bogue, J.; O'Connor, S.; McHugh, C.; Glennon, M. Anodal transcranial direct current stimulation of the left dorsolateral prefrontal cortex enhances emotion recognition in depressed patients and controls. *J. Clin. Exp. Neuropsychol.* **2017**, *39*, 384–395. [CrossRef] [PubMed]
58. Bueno, V.F.; Brunoni, A.R.; Boggio, P.S.; Bensenor, I.M.; Fregni, F. Mood and cognitive effects of transcranial direct current stimulation in post-stroke depression. *Neurocase* **2011**, *17*, 318–322. [CrossRef] [PubMed]
59. Brunoni, A.R.; Tortella, G.; Benseñor, I.M.; Lotufo, P.A.; Carvalho, A.F.; Fregni, F. Cognitive effects of transcranial direct current stimulation in depression: Results from the SELECT-TDCS trial and insights for further clinical trials. *J. Affect. Disord.* **2016**, *202*, 46–52. [CrossRef] [PubMed]
60. Tortella, G.; Casati, R.; Aparicio, L.V.M.; Mantovani, A.; Senço, N.; D'Urso, G.; Brunelin, J.; Guarienti, F.; Selingardi, P.M.L.; Muszkat, D.; et al. Transcranial direct current stimulation in psychiatric disorders. *World J. Psychiatry* **2015**, *5*, 88–102. [CrossRef] [PubMed]
61. Chew, T.; Ho, K.-A.; Loo, C.K. Inter- and intra-individual variability in response to transcranial direct current stimulation (tDCS) at varying current intensities. *Brain Stimul.* **2015**, *8*, 1130–1137. [CrossRef] [PubMed]
62. Martin, D.M.; Alonzo, A.; Mitchell, P.B.; Sachdev, P.; Gálvez, V.; Loo, C.K. Fronto-extracephalic transcranial direct current stimulation as a treatment for major depression: An open-label pilot study. *J. Affect. Disord.* **2011**, *134*, 459–463. [CrossRef] [PubMed]
63. Bai, S.; Dokos, S.; Ho, K.-A.; Loo, C. A computational modelling study of transcranial direct current stimulation montages used in depression. *Neuroimage* **2014**, *87*, 332–344. [CrossRef] [PubMed]
64. Ho, K.-A.; Bai, S.; Martin, D.; Alonzo, A.; Dokos, S.; Loo, C.K. Clinical pilot study and computational modeling of bitemporal transcranial direct current stimulation, and safety of repeated courses of treatment, in major depression. *J. ECT* **2015**, *31*, 226–233. [CrossRef] [PubMed]
65. Ho, K.-A.; Bai, S.; Martin, D.; Alonzo, A.; Dokos, S.; Puras, P.; Loo, C.K. A pilot study of alternative transcranial direct current stimulation electrode montages for the treatment of major depression. *J. Affect. Disord.* **2014**, *167*, 251–258. [CrossRef] [PubMed]
66. Pavlova, E.L.; Menshikova, A.A.; Semenov, R.V.; Bocharnikova, E.N.; Gotovtseva, G.N.; Druzhkova, T.A.; Gersamia, A.G.; Gudkova, A.A.; Guekht, A.B. Transcranial direct current stimulation of 20- and 30-minutes combined with sertraline for the treatment of depression. *Prog. Neuropsychopharmacol. Biol. Psychiatry* **2018**, *82*, 31–38. [CrossRef] [PubMed]
67. Fricke, K.; Seeber, A.A.; Thirugnanasambandam, N.; Paulus, W.; Nitsche, M.A.; Rothwell, J.C. Time course of the induction of homeostatic plasticity generated by repeated transcranial direct current stimulation of the human motor cortex. *J. Neurophysiol.* **2011**, *105*, 1141–1149. [CrossRef] [PubMed]
68. Alonzo, A.; Brassil, J.; Taylor, J.L.; Martin, D.; Loo, C.K. Daily transcranial direct current stimulation (tDCS) leads to greater increases in cortical excitability than second daily transcranial direct current stimulation. *Brain Stimul.* **2012**, *5*, 208–213. [CrossRef] [PubMed]
69. Ferrucci, R.; Bortolomasi, M.; Vergari, M.; Tadini, L.; Salvoro, B.; Giacopuzzi, M.; Barbieri, S.; Priori, A. Transcranial direct current stimulation in severe, drug-resistant major depression. *J. Affect. Disord.* **2009**, *118*, 215–219. [CrossRef] [PubMed]
70. Brunoni, A.R.; Ferrucci, R.; Bortolomasi, M.; Vergari, M.; Tadini, L.; Boggio, P.S.; Giacopuzzi, M.; Barbieri, S.; Priori, A. Transcranial direct current stimulation (tDCS) in unipolar vs. bipolar depressive disorder. *Prog. Neuropsychopharmacol. Biol. Psychiatry* **2011**, *35*, 96–101. [CrossRef] [PubMed]

71. Dondé, C.; Amad, A.; Nieto, I.; Brunoni, A.R.; Neufeld, N.H.; Bellivier, F.; Poulet, E.; Geoffroy, P.-A. Transcranial direct-current stimulation (tDCS) for bipolar depression: A systematic review and meta-analysis. *Prog. Neuropsychopharmacol. Biol. Psychiatry* **2017**, *78*, 123–131. [CrossRef] [PubMed]
72. Minhas, P.; Bikson, M.; Woods, A.J.; Rosen, A.R.; Kessler, S.K. Transcranial direct current stimulation in pediatric brain: A computational modeling study. *Conf. Proc. IEEE Eng. Med. Biol. Soc.* **2012**, *2012*, 859–862. [CrossRef] [PubMed]
73. Moliadze, V.; Schmanke, T.; Andreas, S.; Lyzhko, E.; Freitag, C.M.; Siniatchkin, M. Stimulation intensities of transcranial direct current stimulation have to be adjusted in children and adolescents. *Clin. Neurophysiol.* **2015**, *126*, 1392–1399. [CrossRef] [PubMed]
74. Kessler, S.K.; Minhas, P.; Woods, A.J.; Rosen, A.; Gorman, C.; Bikson, M. Dosage considerations for transcranial direct current stimulation in children: A computational modeling study. *PLoS ONE* **2013**, *8*, e76112. [CrossRef] [PubMed]
75. Brunoni, A.R.; Ferrucci, R.; Bortolomasi, M.; Scelzo, E.; Boggio, P.S.; Fregni, F.; Dell'Osso, B.; Giacopuzzi, M.; Altamura, A.C.; Priori, A. Interactions between transcranial direct current stimulation (tDCS) and pharmacological interventions in the Major Depressive Episode: Findings from a naturalistic study. *Eur. Psychiatry* **2013**, *28*, 356–361. [CrossRef] [PubMed]
76. Segrave, R.A.; Arnold, S.; Hoy, K.; Fitzgerald, P.B. Concurrent cognitive control training augments the antidepressant efficacy of tDCS: A pilot study. *Brain Stimul.* **2014**, *7*, 325–331. [CrossRef] [PubMed]
77. Brunoni, A.R.; Boggio, P.S.; De Raedt, R.; Benseñor, I.M.; Lotufo, P.A.; Namur, V.; Valiengo, L.C.L.; Vanderhasselt, M.A. Cognitive control therapy and transcranial direct current stimulation for depression: A randomized, double-blinded, controlled trial. *J. Affect. Disord.* **2014**, *162*, 43–49. [CrossRef] [PubMed]
78. Martin, D.M.; Teng, J.Z.; Lo, T.Y.; Alonzo, A.; Goh, T.; Iacoviello, B.M.; Hoch, M.M.; Loo, C.K. Clinical pilot study of transcranial direct current stimulation combined with Cognitive Emotional Training for medication resistant depression. *J. Affect. Disord.* **2018**, *232*, 89–95. [CrossRef] [PubMed]
79. Mayur, P.; Howari, R.; Byth, K.; Vannitamby, R. Concomitant transcranial direct current stimulation with ultrabrief electroconvulsive therapy: A 2-week double-blind randomized sham-controlled trial. *J. ECT* **2018**. [CrossRef] [PubMed]

9

Suicide Risk in Bipolar Disorder

Peter Dome [1,2,*], Zoltan Rihmer [1,2] and Xenia Gonda [1,2,3,4]

1 Department of Psychiatry and Psychotherapy, Semmelweis University, Faculty of Medicine, 1125 Budapest, Hungary
2 National Institute of Psychiatry and Addictions, Laboratory for Suicide Research and Prevention, 1135 Budapest, Hungary
3 MTA-SE Neuropsychopharmacology, Neurochemistry Research Group, Hungarian Academy of Sciences, 1089 Budapest, Hungary
4 NAP-2-SE New Antidepressant Target Research Group, Hungarian Brain Research Program, Semmelweis University, 1089 Budapest, Hungary
* Correspondence: dome_peter@yahoo.co.uk;

Abstract: Bipolar disorders (BDs) are prevalent mental health illnesses that affect about 1–5% of the total population, have a chronic course and are associated with a markedly elevated premature mortality. One of the contributors for the decreased life expectancy in BD is suicide. Accordingly, the rate of suicide among BD patients is approximately 10–30 times higher than the corresponding rate in the general population. Extant research found that up to 20% of (mostly untreated) BD subjects end their life by suicide, and 20–60% of them attempt suicide at least one in their lifetime. In our paper we briefly recapitulate the current knowledge on the epidemiological aspects of suicide in BD as well as factors associated with suicidal risk in BD. Furthermore, we also discuss concisely the possible means of suicide prevention in BD.

Keywords: bipolar disorder; mood disorders; suicide; suicidal; mortality

---

1. Introduction

With a lifetime prevalence of 1.3–5.0%, type-I and -II bipolar disorders (BD-I; BD-II) are among the most common psychiatric ailments [1,2]. Patients with BD have poor life expectancies as these patients have a decreased lifespan of about 9–17 years compared with the general population. Furthermore, some studies from different countries (e.g., Denmark and UK) suggest that this mortality gap has become larger over the last decades. Although the largest number of excess death cases in BD may be attributed to natural (e.g., due to cardiovascular diseases or diabetes) and not unnatural causes, suicide is also quite prevalent in the population of subjects with BD [1–5].

At a global scale, approximately 800,000 suicide deaths occur every year (which corresponds to a global suicide rate of 11.4/100,000/year); thus, suicide may be considered a major public health issue [6,7]. Although the great majority (≈90%) of suicide cases occur among subjects with major mental—typically mood–disorders, the majority of patients with mood disorders never become involved in suicidal behaviour. Accordingly, in addition to major mood disorders, other risk factors (including special clinical features of the mental illness as well as some demographic, personality and familial factors) should contribute to suicidality, which therefore should be deemed as a multicausal phenomenon [2,8–10]. Hereinafter, we provide a concise summary of our current knowledge about suicidality in BD based on a review of current literature (mainly review papers, book chapters, meta-analyses, treatment guidelines of international societies, etc.).

2. Epidemiology of Suicidal Behaviour in Bipolar Disorder

Suicidal behaviour is quite frequent among subjects with BD, as up to 4–19% of them ultimately end their life by suicide, while 20–60% of them attempt suicide at least once in their lifetime [2]. In BD, the risk of suicide death is up to 10–30 times higher than that of the general population [2,5,8,10–12]. The estimated annual suicide rate in patients with BD is about 200–400 / 100,000 [8]. BD-associated cases account for about 3–14% of all suicide deaths [13].

It is important to mention that the ratio of suicide attempts to suicide deaths (i.e., the lethality index) is much lower for patients with BD than for the members of the general population (one study, for example, reported that rate as 35:1 and 3:1 for the general population and for BD patients, respectively) [2,8,9]. A possible explanation for this phenomenon may be that BD subjects usually employ more lethal suicide methods compared with members of the general population [2,8,9]. Nevertheless, attempts-to-suicide ratios lower than in the general population are not specific for BD, as it is also observable for instance among patients with schizophrenia or major depressive disorder (MDD) [2,14]. Unsurprisingly, suicidal ideation is also far more frequent in patients with BD (43% past-year prevalence) than in the general population (9.2% life-time prevalence) [7,15].

Though it is indisputable that mood disorders are associated with markedly elevated levels of suicidality, it is hard to pick out from the results of various studies whether there are *relevant* differences in the risk of suicidal behaviour between different kinds of mood disorders. Accordingly, higher, similar or lower levels of suicidality in BD patients compared to MDD patients have also been reported [9,10,16]. In a similar fashion, based on the published information it is hard to disentangle whether any BD subtype (BD-I or BD-II) is associated with a higher level of suicidality than the other [2,8,11,16–19].

It is known that a relatively high proportion (8–55%) of patients with MDD has a history of subthreshold hypomanic symptoms. This so called subthreshold bipolar subgroup of MDD patients differs from MDD patients without subthreshold hypomanic manifestations in several ways. For instance, a wide array of studies demonstrated that subthreshold bipolarity is associated with increased levels of suicidality [20–23].

3. Risk Factors of Suicide in Bipolar Disorder

Several approaches exist to classify risk factors for suicide in BD. One of the most common systems divides risk factors into proximal and distal ones, where proximal (or precipitating) factors are close to suicidal behaviour in time whereas distal factors are rather considered as traits or predispositions and, accordingly, they are enduring [10,24]. Other classifications assign suicide risk factors to conceptual categories (e.g., risk factors associated with genetic or sociodemographic components or illness characteristics or life events) [8,25,26]. Based on different conceptual backgrounds complex models were conceived for the description of the whole process of suicide (e.g., the diathesis-stress model, the bipolar suicidality model, the interpersonal theory of suicide, the three-step theory model or the recently elaborated "neurocognitive model of suicide in the context of bipolar disorders") [10].

In the current paper–without the ambition to be exhaustive–we list and briefly discuss the most relevant risk and protective factors of suicide in BD. In regard to *clinical history, previous suicide attempt(s)* is considered as one of the most powerful single predictors of future attempts and suicide death. The *period soon after hospital discharge* may be characterized by extremely high levels of suicidality. This finding draws attention to the importance of avoiding premature discharges and inappropriate follow-ups. In addition, risk of suicide is increased during the *period immediately after hospital admission*. *Frequent and/or great number of prior hospitalizations* are also associated with heightened risk of suicidal self-harming behaviour. *Early age at onset* is also associated with suicidality in BD. The *early years after the diagnosis* represent a high-risk period for suicide. *Comorbidity* with other psychiatric, addictive or severe somatic disorders also increase the risk of all forms of suicidal behaviour. *Rapid-cycling course* and *predominant depressive polarity* during the prior course are also associated with higher risks of self-destructive behaviour. One of the most important determinants of suicidal behavior in BD is the *type/polarity of the current mood episode/state*: pure major depressive episodes and mixed states carry the highest risk, while suicidal behaviour is rarely present in (euphoric) mania, hypomania and during euthymic periods. However, some recent results indicated that there is no elevated risk of suicidal behaviour during mixed state over the risk attributable to its depressed component. Furthermore, these studies suggest that the majority of suicide risk elevation related to having previous mixed states is not an aftermath of the mixed state itself, but can rather be attributed to a depression-predominant course of the disorder. *Longer duration of untreated illness* (i.e., long time lag from the beginning of the affective symptoms until treatment initiation) is also associated with higher hazards of suicidal behaviour. Regarding *sociodemographic factors*, male *gender* is a risk factor for lethal suicides, while, according to some results, female gender is a risk factor for attempts. These gender differences are similar–but weaker–to those observable in the general population; accordingly, in this otherwise high-risk population gender seems not to be a significant predictor for suicidal behaviour). Suicidality is also more frequent among those bipolar subjects who are *divorced*, *unmarried* or *single-parents* or *living in social isolation*. *Age* is a further important sociodemographic factor: BD subjects under 35 years of age and above 75 years of age are at higher risk for engaging in suicide-related behaviours. *Occupational problems and unemployment* also contribute to elevated levels of suicidality. *Adversities in personal history and acute stressors*, such as experiencing sexual or physical abuse and parental loss in childhood or bereavement, breaking the law/criminal conviction and financial disasters are important precipitants of suicidality as well. Some *personality attributes*, for instance impulsive/aggressive traits, hopelessness and pessimism also increase the risk of suicide. Certain types of *affective temperaments* (first and foremost cyclothymic) have also been demonstrated to be associated with more frequent suicidal behaviour in BD. *Family history* of suicide acts and/or major mood disorders are also strong risk factors for suicide in subjects with BD. Some results also suggest that *living in geographical locations where there are large differences in solar insolation between winter and summer* (i.e., near the poles) may be associated with increased risks of attempted suicide in patients with BD-I [2,7,8,10–12,15,17,19,25–34].

4. Protective Factors of Suicide in Bipolar Disorder

In contrast to the above discussed several risk factors for suicide in BD, only a few protective factors have been identified so far [2]. For instance *good family and social support*, *parenthood* and *the use of adaptive coping strategies* seem to have some protective effects. Furthermore, a strong *perceived meaning of life and hyperthymic affective temperament* are also a protective factors [2,10,24,29]. The possible protective role of religiosity has emerged but results are somewhat inconclusive [2,26,35–37]. Last but not least, it is important to note that treatment (and even more so a good response to treatment) is protective against suicide in BD (see also the section "Suicide prevention in bipolar disorder"). In consonance with the fact that treatment may decrease heightened suicidality, it is not surprising that the majority of suicide victims are *untreated* affective disorder patients [8–11,13,38,39].

5. Suicide Prevention in Bipolar Disorder

From a *pharmacological perspective*, *lithium* seems to possess the greatest suicide-preventive potential in patients with BD. Intriguingly, the suicide protective effect of lithium is not confined to bipolar patients as it has also been demonstrated among patients with MDD (it is not surprising since, as we have discussed it previously, a considerable proportion of "unipolar" MDD patients have subthreshold bipolar features) [5,8,15,40–42]. Overall, compared to placebo, lithium appears to decrease the risk of suicide by more than 60% in mood disorders [8,40,42]. Some results suggest that lithium is protective against suicide, albeit in a decreased manner, even in those BD patients who are moderate/poor responders to the phase-prophylactic effect of it. This finding may suggest that in the case of lithium non-response in a patient who is at high risk for suicide, instead of switching lithium to another mood stabilizer, the clinician should retain lithium (even in a lower dose) and combine it with another mood stabilizer [1,41].

A solid suicide-protective effect related to the administration of *anticonvulsant-type mood stabilizers* (e.g., valproic acid, carbamazepine, lamotrigine) to BD patients has not been proven so far. On the other hand, the concern of the FDA about the potential for an increased risk of suicidality associated with anticonvulsants seems not to be applicable to patients with BD (i.e., in this population the use of these agents is not associated with increased levels of suicidality). According to our current knowledge, in regard to suicide prevention lithium is superior than these agents [2,8,15,41,43,44].

The role of *antidepressants* (ADs) in suicide prevention in individuals with BD seems to be negligible, and, in fact, concerns have been raised that administration of ADs may increase suicidality in BD. It is remarkable that findings are also inconsistent regarding the ability of ADs to prevent suicides in patients with MDD. AD monotherapy should be avoided in BD [2,8,15,41].

Considering their increasing use in BD for instance as maintenance treatment, it is justifiable to ask whether (atypical) *antipsychotics* have any beneficial effects on suicidal behaviour in BD. Unfortunately, there are no high-quality data to answer this question at present, so further studies should elucidate whether treatment with antipsychotics has any benefits in this respect [2,8,15,41].

Ketamin as a possible antidepressant agent has mainly been tested in patients with MDD and only a few studies have been conducted among patients with bipolar depression. According to the results of these small proof-of-concept investigations, ketamin shows similar antidepressive efficacy in bipolar as in unipolar depression. In line with its possible efficacy, ketamin is recommended by the clinical guideline of International College of Neuropsychopharmacology (CINP) for the treatment of bipolar depression, but only as a fourth-line agent and in combination with a mood stabilizer. Similarly, until now, the antisuicidal activity of ketamine was assessed mainly in MDD patients and only a small number of investigations have been conducted in BD patients. These have mainly positive outcomes, but further studies are needed to reveal whether ketamin has a similar antisuicidal effect in BD than in MDD [45–51].

It is well-known that *electroconvulsive therapy* (ECT) shows a similar efficacy in the treatment of depressive episodes in MDD and BPD (and some studies even found it more effective against bipolar than unipolar depression). In line with its antidepressive effects, ECT is also considered as an effective antisuicidal treatment modality, and it has been recently demonstrated that it is superior in this regard to psychopharmacons both in unipolar and bipolar depression (and its antisuicidal efficacy is comparable to the efficacy of psychopharmacons in bipolar mixed states and mania) [2,8,41,52,53].

Unfortunately, only a small number of studies have investigated up to now the efficacy of specific (e.g., dialectical behavior therapy, cognitive-behavioural therapy, interpersonal and social rhythm therapy) or unspecific (e.g., psychoeducation) *psychosocial interventions* against suicide among BD patients. Nonetheless, results of the few existing studies are promising [2,8,54–58].

6. Summary and Clinical Implications

BD is a relatively common psychiatric disorder that is associated with increased mortality due to both natural and unnatural causes. Accordingly, the risk of suicide is highly elevated in this patient population. Because of this, a thorough assessment of suicide risk should take place at all clinical visits. This clinical assessment should include, *inter alia*, the comprehensive examination of the mental state, and the inquiry about the existence and features of current suicidal intents (e.g., duration and intensity), the methods intended to be used, the access to means (e.g., weapons) as well as the compliance to prescribed medications. In addition, it is essential to gain information about previous suicidality. Whenever possible, hetero-anamnestic data should be gathered as well. The management of suicidal behaviour in patients with BD represents a clinical challenge. Appropriate long-term treatment of the disorder seems to be associated with the reduction of suicidality. Furthermore, in acutely suicidal patients the removal of access to obvious means for suicide is essential and, in severe cases, hospitalization may be justifiable as well. Prevention strategies should include the provision of psychoeducation (for example, via information leaflets and/or by the members of the health care staff) to the patients, as well as to relatives and friends, in order that they become able to recognize the warning signs of suicidal behaviour, be aware of the risk periods and the importance of adherence to treatment, avoid isolation and call for help in emergency situations. A written list of sources of support which are available during a suicidal crisis may also be helpful [2,10,15,59].

References

1. Rihmer, Z.; Dome, P. Suicide and Bipolar Disorder. In *Bipolar Depression: Molecular Neurobiology, Clinical Diagnosis, and Pharmacotherapy*, 2nd ed.; Zarate, C.A.J., Manji, H.K., Eds.; Springer: Bern, Switzerland, 2017.
2. Rihmer, Z.; Gonda, X.; Döme, P. The Assessment and Management of SuicideRrisk in Bipolar Disorder. In *The Treatment of Bipolar Disorder: Integrative Clinical Strategies and Future Directions*; Carvalho, A.F., Vieta, E., Eds.; Oxford University Press: Oxford, UK, 2017.
3. Staudt Hansen, P.; Frahm Laursen, M.; Grontved, S.; Puggard Vogt Straszek, S.; Licht, R.W.; Nielsen, R.E. Increasing mortality gap for patients diagnosed with bipolar disorder—A nationwide study with 20 years of follow-up. *Bipolar Disord.* **2019**, *21*, 270–275. [CrossRef] [PubMed]
4. Hayes, J.F.; Marston, L.; Walters, K.; King, M.B.; Osborn, D.P.J. Mortality gap for people with bipolar disorder and schizophrenia: UK-based cohort study 2000–2014. *Br. J. Psychiatry* **2017**, *211*, 175–181. [CrossRef] [PubMed]
5. Bauer, M.; Andreassen, O.A.; Geddes, J.R.; Vedel Kessing, L.; Lewitzka, U.; Schulze, T.G.; Vieta, E. Areas of uncertainties and unmet needs in bipolar disorders: Clinical and research perspectives. *Lancet Psychiatry* **2018**, *5*, 930–939. [CrossRef]
6. World Health Organization. *Preventing Suicide: A Global Imperative*; WHO Press: Geneva, Switzerland, 2014.
7. Turecki, G.; Brent, D.A. Suicide and suicidal behaviour. *Lancet* **2016**, *387*, 1227–1239. [CrossRef]
8. Plans, L.; Barrot, C.; Nieto, E.; Rios, J.; Schulze, T.G.; Papiol, S.; Mitjans, M.; Vieta, E.; Benabarre, A. Association between completed suicide and bipolar disorder: A systematic review of the literature. *J. Affect. Disord.* **2019**, *242*, 111–122. [CrossRef] [PubMed]
9. Rihmer, Z.; Döme, P. Major Mood Disorders and Suicidal Behavior. In *The International Handbook of Suicide Prevention: Research, Policy and Practice*; O'Connor, R.C., Pirkis, J., Eds.; John Wiley and Sons, Ltd.: Chichester, UK, 2016.
10. Malhi, G.S.; Outhred, T.; Das, P.; Morris, G.; Hamilton, A.; Mannie, Z. Modeling suicide in bipolar disorders. *Bipolar Disord.* **2018**, *20*, 334–348. [CrossRef] [PubMed]
11. Vieta, E.; Berk, M.; Schulze, T.G.; Carvalho, A.F.; Suppes, T.; Calabrese, J.R.; Gao, K.; Miskowiak, K.W.; Grande, I. Bipolar disorders. *Nat. Rev. Dis. Primers* **2018**, *4*, 18008. [CrossRef]
12. Pompili, M.; Gonda, X.; Serafini, G.; Innamorati, M.; Sher, L.; Amore, M.; Rihmer, Z.; Girardi, P. Epidemiology of suicide in bipolar disorders: A systematic review of the literature. *Bipolar Disord.* **2013**, *15*, 457–490. [CrossRef]
13. Schaffer, A.; Isometsa, E.T.; Tondo, L.; Moreno, D.H.; Sinyor, M.; Kessing, L.V.; Turecki, G.; Weizman, A.; Azorin, J.-M.; Ha, K.; et al. Epidemiology, neurobiology and pharmacological interventions related to suicide deaths and suicide attempts in bipolar disorder: Part I of a report of the International Society for Bipolar Disorders Task Force on Suicide in Bipolar Disorder. *Aust. N. Z. J. Psychiatry* **2015**, *49*, 785–802. [CrossRef]
14. Desîlets, A.; Labossière, M.; McGirr, A.; Turecki, G. Schizophrenia, Other Psychotic Disorders, and Suicidal Behavior. In *The International Handbook of Suicide Prevention*; O'Connor, R.C., Pirkis, J., Eds.; John Wiley & Sons, Ltd.: Chichester, UK, 2016.
15. Yatham, L.N.; Kennedy, S.H.; Parikh, S.V.; Schaffer, A.; Bond, D.J.; Frey, B.N.; Sharma, V.; I Goldstein, B.; Rej, S.; Beaulieu, S.; et al. Canadian Network for Mood and Anxiety Treatments (CANMAT) and International Society for Bipolar Disorders (ISBD) 2018 guidelines for the management of patients with bipolar disorder. *Bipolar Disord.* **2018**, *20*, 97–170. [CrossRef]
16. Isometsa, E. Suicidal behaviour in mood disorders—Who, when, and why? *Can. J. Psychiatry* **2014**, *59*, 120–130. [CrossRef] [PubMed]
17. Hansson, C.; Joas, E.; Palsson, E.; Hawton, K.; Runeson, B.; Landen, M. Risk factors for suicide in bipolar disorder: A cohort study of 12,850 patients. *Acta Psychiatry Scand.* **2018**, *138*, 456–463. [CrossRef] [PubMed]

18. Tondo, L.; Pompili, M.; Forte, A.; Baldessarini, R.J. Suicide attempts in bipolar disorders: Comprehensive review of 101 reports. *Acta Psychiatry Scand.* **2016**, *133*, 174–186. [CrossRef] [PubMed]
19. Schaffer, A.; Isometsa, E.T.; Tondo, L.; Moreno, D.H.; Turecki, G.; Reis, C.; Cassidy, F.; Sinyor, M.; Azorin, J.-M.; Kessing, L.V.; et al. International Society for Bipolar Disorders Task Force on Suicide: Meta-analyses and meta-regression of correlates of suicide attempts and suicide deaths in bipolar disorder. *Bipolar Disord.* **2015**, *17*, 1–16. [CrossRef] [PubMed]
20. Choi, K.W.; Na, E.J.; Hong, J.P.; Cho, M.J.; Fava, M.; Mischoulon, D.; Jeon, H.J. Comparison of suicide attempts in individuals with major depressive disorder with and without history of subthreshold hypomania: A nationwide community sample of Korean adults. *J. Affect. Disord.* **2019**, *248*, 18–25. [CrossRef] [PubMed]
21. Park, Y.M.; Lee, B.H. Treatment response in relation to subthreshold bipolarity in patients with major depressive disorder receiving antidepressant monotherapy: A post hoc data analysis (KOMDD study). *Neuropsychiatr. Dis. Treat.* **2016**, *12*, 1221–1227. [CrossRef]
22. Koirala, P.; Hu, B.; Altinay, M.; Li, M.; DiVita, A.L.; Bryant, K.A.; Karne, H.S.; Fiedorowicz, J.G.; Anan, A. Sub-threshold bipolar disorder in medication-free young subjects with major depression: Clinical characteristics and antidepressant treatment response. *J. Psychiatr. Res.* **2019**, *110*, 1–8. [CrossRef]
23. Dome, P.; Gonda, X.; Rihmer, Z. Effects of smoking on health outcomes in bipolar disorder with a special focus on suicidal behavior. *Neuropsychiatry* **2012**, *2*, 429–441. [CrossRef]
24. Latalova, K.; Kamaradova, D.; Prasko, J. Suicide in bipolar disorder: A review. *Psychiatr. Danub.* **2014**, *26*, 108–114.
25. Gonda, X.; Pompili, M.; Serafini, G.; Montebovi, F.; Campi, S.; Dome, P.; Duleba, T.; Girardi, P.; Rihmer, Z. Suicidal behavior in bipolar disorder: Epidemiology, characteristics and major risk factors. *J. Affect. Disord.* **2012**, *143*, 16–26. [CrossRef]
26. Da Silva Costa, L.; Alencar, A.P.; Nascimento Neto, P.J.; dos Santos Mdo, S.; da Silva, C.G.; Pinheiro Sde, F.; Silveira, R.T.; Bianco, B.A.V.; Junior, R.F.F.P.; De Lima, M.A.P.; et al. Risk factors for suicide in bipolar disorder: A systematic review. *J. Affect. Disord.* **2015**, *170*, 237–254. [CrossRef] [PubMed]
27. Michaels, M.S.; Balthrop, T.; Pulido, A.; Rudd, M.D.; Joiner, T.E. Is the Higher Number of Suicide Attempts in Bipolar Disorder vs. Major Depressive Disorder Attributable to Illness Severity? *Arch. Suicide Res.* **2018**, *22*, 46–56. [CrossRef] [PubMed]
28. Pallaskorpi, S.; Suominen, K.; Ketokivi, M.; Valtonen, H.; Arvilommi, P.; Mantere, O.; Leppämäki, S.; Isometsä, E. Incidence and predictors of suicide attempts in bipolar I and II disorders: A 5-year follow-up study. *Bipolar Disord.* **2017**, *19*, 13–22. [CrossRef] [PubMed]
29. Vazquez, G.H.; Gonda, X.; Lolich, M.; Tondo, L.; Baldessarini, R.J. Suicidal Risk and Affective Temperaments, Evaluated with the TEMPS-A Scale: A Systematic Review. *Harv. Rev. Psychiatry* **2018**, *26*, 8–18. [CrossRef] [PubMed]
30. Persons, J.E.; Coryell, W.H.; Solomon, D.A.; Keller, M.B.; Endicott, J.; Fiedorowicz, J.G. Mixed state and suicide: Is the effect of mixed state on suicidal behavior more than the sum of its parts? *Bipolar Disord.* **2018**, *20*, 35–41. [CrossRef] [PubMed]
31. Fiedorowicz, J.G.; Persons, J.E.; Assari, S.; Ostacher, M.J.; Zandi, P.; Wang, P.W.; Thase, M.E.; Frye, M.A.; Coryell, W. Depressive symptoms carry an increased risk for suicidal ideation and behavior in bipolar disorder without any additional contribution of mixed symptoms. *J. Affect. Disord.* **2019**, *246*, 775–782. [CrossRef] [PubMed]
32. Tidemalm, D.; Haglund, A.; Karanti, A.; Landen, M.; Runeson, B. Attempted suicide in bipolar disorder: Risk factors in a cohort of 6086 patients. *PLoS ONE* **2014**, *9*, e94097. [CrossRef]
33. Manchia, M.; Hajek, T.; O'Donovan, C.; Deiana, V.; Chillotti, C.; Ruzickova, M.; Del Zompo, M.; Alda, M. Genetic risk of suicidal behavior in bipolar spectrum disorder: Analysis of 737 pedigrees. *Bipolar Disord.* **2013**, *15*, 496–506. [CrossRef]
34. Bauer, M.; Glenn, T.; Alda, M.; Andreassen, O.A.; Angelopoulos, E.; Ardau, R.; Ayhan, Y.; Baethge, C.; Bauer, R.; Baune, B.T.; et al. Association between solar insolation and a history of suicide attempts in bipolar I disorder. *J. Psychiatr. Res.* **2019**, *113*, 1–9. [CrossRef]
35. Caribe, A.C.; Studart, P.; Bezerra-Filho, S.; Brietzke, E.; Nunes Noto, M.; Vianna-Sulzbach, M.; Kapczinski, F.; Neves, F.S.; Corrêa, H.; Miranda-Scippa, A. Is religiosity a protective factor against suicidal behavior in bipolar I outpatients? *J. Affect. Disord.* **2015**, *186*, 156–161. [CrossRef]

36. Gearing, R.E.; Alonzo, D. Religion and Suicide: New Findings. *J. Relig. Health* **2018**, *57*, 2478–2499. [CrossRef] [PubMed]
37. Schaffer, A.; Isometsa, E.T.; Azorin, J.M.; Cassidy, F.; Goldstein, T.; Rihmer, Z.; Sinyor, M.; Tondo, L.; Moreno, D.H.; Turecki, G.; et al. A review of factors associated with greater likelihood of suicide attempts and suicide deaths in bipolar disorder: Part II of a report of the International Society for Bipolar Disorders Task Force on Suicide in Bipolar Disorder. *Aust. N. Z. J. Psychiatry* **2015**, *49*, 1006–1020. [CrossRef] [PubMed]
38. Novick, D.M.; Swartz, H.A.; Frank, E. Suicide attempts in bipolar I and bipolar II disorder: A review and meta-analysis of the evidence. *Bipolar Disord.* **2010**, *12*, 1–9. [CrossRef] [PubMed]
39. Angst, J.; Sellaro, R.; Angst, F. Long-term outcome and mortality of treated versus untreated bipolar and depressed patients: A preliminary report. *Int. J. Psychiatry Clin. Pract.* **1998**, *2*, 115–119. [CrossRef] [PubMed]
40. Smith, K.A.; Cipriani, A. Lithium and suicide in mood disorders: Updated meta-review of the scientific literature. *Bipolar Disord.* **2017**, *19*, 575–586. [CrossRef] [PubMed]
41. Tondo, L.; Baldessarini, R.J. Antisuicidal Effects in Mood Disorders: Are They Unique to Lithium? *Pharmacopsychiatry* **2018**, *51*, 177–188. [CrossRef]
42. Cipriani, A.; Hawton, K.; Stockton, S.; Geddes, J.R. Lithium in the prevention of suicide in mood disorders: Updated systematic review and meta-analysis. *BMJ* **2013**, *346*, f3646. [CrossRef] [PubMed]
43. Chen, T.Y.; Kamali, M.; Chu, C.S.; Yeh, C.B.; Huang, S.Y.; Mao, W.C.; Lin, P.-Y.; Chen, Y.-W.; Tseng, P.-T.; Hsu, C.-Y. Divalproex and its effect on suicide risk in bipolar disorder: A systematic review and meta-analysis of multinational observational studies. *J. Affect. Disord.* **2019**, *245*, 812–818. [CrossRef]
44. Caley, C.F.; Perriello, E.; Golden, J. Antiepileptic drugs and suicide-related outcomes in bipolar disorder: A descriptive review of published data. *Ment. Health Clin.* **2018**, *8*, 138–147. [CrossRef]
45. Alberich, S.; Martinez-Cengotitabengoa, M.; Lopez, P.; Zorrilla, I.; Nunez, N.; Vieta, E.; González-Pinto, A. Efficacy and safety of ketamine in bipolar depression: A systematic review. *Rev. Psiquiatr. Salud Ment.* **2017**, *10*, 104–112. [CrossRef]
46. Lopez-Diaz, A.; Fernandez-Gonzalez, J.L.; Lujan-Jimenez, J.E.; Galiano-Rus, S.; Gutierrez-Rojas, L. Use of repeated intravenous ketamine therapy in treatment-resistant bipolar depression with suicidal behaviour: A case report from Spain. *Ther. Adv. Psychopharmacol.* **2017**, *7*, 137–140. [CrossRef] [PubMed]
47. Andrade, C. Ketamine for Depression, 6: Effects on Suicidal Ideation and Possible Use as Crisis Intervention in Patients at Suicide Risk. *J. Clin. Psychiatry* **2018**, *79*. [CrossRef] [PubMed]
48. Grunebaum, M.F.; Ellis, S.P.; Keilp, J.G.; Moitra, V.K.; Cooper, T.B.; Marver, J.E.; Burke, A.K.; Milak, M.S.; Sublette, M.E.; Oquendo, M.A.; et al. Ketamine versus midazolam in bipolar depression with suicidal thoughts: A pilot midazolam-controlled randomized clinical trial. *Bipolar Disord.* **2017**, *19*, 176–183. [CrossRef] [PubMed]
49. Sanacora, G.; Katz, R. Ketamine: A Review for Clinicians. *Focus* **2018**, *16*, 243–250. [CrossRef]
50. Sanches, M.; Quevedo, J.; Soares, J.C. Treatment Resistance in Bipolar Disorders. In *Treatment Resistance in Psychiatry*; Kim, Y.-K., Ed.; Springer Nature: Singapore, 2019.
51. Fountoulakis, K.N.; Grunze, H.; Vieta, E.; Young, A.; Yatham, L.; Blier, P.; Kasper, S.; Moeller, H.J. The International College of Neuro-Psychopharmacology (CINP) Treatment Guidelines for Bipolar Disorder in Adults (CINP-BD-2017), Part 3: The Clinical Guidelines. *Int. J. Neuropsychopharmacol.* **2017**, *20*, 180–195. [CrossRef] [PubMed]
52. Liang, C.S.; Chung, C.H.; Ho, P.S.; Tsai, C.K.; Chien, W.C. Superior anti-suicidal effects of electroconvulsive therapy in unipolar disorder and bipolar depression. *Bipolar Disord.* **2018**, *20*, 539–546. [CrossRef] [PubMed]
53. Bahji, A.; Hawken, E.R.; Sepehry, A.A.; Cabrera, C.A.; Vazquez, G. ECT beyond unipolar major depression: Systematic review and meta-analysis of electroconvulsive therapy in bipolar depression. *Acta Psychiatr. Scand.* **2019**, *139*, 214–226. [CrossRef] [PubMed]
54. Mendez-Bustos, P.; Calati, R.; Rubio-Ramirez, F.; Olie, E.; Courtet, P.; Lopez-Castroman, J. Effectiveness of Psychotherapy on Suicidal Risk: A Systematic Review of Observational Studies. *Front. Psychol.* **2019**, *10*, 277. [CrossRef]
55. Inder, M.L.; Crowe, M.T.; Luty, S.E.; Carter, J.D.; Moor, S.; Frampton, C.M.; Joyce, P.R. Prospective rates of suicide attempts and nonsuicidal self-injury by young people with bipolar disorder participating in a psychotherapy study. *Aust. N. Z. J. Psychiatry* **2016**, *50*, 167–173. [CrossRef]

56. Rucci, P.; Frank, E.; Kostelnik, B.; Fagiolini, A.; Mallinger, A.G.; Swartz, H.A.; Thase, M.E.; Siegel, L.; Wilson, D.; Kupfer, D.J. Suicide attempts in patients with bipolar I disorder during acute and maintenance phases of intensive treatment with pharmacotherapy and adjunctive psychotherapy. *Am. J. Psychiatry* **2002**, *159*, 1160–1164. [CrossRef]
57. Weinstein, S.M.; Cruz, R.A.; Isaia, A.R.; Peters, A.T.; West, A.E. Child- and Family-Focused Cognitive Behavioral Therapy for Pediatric Bipolar Disorder: Applications for Suicide Prevention. *Suicide Life-Threat Behav.* **2018**, *48*, 797–811. [CrossRef] [PubMed]
58. Goldstein, T.R.; Fersch-Podrat, R.K.; Rivera, M.; Axelson, D.A.; Merranko, J.; Yu, H.; Brent, D.A.; Birmaher, B. Dialectical behavior therapy for adolescents with bipolar disorder: Results from a pilot randomized trial. *J. Child Adolesc. Psychopharmacol.* **2015**, *25*, 140–149. [CrossRef] [PubMed]
59. Wasserman, D.; Rihmer, Z.; Rujescu, D.; Sarchiapone, M.; Sokolowski, M.; Titelman, D.; Zalsman, G.; Zemishlany, Z.; Carli, V. The European Psychiatric Association (EPA) guidance on suicide treatment and prevention. *Eur. Psychiatry* **2012**, *27*, 129–141. [CrossRef] [PubMed]

10

Anhedonia to Gentle Touch in Fibromyalgia: Normal Sensory Processing but Abnormal Evaluation

Rebecca Boehme [1,2,*], Helene van Ettinger-Veenstra [2,3], Håkan Olausson [1,2,4], Björn Gerdle [2,3] and Saad S. Nagi [1,4]

1 Center for Social and Affective Neuroscience, Linköping University, 58185 Linköping, Sweden; hakan.olausson@liu.se (H.O.); saad.nagi@liu.se (S.S.N.)
2 Center for Medical Image Science and Visualization (CMIV), 58185 Linköping, Sweden; helenevanettinger@gmail.com (H.v.E.-V.); bjorn.gerdle@liu.se (B.G.)
3 Pain and Rehabilitation Centre, and Department of Health, Medicine and Caring Sciences, Linköping University, 58185 Linköping, Sweden
4 Department of Clinical Neurophysiology, Linköping University, 58185 Linköping, Sweden
* Correspondence: Rebecca.bohme@liu.se

Abstract: Social touch is important for interpersonal interaction. Gentle touch and slow brushing are typically perceived as pleasant, the degree of pleasantness is linked to the activity of the C-tactile (CT) fibers, a class of unmyelinated nerves in the skin. The inability to experience pleasure in general is called anhedonia, a common phenomenon in the chronic pain condition fibromyalgia. Here, we studied the perception and cortical processing of gentle touch in a well-characterized cohort of fibromyalgia. Patients and controls participated in functional brain imaging while receiving tactile stimuli (brushing) on the forearm. They were asked to provide ratings of pleasantness of the tactile stimulus and ongoing pain. We found high distress, pain catastrophizing, and insomnia, and a low perceived state of health in fibromyalgia. Further, patients rated both slow (CT-optimal) and fast (CT-suboptimal) brushing as less pleasant than healthy participants. While there was no difference in brain activity during touch, patients showed deactivation in the right posterior insula (contralateral to the stimulated arm) during pleasantness rating and activation during pain rating. The opposite pattern was observed in healthy participants. Voxel-based morphometry analysis revealed reduced grey matter density in patients, in the bilateral hippocampus and anterior insula. Our results suggest anhedonia to gentle touch in fibromyalgia with intact early-stage sensory processing but dysfunctional evaluative processing. These findings contribute to our understanding of the mechanisms underlying anhedonia in fibromyalgia.

Keywords: touch; pain; C-tactile afferents; fibromyalgia; anhedonia; fMRI; posterior insula

---

1. Introduction

Fibromyalgia (FM) is a common, debilitating chronic pain condition. According to the American College of Rheumatology 1990 Criteria for the Classification of Fibromyalgia [1], the cardinal features comprise widespread pain and hypersensitivity, i.e., pain evoked by non-painful stimuli and exaggerated pain to painful stimuli. FM includes a myriad of other symptoms, including fatigue, sleep, and affective disturbances (e.g., anxiety and depression). The prevalence of FM is higher among females [2].

Social touch is important for human behavior and communication between individuals [3]. Pleasantness (or pleasure) associated with skin-to-skin contact is linked to a class of nerves in the skin, called C-tactile (CT) fibers. This is of considerable interest for questions about physical and social well-being and the interoceptive system [3]. CTs exhibit a unique 'inverted U-shaped' response pattern to brushing velocities, with slow brushing (1–10 cm/s, 'CT-optimal') producing a robust discharge—a stimulus that is perceived as pleasant and preferred by participants over fast brushing [4]. CTs have also been implicated in pain processing either directly or indirectly, as an allodynic substrate itself or through malfunctioning of this network [5,6].

While unmyelinated nociceptors have been the focus of earlier studies on fibromyalgia [7], less is known about the role of their low-threshold counterparts, the CTs. We have previously shown a blunted affective distinction between slow CT-optimal and fast CT-suboptimal brushing in FM patients, compared to healthy participants [8], suggesting a reduced CT input or processing in FM.

CT-optimal touch produces robust activation of the posterior insula with a somatotopic organization similar to that reported for cutaneous and muscle pain in healthy participants [9,10]. FM patients show higher activity in the insular cortex in response to painful stimuli (5), and have higher levels of glutamate in the posterior insula, an excitatory neurotransmitter associated with clinical pain and mechanical hypersensitivity in FM [11].

In the current study, we hypothesized to find differences in neural processing in the insular cortex, in response to CT-optimal touch in FM. In a group of well-characterized FM patients, we used fMRI to examine the cortical responses to slow and fast brush stroking and compared with matched healthy controls. In parallel, ratings for touch pleasantness and ongoing pain were collected. Grey matter density was also measured.

2. Materials and Methods

2.1. Participants

Female patients with a clinical diagnosis of FM, ranging between 25–55 years old, were recruited through the Pain and Rehabilitation Center at the Linköping University Hospital. These patients were recruited as part of a broader characterization of FM. Age- and gender-matched healthy controls (HC) were recruited through advertisements at the Linköping University and the University Hospital, and in the local news media. The Linköping Regional Ethics Review Board approved the study (Dnr 2016/471-32) and written informed consent was obtained after participants had read the complete study description, in accordance with the Declaration of Helsinki.

On the first visit, all participants underwent a clinical examination. To confirm the patients' eligibility, the eighteen tender points according to the FM classification criteria of the American College of Rheumatology [1] were clinically examined by senior consultants in rheumatology or pain medicine. This was performed in both patients and HC. Revised criteria for FM were recently presented [12,13], but these were not available in the finished form when the current study was designed and ethical approval was sought. The clinical examination also included registration of systolic and diastolic blood pressures. Weight (kg) and height (m) were also registered; body mass index (BMI; kg/m^2) was calculated as weight/height^2. At the time-point of the clinical examination, the subjects answered a health questionnaire covering demographic data as well as pain and psychological characteristics.

Exclusion criteria were MRI-incompatibility (claustrophobia or metal in the body), pregnancy, difficulty understanding Swedish, metabolic disease, neurological disease or severe psychiatric conditions, malignancy, rheumatoid arthritis, unregulated thyroid disease, cardiovascular disease, or lung disease. Another exclusion criterion was the inability to refrain from analgesics, including NSAIDs and sleep medication, for 48 h prior to the fMRI visit (i.e., a 48-h pharmacological washout period). Participants in the HC group reported having no current pain.

Functional imaging data of good quality were obtained for 31 patients (mean age, 39.0 ± 11.4 years) and 29 matched controls (mean age 42.7 ± 10.1 years).

2.2. Background Data

Age and gender were registered. FM patients also reported the duration of their condition in years.

2.2.1. Pain Intensity Aspects

A numeric rating scale (NRS) with anchor points 0 (denoting no pain) and 10 (denoting the worst imaginable pain) was used to capture the current pain (denoted by 'Pain Intensity Current') and the average pain intensity for the previous four weeks (denoted by 'Pain Intensity 4w').

2.2.2. Psychological Distress

The Hospital Anxiety and Depression Scale (HADS) was used to measure symptoms of anxiety and depression. The validated Swedish translation of HADS was chosen to reflect aspects of psychological distress [14,15] and had good psychometric characteristics [15,16]. HADS contains seven items in each of the depression and anxiety subscales (HAD-Depression and HAD-Anxiety). Both subscale scores ranged from 0–21. A score of 7 or less on each subscale was considered normal, a score of 8 to 10 indicated a possible abnormality, and a score of 11 or more indicated a definite abnormality [15]. In the present study, a score ≥ 11 was considered as having severe anxiety and depression symptoms.

2.2.3. Sleeping Problems

The Insomnia Severity Index (ISI) was used to quantify perceived insomnia severity. ISI captures the severity and impact of insomnia symptoms with good validity and internal consistency [17,18]. The seven items of ISI were rated on a five-point Likert scale (0–4). The scores of each item were added to calculate the total score of ISI (max = 28). The score could be divided into four categories–no insomnia (0–7), sub-threshold insomnia (8–14), moderate insomnia (15–21), and severe insomnia (22–28).

2.2.4. Pain Catastrophizing Scale (PCS)

PCS measures three dimensions of catastrophizing—rumination, magnification, and helplessness [19,20]—based on 13 items with anchor points ranging from 0 (not at all) to 4 (all the time). The current study used the total PCS (PCS-total); 52 was the maximum score according to the original scale and a high score represented a worse outcome. This instrument had good internal consistency, test-retest reliability, and validity [21].

2.2.5. Impact of the Pain Aspects

An NRS with anchor points 0 (denoted not at all) and 10 (denoted impossible to perform these activities) was used to capture to what extent the pain hindered daily activities (pain hindrance activities of daily living (ADL)), taking part in leisure activities including social and family activities (pain hindrance leisure), and working, including studies or homework (pain hindrance work). These items were only answered by the FM group.

2.2.6. The European Quality of Life Instrument (EQ-5D)

EQ-5D captured a patient's perceived state of health [22–24]. The first part of the instrument captured five dimensions—mobility, self-care, usual activities, pain/discomfort, and anxiety/depression. In the present study, we used the second part of the instrument and measured the current day's health on a 100-point scale, a thermometer-like scale (EQ-VAS) with defined endpoints (high values indicated good health and low values indicated bad health).

2.2.7. Pharmacological Treatments

Participants were asked to report their ongoing pharmacological treatments. Note that those included in the study were asked to refrain from analgesic use, including NSAIDs and sleep medication, for 48 h prior to the fMRI visit.

2.3. *Stimuli and Procedures*

2.3.1. Task

Before entering the MRI scanner, participants were instructed that they will be brushed on the forearm and were shown the rating scales. They were also brushed once on the forearm. During MRI, participants were brushed on the left forearm at two different velocities—3 cm/s (CT-optimal) and 30 cm/s (CT-suboptimal). The brusher, who was trained in the delivery of these stimuli, stood next to the scanner bore and received auditory cues over headphones. A 9-cm long line with 3-cm increments, was marked on the left forearm to aid the brusher to maintain the correct speed. The task consisted of three runs of 6 min each. In between runs, the participants were asked if they were alright in the scanner and okay to continue with the next run. In total, there were 15 repetitions of slow and fast brushing blocks, each lasting 12 s. The intertrial interval (ITI) between blocks was 10 to 12 s. The order of brushing velocities was randomized. During ITIs, participants looked at a fixation cross. Three times per condition (slow or fast), following a 10 to 12-s ITI, a question appeared on the screen asking the participant to rate the pleasantness of the brushing ("How pleasant is the stimulus?") and if they felt any pain ("Do you feel any pain?"). We formulated the latter question in this specific way because we assumed it might be difficult for the FM group to disentangle ongoing pain and specific pain related to the stimulus. This rating was therefore to be understood as rating of any ongoing pain. Using a button box in their right hand, participants moved a cursor on a visual analog scale (VAS) between the endpoints "unpleasant–pleasant" or "no pain–intense pain" (in Swedish). During analysis, the cursor positions were converted to their numerical values, ranging from −10 to +10 for pleasantness and 0 to 20 for pain. The pain ratings were not specifically related to brush-evoked sensation but to the subjects' general pain level.

2.3.2. MRI

Participants laid comfortably in a 3.0 Tesla Siemens scanner (Prisma, Siemens, Erlangen, Germany). Their left arm was placed on their belly and propped up by pillows. A 12-channel head coil was used to acquire 295 T2-weighted echo-planar images (EPI) per run, containing 48 multiband slices (TR = 1030 ms, TE = 30 ms, slice thickness = 3 mm, matrix size = 64 × 64, field of view = 488 × 488 mm, in-plane voxel resolution = 3 mm^2, flip angle = 63°). T1-weighted anatomical images were also acquired.

2.3.3. Analysis

Behavioral data were analyzed using SPSS (IBM Corp., Armonk, NY, USA). Ratings for slow and fast blocks were averaged. Ratings of the patient group were normally distributed; ratings of the control group were not due to a strong ceiling effect. Ratings were compared between conditions using paired t-test (FM) and Wilcoxon test (HC), and between groups, using Mann–Whitney U test. p-values < 0.05 were considered significant.

Functional MRI data were analyzed using statistical parametric mapping (SPM12, Wellcome Department of Imaging Neuroscience, London, UK; http://www.fil.ion.ucl.ac.uk/spm) in Matlab R2016a (The MathWorks, Natick, MA, USA). The following steps were performed—motion correction, co-registration of the mean EPI and the anatomical image, spatial normalization to the MNI T1 template, and segmentation of the T1 image, using the unified segmentation approach [25]. Normalization parameters were applied to all EPIs. All images were spatially smoothed with an isotropic Gaussian kernel of 6 mm full width, at half maximum. For statistical analysis of the BOLD response, the general linear model approach was used as implemented in SPM12. Using a block-design, the conditions (slow and fast) and the rating phase were convolved with the hemodynamic response function. Motion parameters were added as regressors of no interest. Family-wise-error (FWE) correction on the voxel level was used to correct for multiple comparisons on the whole-brain level and using small volume correction based on our a priori regions of interest (ROI). Based on previous studies [10,26], we were specifically interested in posterior insula activations, therefore, a posterior insula mask was used for small volume corrections (SVC) [27].

2.3.4. VBM

Voxel-based morphometry (VBM) was estimated using the VBM routine provided by the CAT12 toolbox (Gaser & Dahnke, Jena University Hospital, Departments of Psychiatry and Neurology) in SPM12. Total intracranial volume was included as a covariate. Groups were compared using a *t*-test at the whole brain level.

3. Results

3.1. Clinical Characteristics

The disease duration in the FM cohort was 4.4 years, on average, since diagnosis and as expected, they had a high number of tender points, i.e., at the group level, >16 out of 18. In HC, the tender points were scarcely found. FM patients had significantly higher blood pressure and BMI than HC. While HC reported no pain, both pain intensity measures (current and at 4 weeks) in FM patients were above 5 on the NRS. Distress, pain catastrophizing, and insomnia (HADS, PCS, and ISI) were significantly higher and overall health (EQ-VAS) was significantly lower in FM patients (Table 1).

Table 1. Age, pain characteristics, psychological variables, the impact of pain and health aspects in the fibromyalgia group (FM) and in the healthy controls (HC); mean and one standard deviation (SD).

Group	HC	$n = 29$	FM	$n = 31$	Statistics
Variables	**Mean**	**SD**	**Mean**	**SD**	***p*-Value**
Age (years)	42.7	10.1	39.2	11.4	0.219
Systolic BP (mm Hg)	113.2	8.8	121.5	12.9	0.006
Diastolic BP (mm Hg)	75.3	8.5	80.6	10.6	0.040
Number of tender points	0.3	0.9	16.7	1.5	<0.001
FM duration (years)			4.4	5.0	NA
Height (m)	1.69	0.06	1.66	0.06	0.090
Weight (kg)	68.4	10.9	81.4	19.2	0.002
BMI (kg/m^2)	23.8	3.1	29.3	6.3	<0.001
Pain intensity current	0.0	0.0	5.7	1.8	<0.001
Pain intensity 4w	0.0	0.0	5.9	1.8	<0.001
HADS-Depression	1.4	1.7	6.0	3.6	<0.001
HADS-Anxiety	2.6	2.3	7.8	4.0	<0.001
PCS	11.8	9.2	20.3	10.5	0.001
ISI	4.5	4.5	13.4	5.9	<0.001
Pain hindrance ADL			5.7	2.3	NA
Pain hindrance leisure			5.7	2.5	NA
Pain hindrance work			4.9	2.7	NA
EQ-VAS	86.8	7.8	53.3	19.5	<0.001

BP = blood pressure; HADS = Hospital Anxiety and Depression Scale; PCS = Pain Catastrophizing Scale; ISI = Insomnia Severity Index; EQ-VAS = the health scale of EQ-5D (European Quality of Life instrument); w = weeks; NA = not applicable.

Four FM patients had more severe symptoms (≥11) according to the HADS-Depression subscale, compared to none in the HC. Corresponding figures for the HADS-Anxiety were eight patients in FM and none in HC. At least moderate insomnia (≥15) was found in 14 FM patients and in one HC.

Three FM patients and 26 HC did not use any pharmacological drugs. Those using medication among the FM cohort were often on several substances (range 1–5), including paracetamol ($n = 19$), antidepressant medication (selective serotonin reuptake inhibitor and serotonin-norepinephrine reuptake inhibitor, $n = 12$), tricyclic antidepressants ($n = 9$), opioids ($n = 7$), vitamins (e.g., B12, $n = 5$), medication for high blood pressure ($n = 3$), proton-pump inhibitors ($n = 3$), gabapentin ($n = 2$), antihistamine ($n = 2$), and other medications ($n = 9$). HC reported sumatriptan ($n = 1$), tricyclic antidepressant ($n = 1$), methotrexate ($n = 1$), and metoprolol ($n = 1$). All participants refrained from analgesics including NSAIDs and sleep medication for 48 h prior to the fMRI visit (cf. Methods).

3.2. Behavior

HC rated slow and fast brushing as similarly pleasant (Figure 1, top panel). Within the FM patient group, slow brushing was rated as pleasant, while fast brushing was rated as unpleasant. Affective ratings to slow and fast brushing were lower in FM patients than HC. Pain was rated very low in HC, as expected (Figure 1, bottom panel). Notwithstanding, HC reported less pain to slow than to fast brushing. In FM, pain was also rated somewhat lower after slow than after fast brushing. As described in the Methods, the pain ratings were not specifically related to brush-evoked sensation but to the subjects' general pain level. In summary, the HC and FM groups differed in their ratings of touch pleasantness and ongoing pain. FM rated both slow and fast brushing as less pleasant than HC. In addition, pain ratings in FM were higher than HC.

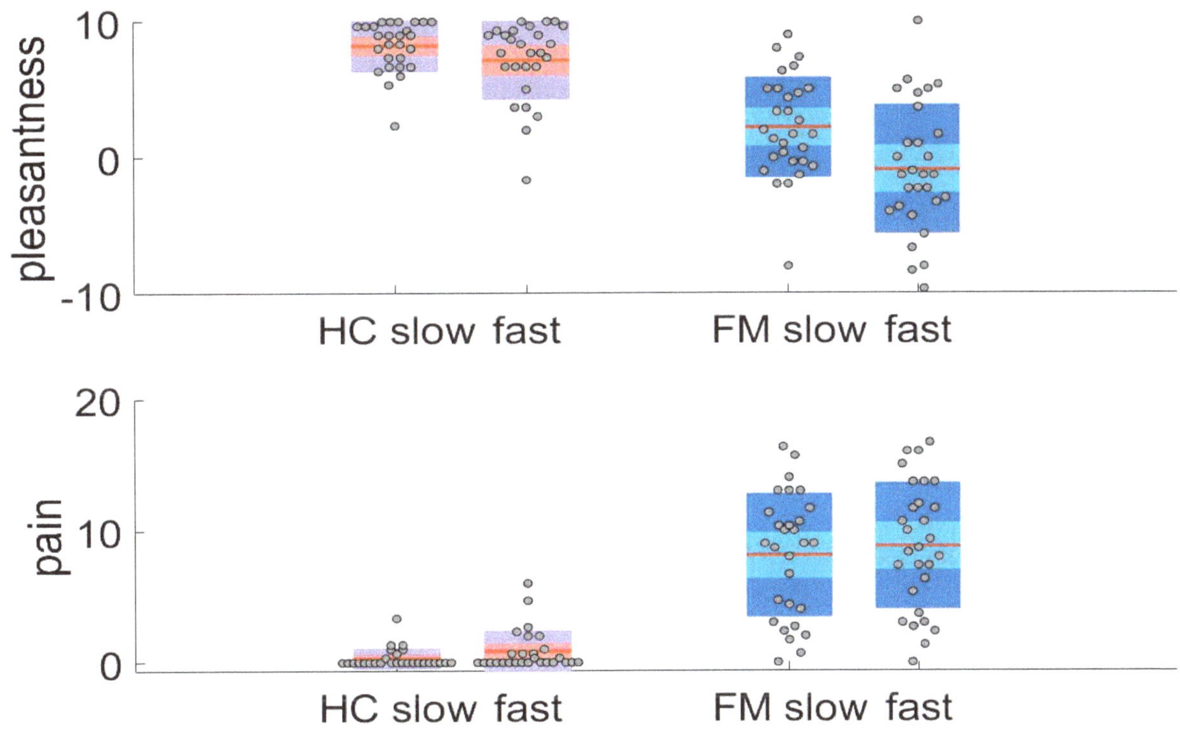

Figure 1. Ratings of touch pleasantness and pain during fMRI. Top: HC rated slow and fast brushing as similarly pleasant on a VAS (mean slow = 8.2 ± 1.9, mean fast = 7.2 ± 3, $Z = -1.6$, $p < 0.103$). FM rated slow brushing as significantly more pleasant than fast (mean slow = 2.1 ± 3.7, mean fast = −0.9 ± 4.7, $t = 4.9$, $p < 0.001$). Groups differed in their ratings of the different conditions (Mann–Whitney U test, pleasantness ratings: slow $Z = -5.7$, $p < 0.001$, fast $Z = -5.4$, $p < 0.001$). Bottom: HC rated less pain after slow than after fast brushing on a VAS (mean slow = 0.33 ± 0.04, mean fast = 0.86 ± 1.53, $Z = -2.4$, $p < 0.017$). FM rated less pain after slow than after fast brushing (mean slow = 8.3 ± 4.7, mean fast = 9 ± 4.9, $t = -2.7$, $p < 0.011$). The groups differed in their ratings of the different conditions (Mann–Whitney U test, pain ratings: slow $Z = -6.2$, $p < 0.001$, fast $Z = -5.9$, $p < 0.001$). Note that the pain ratings were not specifically related to brush-evoked sensation but to the subjects´ general pain level.

3.3. Functional Imaging

Across all participants, we found a significantly stronger activation for slow compared to fast brushing in the right posterior insula (contralateral to the stimulated forearm) (Figure 2). There was no main effect of group and no difference between groups for separate slow or fast brushing.

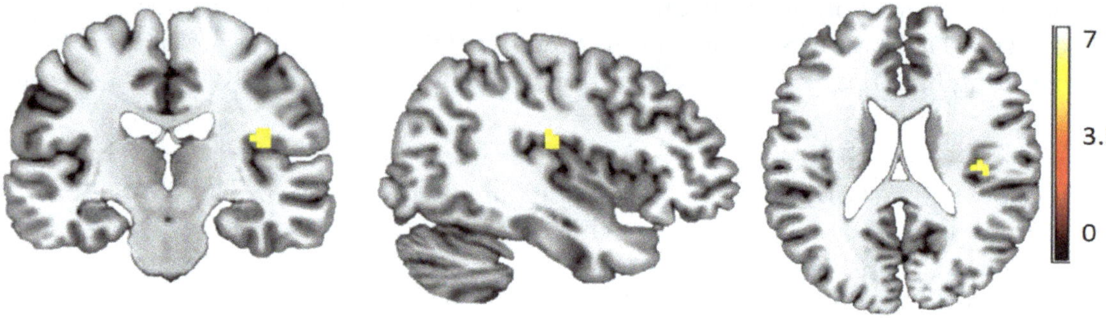

Figure 2. More activation in the posterior insula during slow brushing compared to fast brushing. In all participants, [39–1920] $t = 6.25$, $Z = 5.79$, FWE corrected at the whole-brain level $p < 0.05$, color scale depicts t-values for the contrast slow > fast.

Since we found a difference in ratings between HC and FM, we also explored group differences during the rating period. Activation in posterior insula was related to whether the subjects were rating on the pleasantness or the pain scale (Figure 3A). While HC showed activation in this area during pleasantness ratings and deactivation during pain ratings, patients showed the opposite pattern, i.e., deactivation during pleasantness ratings and activation during pain ratings (Figure 3B).

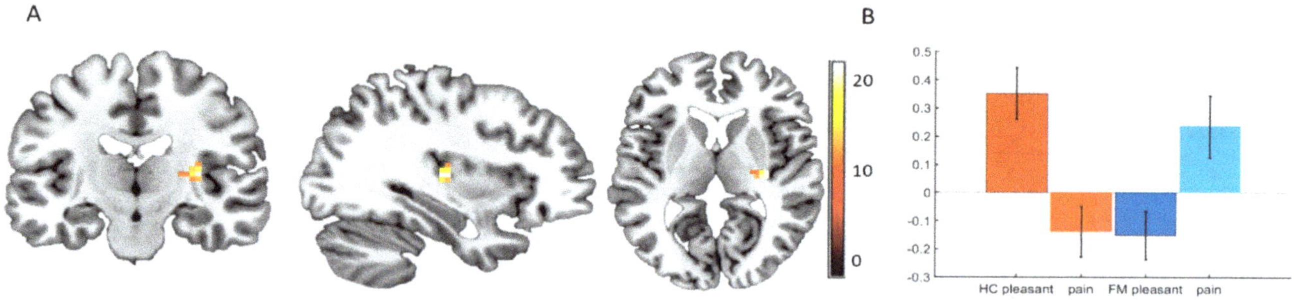

Figure 3. Insula activity differs between FM patients and HC during rating period. (**A**) Interaction group*ratings type (pleasantness and pain). During the rating period, we found a group*rating-type interaction in the posterior insula ([33–198], F = 22.67, Z = 4.39 p = 0.001 FWE, SVC for posterior insula), color scale depicts the F-values. (**B**) Beta values extracted from a 6 mm radius sphere around the peak of the interaction in the posterior insula [33–198].

3.4. Voxel-Based Morphometry

VBM analysis comparing HC and FM revealed reduced grey matter density in patients in the bilateral hippocampus and anterior insula. This difference was even stronger when including age as a covariate of no interest (Figure 4 and Table 2). There was no area where FM had a higher grey matter density than HC.

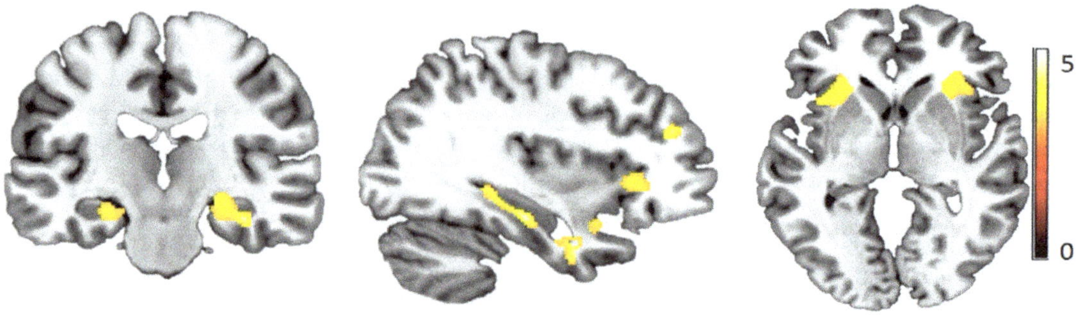

Figure 4. Reduced grey matter in FM. FM showed reduced grey matter density in bilateral insula and hippocampus ([35–19–1], $p < 0.001$, cluster size = 50), color scale depicts the t-values.

Table 2. Regions with reduced grey matter density in FM compared to HC. Age was included as covariate of no interest. *t*-test at the whole brain level, thresholded at $p < 0.001$ uncorrected.

Region	x	y	z	Hemi-Sphere	Cluster Size	*t*	*p*
Hippocampus	36	−22.5	−18	Right	469	4.98	>0.0001
Parahippocampal Gyrus	37.5	−31.5	−12	Right		4.68	>0.0001
	24	−19.5	−9			3.91	0.0001
	−24	−19.5	−16.5	Left	146	3.94	0.0002
Middle Frontal Gyrus	31.5	45	22.5	Right	233	4.69	>0.0001
Rectal Gyrus	3	37.5	−28.5	Right	339	4.51	>0.0001
Uncus	34.5	0	−34.5	Right	505	4.43	>0.0001
	−34.5	1.5	−28.5	Left	215	3.69	0.0003
Superior Temporal Gyrus	46.5	0	−16.5	Right		3.91	0.0001
	−40.5	6	−18	Left		3.49	0.0005
Subcallosal Gyrus	13.5	6	−19.5	Right	288	4.29	>0.0001
Anterior Cingulate	9	18	−12	Right		3.51	0.0004
Anterior Insula	−28.5	21	1.5	Left	764	4.20	>0.0001
	27	25.5	0	Right	430	4.13	0.0001
Middle Occipital Gyrus	−22.5	−88.5	4.5	Left	175	4.18	0.0001
Inferior Frontal Gyrus	37.5	24	−1.5	Right		3.77	0.0002
Cingulate Gyrus	−6	−10.5	43.5	Left	131	4.07	0.0001
	−9	−10.5	36			3.72	0.0001
Cerebellum	−22.5	−31.5	−33	Left	72	3.69	0.0003

4. Discussion

In the current study, we found intact neural processing of positive affective touch in FM patients. However, slow soft brushing was reported as less pleasant by FM patients than healthy controls. We found that FM patients differed from HC during the rating of perceived pleasantness and pain. FM patients showed deactivation in the right posterior insula during the pleasantness rating and activation during the pain rating, the opposite pattern of what was observed in the HC.

4.1. Behavior

The pathophysiology of FM is not well-understood. Both peripheral and central nervous system alterations are involved in the development and maintenance of FM. Hence, alterations in the brain including neuroinflammation and activation of glial cells, nociception-driven amplification of neural signaling (central sensitization), opioidergic dysregulation, and impaired top-down modulation were found, as well as signs of systemic low-grade inflammation (e.g., regarding cytokine profile and inflammatory lipids) and nociceptor and muscle protein changes [28–40]. In an earlier psychophysical study in FM patients, we found that pleasantness ratings to brushing were normal, but the distinction between slow CT-optimal and fast CT-suboptimal brushing was diminished [8]. In the current study, we found that while the affective touch sensitivity (slow versus fast) was preserved, the pleasantness ratings were significantly lower in FM. Despite these differences which, in part at least, could be due to the heterogeneity of the condition [41], there is likely a disturbance in the affective touch system. To confirm whether this has a peripheral involvement would require electrophysiological recordings (microneurography) from CT afferents in FM patients.

The finding that HC did not rate the pleasantness of slow and fast brushing differently needs further consideration. Although average pleasantness ratings were descriptively higher for slow than for fast brushing, they were not statistically different. Previous studies have reported that people rate slow, CT-optimal brushing velocities as more pleasant than fast, CT-non-optimal brushing [3,26,42]. However, a recent study challenged the view of an inverted U-shaped curve for pleasantness ratings that peaks at the CT-optimal velocity, suggesting that the inverted U-shape can only be found as a group average [43]. Our sample might have contained healthy individuals who did not differentiate as much between a slow and fast touch. Another, possibly complementary explanation, might be a ceiling effect. This might be driven by a number of factors; the MRI-scanner environment was loud, uncomfortable, and boring, so any positive stimulus might be evaluated as especially pleasant. In addition, the combination with a question on pain experience might drive an overly positive evaluation of the brushing stimuli.

4.2. Functional Imaging

We found differential processing during the evaluative period for the two groups and conditions. While HC showed activation in posterior insula during pleasantness evaluation and deactivation during pain evaluation, FM showed deactivation during pleasantness evaluation and activation during pain evaluation. This result should be considered preliminary as it was the result of an exploratory analysis. That the cluster of the interaction effect did not directly overlap with the main effect of slow versus fast touch was not surprising, since the evaluative processing of the current experience was a different, hierarchically higher processing, and might therefore have involved different clusters within the insula [44–48].

FM patients display hyper-sensitivity to a range of sensory stimuli [49], so it has been suggested that this might be a general hypersensitivity syndrome [50]. Our results suggest that FM patients do not exhibit hypersensitivity to pleasant touch at an early processing stage, as we found no difference in neural activation in the posterior insula. However, we found altered activation patterns during the evaluation of positive stimuli and reporting of current pain levels, suggesting dysfunctional evaluative processes. This was in line with other studies; for instance, a study in which FM patients were compared to subjects with masochistic behavior found an alteration in the late response to tactile stimulation in the primary somatosensory cortex, as measured by magnetoencephalography [51]. The amplitude of this cortical response was inversely correlated with pain catastrophizing. Dysfunctional evaluative processing of a pleasant stimulus might be associated with anhedonia in FM. FM patients are less efficient at modulating their pain perception through concomitant positive stimuli [52], however, we found a small but significant reduction in pain ratings after slow brushing (rated as pleasant by the patients). Pain catastrophizing affects pain sensitivity (i.e., pain thresholds for pressure, cold, or heat) as reported in various cohorts of patients with chronic pain [53,54]. However, correlations are moderate, and the pain sensitivity is not solely explained by psychological aspects. Moreover, catastrophizing is related to fear of pain but also these correlations are moderate [55–57].

4.3. VBM

Alterations in grey matter in many brain regions related to pain processing have been reported in several studies (for review see [58]). These include grey matter increases in the cerebellum and the striatum [59] and decreases in the brainstem, anterior and posterior cingulate cortices, prefrontal cortex, parahippocampal gyrus, and hippocampus [60,61]. For certain areas, interaction with age was also reported, e.g., increased grey matter in the insula of patients younger than 50 years [62]. In the current study, we found decreased grey matter density in FM, in the bilateral hippocampus and insula—a reduction that was more pronounced when age was included (as a covariate of no interest). However, we found no brain region where FM patients had higher grey matter density than HC.

The hippocampal grey matter is decreased in people suffering from stress [63] and post-traumatic stress disorder [64]. This is consistent with a high prevalence of early life stress and adverse events in FM [65,66]. In our FM cohort, we found high distress, pain catastrophizing and insomnia, and a low perceived state of health. The insula plays an important role in the perception of one's own body and sensations created within [48], specifically pain [67]. The anterior insula is involved in stratifying sensations into painful and non-painful [68]. The reduction in the anterior insular grey matter observed here might relate to alterations in the pain network in FM, as has been suggested previously [69].

4.4. Limitations and Future Direction

There are several limitations that need to be considered when interpreting our results. FM is a condition of highly varied symptoms and severity; therefore, patient samples tend to be heterogeneous. Larger and longitudinal studies are needed to distinguish subgroups within FM. Here, we focused on brushing for its affective attribute and link to C-tactile fibers, and questionnaires to capture the clinical characteristics, but we did not perform a detailed battery of quantitative somatosensory tests [70–72]; the combination of these could provide important insights into the peripheral nerve function, the role of top-down modulation, and the broader interplay between somatosensory and affective systems in aberrant pain states. To further disentangle perception and evaluation of sensory inputs, future studies could compare measures of hypersensitivity in the tactile domain with other sensory domains [73]. Physical activity is another important factor—while exercise leads to hypoalgesia in healthy individuals, it leads to hyperalgesia in patients with FM [74]. Further, FM patients have a heightened sensitivity to activity-related increases in pain [56]. Here, we simply asked patients to rate the extent to which pain affected their activities of daily living, leisure, and work. In future studies it would be interesting to explore this in detail using, for instance, the Sensitivity to Physical Activity (SPA) measures that are associated with clinical indices of pain hypersensitivity [75]. Another interesting future direction would be to focus on neurotransmitters such as glutamate, which is elevated in the insula in FM [11]. Glutamate could be tracked using biosensors [76] or could be measured in the brain using magnetic resonance spectroscopy [77], and these measures could then be related to behavioral and functional differences in FM patients.

Taken together, our results suggest intact early-stage sensory processing of positive tactile stimuli but dysfunctional evaluative processing. These findings contribute to our understanding of the mechanisms underlying anhedonia in FM.

Author Contributions: Conceptualization, B.G., H.O., and H.v.E.-V.; methodology, B.G., H.O., S.S.N.; software, R.B. and H.v.E.-V.; formal analysis, R.B.; investigation, S.S.N., R.B., and H.v.E.-V., B.G.; resources, B.G. and H.O.; data curation, R.B., S.S.N., H.v.E.-V., and B.G.; writing—original draft preparation, R.B.; writing—review and editing, R.B., S.S.N., H.O., and B.G.; visualization, R.B.; supervision, H.O. and B.G.; project administration, B.G.; funding acquisition, R.B., B.G., H.O., and S.S.N. All authors have read and agreed to the published version of the manuscript.

Acknowledgments: We would like to thank research nurse Eva-Britt Lind and research physiotherapist Ulrika Wentzel Olausson at the Pain and Rehabilitation Centre, University hospital, Linköping, for valuable help during the recruitment process and sample collection.

References

1. Wolfe, F.; Smythe, H.A.; Yunus, M.B.; Bennett, R.M.; Bombardier, C.; Goldenberg, D.L.; Tugwell, P.; Campbell, S.M.; Abeles, M.; Clark, P.; et al. The American College of Rheumatology 1990 Criteria for the Classification of Fibromyalgia. Report of the Multicenter Criteria Committee. *Arthritis Rheum.* **1990**, *33*, 160–172. [CrossRef] [PubMed]
2. Wolfe, F.; Ross, K.; Anderson, J.; Russell, I.J.; Hebert, L. The prevalence and characteristics of fibromyalgia in the general population. *Arthritis Rheum.* **1995**, *38*, 19–28. [CrossRef] [PubMed]
3. McGlone, F.; Wessberg, J.; Olausson, H. Discriminative and affective touch: Sensing and feeling. *Neuron* **2014**, *82*, 737–755. [CrossRef] [PubMed]
4. Löken, L.S.; Wessberg, J.; McGlone, F.; Olausson, H. Coding of pleasant touch by unmyelinated afferents in humans. *Nat. Neurosci.* **2009**, *12*, 547. [CrossRef]
5. Liljencrantz, J.; Strigo, I.; Ellingsen, D.; Krämer, H.; Lundblad, L.; Nagi, S.; Leknes, S.; Olausson, H. Slow brushing reduces heat pain in humans. *Eur. J. Pain* **2017**, *21*, 1173–1185. [CrossRef] [PubMed]
6. Nagi, S.S.; Rubin, T.K.; Chelvanayagam, D.K.; Macefield, V.G.; Mahns, D.A. Allodynia mediated by C-tactile afferents in human hairy skin. *J. Physiol.* **2011**, *589*, 4065–4075. [CrossRef]

7. Serra, J.; Collado, A.; Solà, R.; Antonelli, F.; Torres, X.; Salgueiro, M.; Quiles, C.; Bostock, H. Hyperexcitable C nociceptors in fibromyalgia. *Ann. Neurol.* **2014**, *75*, 196–208. [CrossRef]
8. Case, L.K.; Ceko, M.; Gracely, J.L.; Richards, E.A.; Olausson, H.; Bushnell, M.C. Touch Perception Altered by Chronic Pain and by Opioid Blockade. *eNeuro* **2016**, *3*, ENEURO.0138-15.2016. [CrossRef]
9. Henderson, L.A.; Gandevia, S.C.; Macefield, V.G. Somatotopic organization of the processing of muscle and cutaneous pain in the left and right insula cortex: A single-trial fMRI study. *Pain* **2007**, *128*, 20–30. [CrossRef]
10. Bjornsdotter, M.; Loken, L.; Olausson, H.; Vallbo, A.; Wessberg, J. Somatotopic organization of gentle touch processing in the posterior insular cortex. *J. Neurosci.* **2009**, *29*, 9314–9320. [CrossRef]
11. Harris, R.E.; Sundgren, P.C.; Pang, Y.; Hsu, M.; Petrou, M.; Kim, S.H.; McLean, S.A.; Gracely, R.H.; Clauw, D.J. Dynamic levels of glutamate within the insula are associated with improvements in multiple pain domains in fibromyalgia. *Arthritis Rheum.* **2008**, *58*, 903–907. [CrossRef] [PubMed]
12. Wolfe, F.; Clauw, D.J.; Fitzcharles, M.A.; Goldenberg, D.L.; Hauser, W.; Katz, R.L.; Mease, P.J.; Russell, A.S.; Russell, I.J.; Walitt, B. 2016 Revisions to the 2010/2011 fibromyalgia diagnostic criteria. *Semin. Arthritis Rheum.* **2016**, *46*, 319–329. [CrossRef] [PubMed]
13. Arnold, L.M.; Bennett, R.M.; Crofford, L.J.; Dean, L.E.; Clauw, D.J.; Goldenberg, D.L.; Fitzcharles, M.A.; Paiva, E.S.; Staud, R.; Sarzi-Puttini, P.; et al. AAPT Diagnostic Criteria for Fibromyalgia. *J. Pain* **2019**, *20*, 611–628. [CrossRef]
14. Lisspers, J.; Nygren, A.; Söderman, E. Hospital Anxiety and Depression Scale (HAD): Some psychometric data for a Swedish sample. *Acta Psychiatr. Scand.* **1997**, *96*, 281–286. [CrossRef] [PubMed]
15. Zigmond, A.S.; Snaith, R.P. The hospital anxiety and depression scale. *Acta Psychiatr. Scand.* **1983**, *67*, 361–370. [CrossRef] [PubMed]
16. Bjelland, I.; Dahl, A.A.; Haug, T.T.; Neckelmann, D. The validity of the Hospital Anxiety and Depression Scale. An updated literature review. *J. Psychosom. Res.* **2002**, *52*, 69–77. [CrossRef]
17. Bastien, C.H.; Vallieres, A.; Morin, C.M. Validation of the Insomnia Severity Index as an outcome measure for insomnia research. *Sleep Med.* **2001**, *2*, 297–307. [CrossRef]
18. Morin, C.M.; Belleville, G.; Belanger, L.; Ivers, H. The Insomnia Severity Index: Psychometric indicators to detect insomnia cases and evaluate treatment response. *Sleep* **2011**, *34*, 601–608. [CrossRef]
19. Miro, J.; Nieto, R.; Huguet, A. The Catalan version of the Pain Catastrophizing Scale: A useful instrument to assess catastrophic thinking in whiplash patients. *J. Pain* **2008**, *9*, 397–406. [CrossRef]
20. Sullivan, M.; Bishop, S.; Pivik, J. The Pain catastrophizing scale: Development and validation. *Psychol. Assess.* **1995**, *7*, 524–532. [CrossRef]
21. Kemani, M.K.; Grimby-Ekman, A.; Lundgren, J.; Sullivan, M.; Lundberg, M. Factor structure and internal consistency of a Swedish version of the Pain Catastrophizing Scale. *Acta Anaesthesiol. Scand.* **2019**, *63*, 259–266. [CrossRef] [PubMed]
22. EuroQol. EuroQol: A new facility for the measurement of health-related quality of life. *Health Policy* **1990**, *16*, 199–208. [CrossRef]
23. Brooks, R. EuroQol: The current state of play. *Health Policy* **1996**, *37*, 53–72. [CrossRef]
24. Dolan, P.; Sutton, M. Mapping visual analogue scale health state valuations onto standard gamble and time trade-off values. *Soc. Sci. Med.* **1997**, *44*, 1519–1530. [CrossRef]
25. Ashburner, J.; Friston, K.J. Unified segmentation. *Neuroimage* **2005**, *26*, 839–851. [CrossRef]
26. Morrison, I.; Bjornsdotter, M.; Olausson, H. Vicarious responses to social touch in posterior insular cortex are tuned to pleasant caressing speeds. *J. Neurosci.* **2011**, *31*, 9554–9562. [CrossRef]
27. Larsson, M.B.; Tillisch, K.; Craig, A.; Engström, M.; Labus, J.; Naliboff, B.; Lundberg, P.; Ström, M.; Mayer, E.A.; Walter, S.A. Brain responses to visceral stimuli reflect visceral sensitivity thresholds in patients with irritable bowel syndrome. *Gastroenterology* **2012**, *142*, 463–472.e3. [CrossRef]
28. Backryd, E.; Tanum, L.; Lind, A.L.; Larsson, A.; Gordh, T. Evidence of both systemic inflammation and neuroinflammation in fibromyalgia patients, as assessed by a multiplex protein panel applied to the cerebrospinal fluid and to plasma. *J. Pain Res.* **2017**, *10*, 515–525. [CrossRef]
29. Furer, V.; Hazan, E.; Mor, A.; Segal, M.; Katav, A.; Aloush, V.; Elkayam, O.; George, J.; Ablin, J.N. Elevated Levels of Eotaxin-2 in Serum of Fibromyalgia Patients. *Pain Res. Manag.* **2018**, *2018*, 7257681. [CrossRef]
30. Rodriguez-Pinto, I.; Agmon-Levin, N.; Howard, A.; Shoenfeld, Y. Fibromyalgia and cytokines. *Immunol. Lett.* **2014**, *161*, 200–203. [CrossRef]

31. Stensson, N.; Ghafouri, N.; Ernberg, M.; Mannerkorpi, K.; Kosek, E.; Gerdle, B.; Ghafouri, B. The Relationship of Endocannabinoidome Lipid Mediators With Pain and Psychological Stress in Women With Fibromyalgia: A Case-Control Study. *J. Pain* **2018**, *19*, 1318–1328. [CrossRef] [PubMed]
32. Sluka, K.A.; Clauw, D.J. Neurobiology of fibromyalgia and chronic widespread pain. *Neuroscience* **2016**, *338*, 114–129. [CrossRef] [PubMed]
33. Schrepf, A.; Harper, D.E.; Harte, S.E.; Wang, H.; Ichesco, E.; Hampson, J.P.; Zubieta, J.K.; Clauw, D.J.; Harris, R.E. Endogenous opioidergic dysregulation of pain in fibromyalgia: A PET and fMRI study. *Pain* **2016**, *157*, 2217–2225. [CrossRef] [PubMed]
34. Üçeyler, N.; Sommer, C. Small nerve fiber pathology. In *Fibromylagia Syndrome and Widespread Pain—From Construction to Relevant Recognition*; Häuser, W., Perrot, S., Eds.; Wolters Kluwer: Philadelphia, PA, USA, 2018; pp. 204–214.
35. Gerdle, B.; Larsson, B. Muscle. In *Fibromyalgia Syndrome and Widespread Pain—From Construction to Relevant Recognition*; Häuser, W., Perrot, S., Eds.; Wolters Kluwer: Philadelphia, PA, USA, 2018; pp. 215–231.
36. Albrecht, D.S.; Forsberg, A.; Sandstrom, A.; Bergan, C.; Kadetoff, D.; Protsenko, E.; Lampa, J.; Lee, Y.C.; Hoglund, C.O.; Catana, C.; et al. Brain glial activation in fibromyalgia—A multi-site positron emission tomography investigation. *Brain Behav. Immun.* **2019**, *75*, 72–83. [CrossRef]
37. Jensen, K.B.; Kosek, E.; Petzke, F.; Carville, S.; Fransson, P.; Marcus, H.; Williams, S.C.R.; Choy, E.; Giesecke, T.; Mainguy, Y.; et al. Evidence of dysfunctional pain inhibition in Fibromyalgia reflected in rACC during provoked pain. *Pain* **2009**, *144*, 95–100. [CrossRef]
38. Olausson, P.; Gerdle, B.; Ghafouri, N.; Larsson, B.; Ghafouri, B. Identification of proteins from interstitium of trapezius muscle in women with chronic myalgia using microdialysis in combination with proteomics. *PLoS ONE* **2012**, *7*, e52560. [CrossRef]
39. Olausson, P.; Gerdle, B.; Ghafouri, N.; Sjostrom, D.; Blixt, E.; Ghafouri, B. Protein alterations in women with chronic widespread pain—An explorative proteomic study of the trapezius muscle. *Sci. Rep.* **2015**, *5*, 11894. [CrossRef]
40. Hadrevi, J.; Ghafouri, B.; Larsson, B.; Gerdle, B.; Hellstrom, F. Multivariate modeling of proteins related to trapezius myalgia, a comparative study of female cleaners with or without pain. *PLoS ONE* **2013**, *8*, e73285. [CrossRef]
41. Hurtig, I.M.; Raak, R.I.; Kendall, S.A.; Gerdle, B.; Wahren, L.K. Quantitative sensory testing in fibromyalgia patients and in healthy subjects: Identification of subgroups. *Clin. J. Pain* **2001**, *17*, 316–322. [CrossRef]
42. Olausson, H.; Wessberg, J.; Morrison, I.; McGlone, F.; Vallbo, A. The neurophysiology of unmyelinated tactile afferents. *Neurosci. Biobehav. Rev.* **2010**, *34*, 185–191. [CrossRef]
43. Croy, I.; Bierling, A.; Sailer, U.; Ackerley, R. Individual variability of pleasantness ratings to stroking touch over different velocities. *Neuroscience* **2020**, in press. [CrossRef] [PubMed]
44. Frot, M.; Faillenot, I.; Mauguière, F. Processing of nociceptive input from posterior to anterior insula in humans. *Hum. Brain Mapp.* **2014**, *35*, 5486–5499. [CrossRef] [PubMed]
45. Kurth, F.; Zilles, K.; Fox, P.T.; Laird, A.R.; Eickhoff, S.B. A link between the systems: Functional differentiation and integration within the human insula revealed by meta-analysis. *Brain Struct. Funct.* **2010**, *214*, 519–534. [CrossRef] [PubMed]
46. Uddin, L.Q.; Kinnison, J.; Pessoa, L.; Anderson, M.L. Beyond the tripartite cognition–emotion–interoception model of the human insular cortex. *J. Cognit. Neurosci.* **2014**, *26*, 16–27. [CrossRef]
47. Evrard, H.C. The organization of the primate insular cortex. *Front. Neuroanat.* **2019**, *13*, 43. [CrossRef]
48. Craig, A.D. How do you feel—Now? The anterior insula and human awareness. *Nat. Rev. Neurosci.* **2009**, *10*, 59–70. [CrossRef]
49. Geisser, M.E.; Glass, J.M.; Rajcevska, L.D.; Clauw, D.J.; Williams, D.A.; Kileny, P.R.; Gracely, R.H. A psychophysical study of auditory and pressure sensitivity in patients with fibromyalgia and healthy controls. *J. Pain* **2008**, *9*, 417–422. [CrossRef]
50. B Yunus, M. Editorial review (thematic issue: An update on central sensitivity syndromes and the issues of nosology and psychobiology). *Curr. Rheumatol. Rev.* **2015**, *11*, 70–85. [CrossRef]
51. Pollok, B.; Krause, V.; Legrain, V.; Ploner, M.; Freynhagen, R.; Melchior, I.; Schnitzler, A. Differential effects of painful and non-painful stimulation on tactile processing in fibromyalgia syndrome and subjects with masochistic behaviour. *PLoS ONE* **2010**, *5*, e15804. [CrossRef]

52. Kamping, S.; Bomba, I.C.; Kanske, P.; Diesch, E.; Flor, H. Deficient modulation of pain by a positive emotional context in fibromyalgia patients. *PAIN®* **2013**, *154*, 1846–1855. [CrossRef]
53. Wallin, M.; Liedberg, G.; Börsbo, B.; Gerdle, B. Thermal detection and pain thresholds but not pressure pain thresholds are correlated with psychological factors in women with chronic whiplash-associated pain. *Clin. J. Pain* **2012**, *28*, 211–221. [CrossRef] [PubMed]
54. Grundström, H.; Larsson, B.; Arendt-Nielsen, L.; Gerdle, B.; Kjølhede, P. Pain catastrophizing is associated with pain thresholds for heat, cold and pressure in women with chronic pelvic pain. *Scand. J. Pain* **2020**, in press.
55. Martínez, M.P.; Sánchez, A.I.; Miró, E.; Medina, A.; Lami, M.J. The relationship between the fear-avoidance model of pain and personality traits in fibromyalgia patients. *J. Clin. Psychol. Med. Settings* **2011**, *18*, 380–391. [CrossRef]
56. Lambin, D.I.; Thibault, P.; Simmonds, M.; Lariviere, C.; Sullivan, M.J. Repetition-induced activity-related summation of pain in patients with fibromyalgia. *Pain* **2011**, *152*, 1424–1430. [CrossRef]
57. Burri, A.; Ogata, S.; Rice, D.; Williams, F. Pain catastrophizing, neuroticism, fear of pain, and anxiety: Defining the genetic and environmental factors in a sample of female twins. *PLoS ONE* **2018**, *13*, e0194562. [CrossRef]
58. Shi, H.; Yuan, C.; Dai, Z.; Ma, H.; Sheng, L. Gray matter abnormalities associated with fibromyalgia: A meta-analysis of voxel-based morphometric studies. *Semin. Arthritis Rheum.* **2016**, *46*, 330–337. [CrossRef]
59. Schmidt-Wilcke, T.; Luerding, R.; Weigand, T.; Jürgens, T.; Schuierer, G.; Leinisch, E.; Bogdahn, U. Striatal grey matter increase in patients suffering from fibromyalgia—A voxel-based morphometry study. *Pain* **2007**, *132*, S109–S116. [CrossRef]
60. Burgmer, M.; Gaubitz, M.; Konrad, C.; Wrenger, M.; Hilgart, S.; Heuft, G.; Pfleiderer, B. Decreased gray matter volumes in the cingulo-frontal cortex and the amygdala in patients with fibromyalgia. *Psychosom. Med.* **2009**, *71*, 566–573. [CrossRef]
61. Fallon, N.; Alghamdi, J.; Chiu, Y.; Sluming, V.; Nurmikko, T.; Stancak, A. Structural alterations in brainstem of fibromyalgia syndrome patients correlate with sensitivity to mechanical pressure. *NeuroImage Clin.* **2013**, *3*, 163–170. [CrossRef]
62. Ceko, M.; Bushnell, M.C.; Fitzcharles, M.-A.; Schweinhardt, P. Fibromyalgia interacts with age to change the brain. *NeuroImage Clin.* **2013**, *3*, 249–260. [CrossRef]
63. Gianaros, P.J.; Jennings, J.R.; Sheu, L.K.; Greer, P.J.; Kuller, L.H.; Matthews, K.A. Prospective reports of chronic life stress predict decreased grey matter volume in the hippocampus. *Neuroimage* **2007**, *35*, 795–803. [CrossRef]
64. Felmingham, K.; Williams, L.M.; Whitford, T.J.; Falconer, E.; Kemp, A.H.; Peduto, A.; Bryant, R.A. Duration of posttraumatic stress disorder predicts hippocampal grey matter loss. *Neuroreport* **2009**, *20*, 1402–1406. [CrossRef]
65. Haviland, M.G.; Morton, K.R.; Oda, K.; Fraser, G.E. Traumatic experiences, major life stressors, and self-reporting a physician-given fibromyalgia diagnosis. *Psychiatry Res.* **2010**, *177*, 335–341. [CrossRef]
66. Anderberg, U.; Marteinsdottir, I.; Theorell, T.; Von Knorring, L. The impact of life events in female patients with fibromyalgia and in female healthy controls. *Eur. Psychiatry* **2000**, *15*, 295–301. [CrossRef]
67. Segerdahl, A.R.; Mezue, M.; Okell, T.W.; Farrar, J.T.; Tracey, I. The dorsal posterior insula subserves a fundamental role in human pain. *Nat. Neurosci.* **2015**, *18*, 499–500. [CrossRef]
68. Wiech, K.; Lin, C.-s.; Brodersen, K.H.; Bingel, U.; Ploner, M.; Tracey, I. Anterior insula integrates information about salience into perceptual decisions about pain. *J. Neurosci.* **2010**, *30*, 16324–16331. [CrossRef]
69. Cagnie, B.; Coppieters, I.; Denecker, S.; Six, J.; Danneels, L.; Meeus, M. Central sensitization in fibromyalgia? A systematic review on structural and functional brain MRI. *Semin. Arthritis Rheum.* **2014**, *44*, 68–75. [CrossRef]
70. Uddin, Z.; MacDermid, J.C.; Ham, H.H. Test–retest reliability and validity of normative cut-offs of the two devices measuring touch threshold: Weinstein Enhanced Sensory Test and Pressure-Specified Sensory Device. *Hand Ther.* **2014**, *19*, 3–10. [CrossRef]
71. Rolke, R.; Baron, R.; Maier, C.A.; Tölle, T.; Treede, R.-D.; Beyer, A.; Binder, A.; Birbaumer, N.; Birklein, F.; Bötefür, I. Quantitative sensory testing in the German Research Network on Neuropathic Pain (DFNS): Standardized protocol and reference values. *Pain* **2006**, *123*, 231–243. [CrossRef]

72. Pickering, G.; Achard, A.; Corriger, A.; Sickout-Arondo, S.; Macian, N.; Leray, V.; Lucchini, C.; Cardot, J.M.; Pereira, B. Electrochemical Skin Conductance and Quantitative Sensory Testing on Fibromyalgia. *Pain Pract.* **2020**, *20*, 348–356. [CrossRef]
73. Wilbarger, J.L.; Cook, D.B. Multisensory hypersensitivity in women with fibromyalgia: Implications for well being and intervention. *Arch. Phys. Med. Rehabilit.* **2011**, *92*, 653–656. [CrossRef]
74. Vierck, C.J., Jr.; Staud, R.; Price, D.D.; Cannon, R.L.; Mauderli, A.P.; Martin, A.D. The effect of maximal exercise on temporal summation of second pain (windup) in patients with fibromyalgia syndrome. *J. Pain* **2001**, *2*, 334–344. [CrossRef]
75. Woznowski-Vu, A.; Uddin, Z.; Flegg, D.; Aternali, A.; Wickens, R.; Sullivan, M.J.; Sweet, S.N.; Skou, S.T.; Wideman, T.H. Comparing Novel and Existing Measures of Sensitivity to Physical Activity Among People With Chronic Musculoskeletal Pain. *Clin. J. Pain* **2019**, *35*, 656–667. [CrossRef]
76. Schultz, J.; Uddin, Z.; Singh, G.; Howlader, M.M. Glutamate sensing in biofluids: Recent advances and research challenges of electrochemical sensors. *Analyst* **2020**, *145*, 321–347. [CrossRef]
77. Gleich, T.; Deserno, L.; Lorenz, R.C.; Boehme, R.; Pankow, A.; Buchert, R.; Kühn, S.; Heinz, A.; Schlagenhauf, F.; Gallinat, J. Prefrontal and striatal glutamate differently relate to striatal dopamine: Potential regulatory mechanisms of striatal presynaptic dopamine function? *J. Neurosci.* **2015**, *35*, 9615–9621. [CrossRef]

11

The Role of Demoralization and Hopelessness in Suicide Risk in Schizophrenia

Isabella Berardelli [1,*], Salvatore Sarubbi [2], Elena Rogante [2], Michael Hawkins [3], Gabriele Cocco [4], Denise Erbuto [1], David Lester [5] and Maurizio Pompili [1]

1 Department of Neurosciences, Mental Health and Sensory Organs, Suicide Prevention Center, Sant'Andrea Hospital, Sapienza University of Rome, 00185 Rome, Italy; denise.erbuto@uniroma1.it (D.E.); maurizio.pompili@uniroma1.it (M.P.)
2 Department of Psychology, Sapienza University of Rome, 00185 Rome, Italy; salvatore.sarubbi@uniroma1.it (S.S.); elena.rogante@gmail.com (E.R.)
3 Department of Psychiatry, University of Toronto, Toronto, ON M4B 1B4, Canada; michael.hawkins@mail.utoronto.ca
4 Faculty of Medicine and Psychology, Sapienza University of Rome, 00185 Rome, Italy; gabri.cocco84@hotmail.it
5 Psychology Program, Stockton University, Galloway, NJ 08205, USA; David.Lester@stockton.edu
* Correspondence: isabella.berardelli@uniroma1.it

Abstract: *Background and Objectives:* Demoralization has been defined by hopelessness and helplessness attributable to a loss of purpose and meaning in life. Demoralization is a meaningful mental health concern, frequently associated with suicide risk in medical and psychiatric patients. The aim of this systematic review was to synthesize the recent empirical evidence on demoralization in patients with schizophrenia and to better understand the relationship between demoralization and suicide risk in patients with schizophrenia. *Methods:* A comprehensive literature search using key words and subject headings was performed following PRISMA guidelines with several bibliographic databases, resulting in the identification of 27 studies. *Results:* The findings suggested that demoralization is prevalent in patients with schizophrenia and supported the hypothesis that the association between depression and suicide is moderated by hopelessness. In clinical practice, it is important to recognize symptoms of demoralization using appropriate psychological tools to better understand the suffering of patients with schizophrenia and to implement suicide prevention programs.

Keywords: demoralization; schizophrenia; suicide risk

1. Introduction

Jerome Frank [1], more than forty years ago, defined demoralization as "a syndrome of existential distress occurring in patients with severe conditions that threaten life or integrity of being, such as physical illness or mental disorders." Demoralization is characterized by "feelings of impotence, isolation, and despair." Frank interpreted demoralization as an outcome caused by someone's failure to cope when faced with an event generally described as easy to manage [2]. In those who are demoralized, self-esteem suffers, and rejection is felt as a result of individuals believing they have failed to meet the expectations of others [1–3]. This highlights the salience that stressful events may have on the human psyche [4].

In more recent years, Irvin Yalom, an existential psychotherapist [5], noted how demoralization represents the outcome of a conflict between the individual and his personal existence. When a person is unable to face this conflict, demoralization can develop. Based on this, the definition of demoralization was subsequently enriched with new concepts [6], with the link between distress and subjective incompetence at the base of the construct of demoralization.

In the following years, several authors attempted to describe the demoralization syndrome. Fava et al. [7] used three diagnostic criteria for demoralization, including the failure of individuals to meet expectations set by themselves, those set by others, and their general inability to cope with demands. This results in feelings of helplessness, hopelessness, and a desire to give up. According to a psychosomatic perspective, demoralization is a predictor for the development of a medical illness [7].

A recent definition of demoralization was proposed by Kissane and Clarke [8,9] at the beginning of the 2000s. Demoralization was defined as a clinical entity characterized by symptoms such as existential distress, hopelessness, loss of meaning and purpose in life, a sense of being trapped, personal failure, and difficulty coping. Kissane focused on demoralization as a predictive variable for suicidal ideation in terminally ill patients [2]. Kissane described demoralization as an abnormal response characterized by two key aspects: loss of meaning in life and loss of hope. Considering that hopelessness is one of the most important predictors of suicide, patients with the demoralization syndrome may have a higher risk of suicide than patients without the demoralization syndrome [2].

The debate on demoralization as a syndrome is still controversial. The categorization of demoralization as an "abnormal response" has been criticized by different authors. Several authors emphasized that demoralization is a normal psychological response in patients affected by a medical illness [10] and compared demoralization to the Adjustment Disorders, described in DSM-5, or as a normal response to loss [11,12]. Furthermore, the main controversy centers on whether demoralization constitutes a syndrome of despair, distress, and hopelessness separate from depression. Kissane saw the concept of demoralization as a syndrome, contextualizing it on a spectrum where the end of this spectrum warrants a "psychiatric alert". Demoralization becomes clinically relevant when there is a significant loss of meaning and purpose in life, and suicidal thinking appears [13]. It has been argued that the critical feature distinguishing depression from demoralization is the presence or absence of anhedonia [14]. However, depression and anxiety are symptoms that are often present in the demoralization syndrome [8].

Although demoralization can occur in response to many distressing circumstances, much of the literature about demoralization focuses on people who have a terminal or severely disabling physical illness [15,16], but only a few studies have focused on psychiatric patients, such as patients with schizophrenia [17].

Patients with schizophrenia often die prematurely [18]. Though the lifetime risk for suicide for people with schizophrenia is estimated to be about 4.9% [19], up to 40% [20] of their premature mortality can be attributed to suicide and unnatural deaths. Several psychological features seem to contribute to suicide in this population, including hopelessness, recent loss or rejection, fear of further illness deterioration, awareness of their illness, loss of faith in treatment, post-psychotic depression, or failure in interpersonal relationships [21]. A number of clinical features have been associated with completed suicide in people with schizophrenia, including being young, male, Caucasian, and never married, and having good premorbid function and a history of substance abuse and suicide attempts [21,22]. Hopelessness, social isolation, and hospitalization are also important risk factors for completed suicide in individuals with schizophrenia. Among these features, hopelessness plays a large role in affecting the suicide risk of these patients. Higher hopelessness scores, regardless of the presence of only depressive symptoms, predicted a worse short-term outcome and worse global functioning, which are considered important risks factor for suicidal behavior [23]. Furthermore, a greater surveillance for suicide is required in the period after discharge from hospital and after periods of remission. Patients with schizophrenia usually experience hopelessness and demoralization after discharge from hospital which increases their suicide risk. During periods of remission, they can develop a painful awareness of their illness. At this point, their expectations contrast sharply with their declining functioning, leading to feelings of inadequacy, depression, and hopelessness. It has been suggested that hopelessness and greater insight are associated with current and lifetime risk of suicide [24].

Drake has described a demoralization syndrome in individuals with schizophrenia, in which repeated exacerbations of psychotic symptoms, functional deterioration, and a non-delusional awareness of the effects of the illness can lead to feelings of hopelessness, depression, and ultimately suicide [25].

In this view, premorbid adjustment and insight interact, resulting in demoralization and depression, potentially culminating in suicidal behavior. Interestingly, on the one hand, depression has been recognized as a major risk factor for suicide attempt among patients with schizophrenia [26]. On the other hand, depression is difficult to diagnose in patients with schizophrenia. In clinical practice, nonspecific sadness is more often observed than major depressive episodes. In the 1980s, Bartels and Drake [27] considered chronic demoralization to be a variable that predicted the risk of suicide in patients with schizophrenia. This hypothesis was then validated in several studies that have shown how the presence of depression, hopelessness, negative self-thoughts, anxiety, insomnia, self-devaluation, low self-esteem, and a feeling of guilt were strongly associated with a higher risk of suicide in patients with schizophrenia [21–28]. Research on this topic was then enriched with papers on patients with schizophrenia linking hopelessness with social and vocational dysfunction [29–31], suicide risk [25–32], avoidant coping [33,34], and stigma [35–37].

In line with the hypothesis that the demoralization syndrome and hopelessness are important risk factors for suicide in patients with schizophrenia, and on the basis that these two constructs are related to both patient insight and stigma, variables involved in suicide risk, we reviewed those studies investigating the presence of demoralization (and its constructs) and suicide, in patients with schizophrenia.

The principal aim of this review was to clarify the role of demoralization and hopelessness in affecting suicide risk in patients with schizophrenia. The second aim of this review paper was to better understand the complex relationship between demoralization and hopelessness, along with patient insight and stigma, and suicide risk in patients with schizophrenia.

2. Methods

We performed a systematic review of demoralization (according to a definition of demoralization that includes the inability to cope, helplessness, hopelessness, and low self-esteem) and suicidal risk in schizophrenia using MedLine, Excerpta Medica, PsycLit, PsycInfo, and Index Medicus search to identify all papers published between 1970 and 2018. The PRISMA statement for reporting systematic reviews was followed. Search terms used were: demoralization OR demoralization syndrome OR helplessness OR hopelessness AND suicide risk AND Schizophrenia, Psychosis. We first reviewed the titles and abstracts and applied the selection criteria outlined above with the exception of study design (Figure 1). Only articles published in English peer-reviewed journals were considered, and the articles were examined to for their relevance based on the inclusion criteria. Possible discrepancies between the reviewers with regard to inclusion criteria were resolved through consultation with the senior authors. In addition, reference lists were also examined. In the results section, we excluded case reports, meta-analyses, and systematic reviews, and studies that did not clearly report statistical analysis, diagnostic criteria, or the number of patients included. We found 27 articles on demoralization and schizophrenia that met these criteria and we discussed them in the two sections of the results (Clinical Studies included in qualitative synthesis). We have included three systematic reviews exclusively in the discussion section but not in the results section. The principal reviewer (IB) checked all items. Then, three reviewers independently inspected all citations of the studies identified by the search and grouped them according to topic.

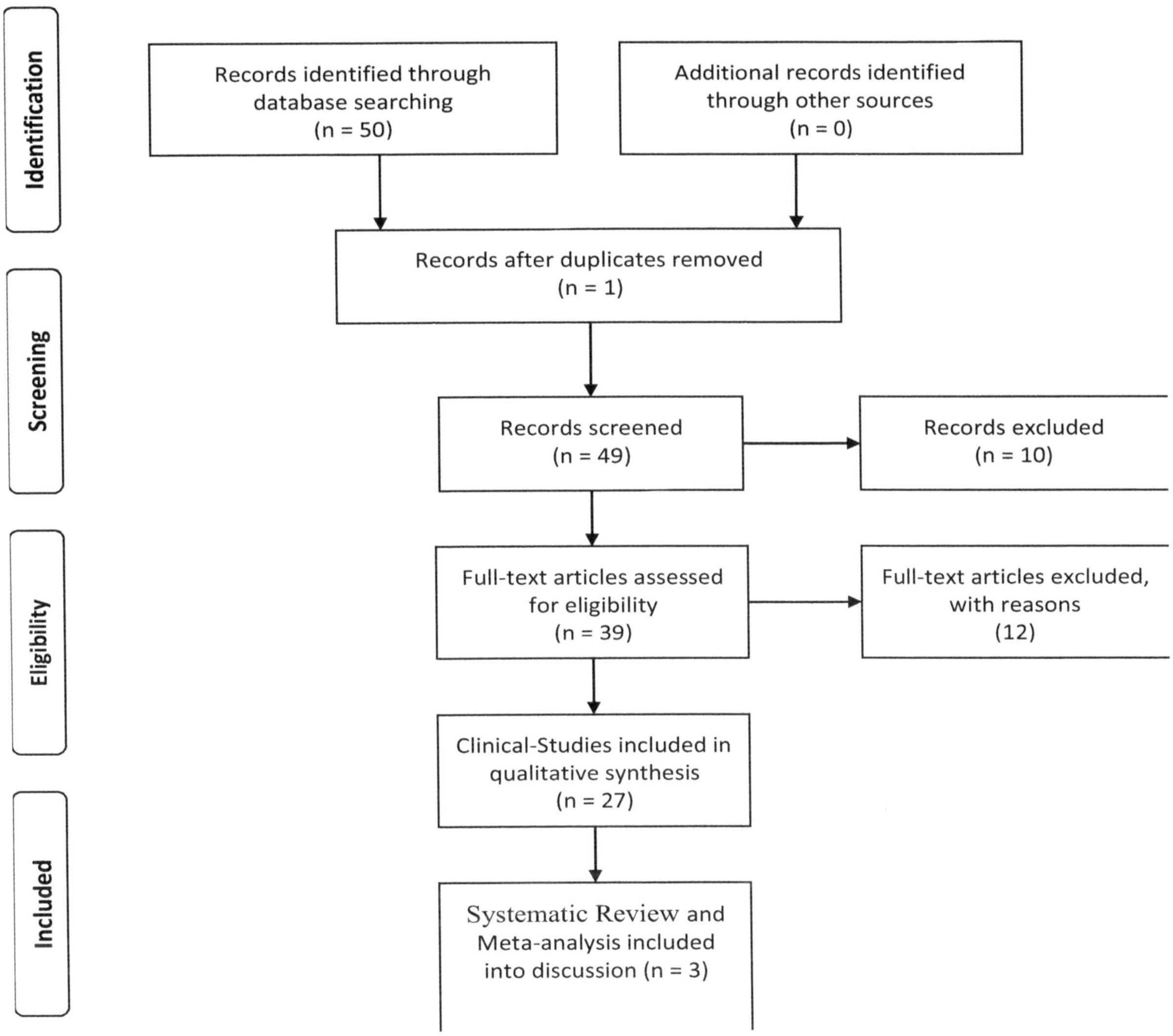

Figure 1. Flowchart of the search and selection process.

3. Results

3.1. Demoralization and Suicide Risk in Schizophrenia

Depressive features, including demoralization and hopelessness, are common in schizophrenia and are often intertwined with psychotic symptoms, becoming a significant mediator of disability and suicidality. Cotton et al. [38] interviewed 20 therapists who had clinically followed 20 patients with schizophrenia who completed suicide. These interviews indicated that the profile of the patients was of young men in their thirties with a chronic history of illness with exacerbations. From the interviews, it emerged that patients expressed hopelessness at the time of their suicide. The patients had a strong desire to escape through death, and most of them had a previous history of suicidal behavior. Cotton then showed how different clinical features resulted in guidelines for the treatment of these patients. For example, it is important to assess the patient's self-esteem, the protective function that psychosis may have in regard to suicide, and the importance of differentiating an inability to function from an unwillingness to function (i.e., unwillingness to share their thoughts of life and death or share the burden of despair resulting from their illness).

Drake et al. [39] examined risk factors for suicide in patients with schizophrenia, noting that the risk factors for suicide included demoralization and feelings of hopelessness and inadequacy. A few years later, the same authors investigated the clinical features of depression, hopelessness, and their relationship to major depressive episodes and suicides in 104 patients with schizophrenia, 15 of whom died by suicide [40]. Most patients (54%) endorsed "depressed mood", and 21% of these patients met DSM criteria for a depressive disorder. Although the presence of depressed mood increased their risk of suicide, the severity of depression did not increase the risk of suicide. In contrast, the development of hopelessness, in addition to depressed mood, significantly increased the probability of suicide. In absence of hopelessness, depressed patients with schizophrenia presented a similar risk for suicide to that of non-depressed patients with schizophrenia. Thus, these results suggest that hopelessness mediates the relationship between depression and suicide risk in patients with schizophrenia.

Data from a prospective community treatment study on suicide in patients with schizophrenia showed that the group of patients who died by suicide were younger, with an earlier onset of illness compared to patients who did not complete suicide, and suicide occurred very early in the course of illness [32]. Furthermore, hopelessness was a very discriminative feature between the two groups ($z = 3.27$, $p < 0.05$), and patients who completed suicide showed a significant increase in hopelessness and depression.

Fenton et al. [41] studied the relationship between positive and negative symptoms, illness subtype, and suicidal behavior in 187 patients with schizophrenia, 87 patients with schizoaffective disorder, 15 patients with schizophreniform disorder, and 33 patients with schizotypal personality disorder. The authors demonstrated that the progressive loss of social drive, the diminished capacity to experience affect, and an indifference toward the future may preclude the painful self-awareness associated with suicide.

Nordentoft et al. [42] investigated predictive factors for suicidal behavior in 321 patients with first-episode psychosis. Their results demonstrated that a suicide attempt was associated with younger age, depression, hopelessness, and hallucinations. Being female, reported hopelessness at baseline, the presence of hallucinations, and a suicide attempt reported at the initial interview were associated with a suicide attempt by the one-year follow up.

Kim et al. [43] enrolled 333 patients with schizophrenia to clarify the clinical role of hopelessness, insight, and cognitive dysfunction for suicide risk. They found that hopelessness was significantly higher in patients with lifetime suicidality and in those with current suicide risk compared to patients without history of suicidal behavior, thereby supporting the role of hopelessness as a predictor of the lifetime risk of suicide.

Montross et al. [44] examined the prevalence of suicidal behavior in 132 patients with schizophrenia. Depression and hopelessness were significantly higher in the group with suicidal ideation. Predictive features for current suicidal ideation included depression, hopelessness, gender, general psychopathology, and the presence of a past suicide attempt. They also found that hopelessness and a past history of suicide attempts were the only variables associated with current suicidal ideation.

Restifo et al. [45] tested the demoralization hypothesis as an independent risk factor for suicidal behaviors in 164 patients, 115 of whom had a diagnosis of schizophrenia and 49 a diagnosis of schizoaffective disorder. The sample was divided in two groups: patients with a history of a previous suicide attempt ($N = 59$) and patients without a history of previous suicide attempts ($N = 105$). The authors observed that premorbid functioning and insight were associated with more depressive symptoms. Furthermore, cognitive symptoms of depression (poor concentration, indecisiveness, forgetfulness) and subclinical symptoms of depression were linked with past suicide attempts, while hopelessness predicted current and lifetime risk of suicide among these patients with schizophrenia. In support of these results, a case-control study [46] confirmed that a history of suicide attempts, hopelessness, and self-devaluation were the three variables that had the strongest association with completed suicide in patients with schizophrenia.

More recently Klonsky, et al. [47], in a 10-year longitudinal study of 414 patients with first-admission psychosis, clarified the relationship between hopelessness and suicide attempt. Both hopelessness and recent suicide attempts were assessed at multiple time-points. The results demonstrated that hopelessness at baseline predicted a suicide attempt during the subsequent 10 years independent of the presence of depression.

A few studies have investigated the association between self-esteem and suicide risk in patients with schizophrenia [48] (Table 1). Tarrier et al. [49] examined 59 patients with recent onset schizophrenia, reporting that greater hopelessness (odds ratio (OR) 1.22) and a longer duration of illness (OR 1.13) increased the risk of suicide in these patients. Hopelessness was associated with higher negative self-evaluation and social isolation, while negative self-evaluation was associated with self-criticism and negative symptoms. Acosta et al. [50], in a study of 60 patients with schizophrenia showed that negative cognitions about the psychiatric diagnosis were associated with depressive symptoms and hopelessness. Interestingly, negative cognition did not differ in patients with and without a history of previous suicide attempts. Yoo et al. [51] studied 87 patients with schizophrenia, of whom 20 (23.0%) had a history of suicide attempts. Their results revealed that patients with a history of suicide attempts had significantly higher scores on the Beck Depression Inventory ($p = 0.036$) and on the Korean version of the Internalized Stigma of Mental Illness scale ($p = 0.009$), and significantly lower scores on the Rosenberg Self-Esteem Scale ($p = 0.001$), demonstrating that low self-esteem represents a psychological feature of those who attempt suicide, thereby increasing their risk of suicide.

Table 1. Demoralization and Suicide Risk in Schizophrenia.

Authors	Purpose	Measures	Results/Discussion
Drake et al. (1984)	Risk factors for suicide in patients with schizophrenia N = 104 (15 clinical vs. 89 controls; all met DSM-III diagnostic criteria for Schizophrenia)	3d edition of the Diagnostic and Statistical Manual of Mental Disorders from the American Psychiatric Association (DSM-III)	Depressed mental status is more frequently observed in suicide group vs. non-suicide group (80% vs. 48%; $p < 0.01$).
Cotton et al. (1985)	Psychotherapy of suicidal schizophrenic patients. N = 20 (schizophrenia)	Semi-structured interviews	Patients with schizophrenia reported hopelessness and a strong desire to escape through death at the time of suicide. It is important to assess self-esteem, the presence of psychosis, and distinguish inability to function from unwillingness to function
Drake & Cotton (1986)	DSM-III depressive symptoms vs. hopelessness in schizophrenic suicides and non-suicides patients N = 104 (15 = s; 89 = n-s)	3d edition of the Diagnostic and Statistical Manual of Mental Disorders from the American Psychiatric Association (DSM-III); Beck Hopelessness Scale (BHS)	Suicide ideas, depressive mood, and hopelessness rather than depression increases risk of suicide (respectively 87%, 80%, and 67% vs. 33% of depression in suicide sample); $p < 0.01$
Cohen et al. (1990)	Suicide in long-term treatment schizophrenia. N = 122 (67.2% male) with Schizophrenia, schizoaffective disorder (research diagnostic criteria), or schizotypal personality disorder (DSM-III)	Symptom Checklist 90-R (SCL-90-R); Brief Psychiatric Rating Scale (BPRS); Self-report measure of satisfaction	Baseline SCL-90-R scores for: hopelessness (6.30 vs. 2.96), hostility (3.53 vs. 1.63), depression (5.89 vs. 3.52), paranoid ideation (4.51 vs. 2.71), and obsessive-compulsive (3.73 vs. 2.23) were very discriminative between suicides (N = 8) and non-suicides (N = 74)

Table 1. *Cont.*

Authors	Purpose	Measures	Results/Discussion
Fenton et al. (1997)	Suicidality in schizophrenia and its relationship with subtypes N = 322 (schizophrenia n =187; schizoaffective disorder n = 87; schizophreniform disorder N = 15; schizotypal personality disorder n = 33)	3d edition of the Diagnostic and Statistical Manual of Mental Disorders from the American Psychiatric Association (DSM-III); Positive and Negative Symptoms Scale (PANSS); self-report interviews	Negative symptoms: blunted affect ($p = 0.03$), poverty of speech ($p = 0.02$), stereotyped thinking ($p = 0.005$), and only one of positive symptoms (grandiosity ($p < 0.05$)) were correlated with suicide behavior.
Nordentoft et al. (2002)	Suicidal behavior and treatment in first-episode schizophrenia (FEP) N = 341 (FEP disorder); attempts reported at baseline (N = 321); attempts during first year of treatment (N = 275) Diagnosis: schizophrenia, schizotypal disorder, delusional disorder, acute or transient psychosis, schizoaffective psychosis, induced psychosis, or unspecific non-organic psychosis according to ICD–10	Schedules for Clinical Assessment in Neuropsychiatry (SCAN 2.0), Scale for the Assessment of Negative Symptoms (SANS), Scale for the Assessment of Positive Symptoms (SAPS)	Baseline period: being male ($p = 0.001$) and suicidal plans the week prior ($p = 0.001$) were significant predictors of suicide; Follow up period: being male ($p = 0.002$), suicidal plans the week prior ($p < 0.001$), and previous suicide attempts ($p = 0.001$) were significantly associated with suicide. There was a weak association between hopelessness and suicide in the integrated treatment's group one year after treatment compared to the standard treatment's group ($p < 0.01$)
Kim et al. (2002)	Hopelessness, insight, cognitive dysfunction, and suicidality in schizophrenia N = 333 (schizophrenia)	Schedule for Affective Disorders and Schizophrenia (SADS), Hamilton Depression Rating Scale (HDRS), Brief Psychiatric Rating Scale (BPRS)	Regression analysis predicted Hopelessness as the most important predictor of current and lifetime suicidality ($\beta = 0.41$, $p = 0.0001$; $\beta = 0.35$, $p = 0.01$, respectively). Further, insight and substance abuse were predictors for lifetime and current suicidality ($p = 0.001$ and $p = 0.004$; $p = 0.001$ and $p = 0.033$, respectively).
Tarrier et al. (2004)	Factors (self-esteem, relatives' expressed emotions, demographic, social, clinical) associated with suicidal ideation and/or previous suicide attempts as proxy measures of suicide risk N = 59 (DSM-IV diagnosis of recent onset schizophrenia)	4d edition of the Diagnostic and Statistical Manual of Mental Disorders from the American Psychiatric Association (DSM-IV); Modified Self-Evaluation and Social Support for Schizophrenia (SESS-sv); Positive and Negative Symptoms Scale (PANSS); Beck Depression Inventory (BDI); Beck Hopelessness Scale (BHS); Insight Scale (IS)	Greater hopelessness (OR 1.22) and longer duration of illness (OR 1.13) increase suicide risk. Hopelessness was also associated with higher negative self-evaluation and social isolation.

Table 1. *Cont.*

Authors	Purpose	Measures	Results/Discussion
Ran et al. (2005)	Suicide attempters' (N = 38) vs. non-attempters' (N = 472) clinical features. N = 510 (schizophrenia)	Screening schedule for Psychosis, Present State Examination, Chinese version (PSE-9), Social Disability Screening Schedule (SDSS), General Psychiatric Interview Schedule and Summary Form	Hopelessness and depressed mood were present in 60.5% of the patients with a history of lifetime suicide attempt ($p < 0.001$).
Montross et al. (2008)	Prevalence and correlates of suicide in 40-year-old and older schizophrenic patients N = 132 (schizophrenia spectrum disorder and concurrent depressive symptoms)	SCID, Beck Scale for Suicidal Ideation (BSSI), Hamilton Depression Rating Scale (HAM-D), Calgary Depression Rating Scale (CDRS), Positive and Negative Symptoms Scale (PANSS), Clinical Global Impression Scale (CGI), Cumulative Illness Rating Scale-Geriatrics version C(IRS-G), Beck Hopelessness Scale (BHS)	Hopelessness rated by BHS (5.8; $p = 0.001$), and level of depression rated by HAM-D (13; $p = 0.000$) and CDR (6.4; $p = 0.001$) significantly differentiated the suicidal ideation and non-suicidal ideation groups.
Restifo et al. (2009)	Demoralization model (premorbid adjustment x insight) N = 164 (schizophrenia, N = 115; schizoaffective, N = 49)	Diagnostic Interview of Genetic Studies (DIGS), Premorbid Adjustment Scale (PAS)	Interaction between premorbid adjustment and insight did not significantly predict suicide attempt ($p = 0.88$, $p = 0.91$)
Pompili et al. (2009)	Understanding suicide risk in 20 patients with schizophrenia who died by suicide vs. C 20 controls	Beck Hopelessness Scale (BHS)	Hopelessness (OR = 51.00; 95%CI = 7.56–343.72) was a risk factor for suicide
Klonsky et al. (2012)	Longitudinal relationship of hopelessness and attempted suicide in DSM-III-R psychotic disorders N = 414	3d edition of the Diagnostic and Statistical Manual of Mental Disorders from the American Psychiatric Association DSM-III-R; Beck Hopelessness Scale (BHS); Hamilton Depression Rating Scale (HAM-D)	Hopelessness in psychotic disorders provides information about suicide risk. In comparison to non-psychotic population, even relatively modest levels of hopelessness increase risk for suicide in psychotic patients.
Acosta et al. (2012)	Relationship between schizophrenic patients' cognitions about their illness and past suicidal behaviors Relationship between patients' beliefs about the illness with potential mediators of suicidal behaviors such as depressive symptoms, hopelessness, and insight N = 60 (ICD-10 diagnosis of schizophrenia)	International Classification of Diseases 10th Revision); (ICD-10); Calgary Depression Scale (CDS); Beck Hopelessness Scale (BHS);	Negative appraisals were associated with hopelessness and depressive symptoms (negative expectations and stigma showed the strongest associations). No differences between patients with and without past suicidal behaviors

Table 1. *Cont.*

Authors	Purpose	Measures	Results/Discussion
Fulginiti & Brekke (2015)	Association between discrepancy factors (self-esteem and quality of life) and suicidal ideation in DSM-IV schizophrenia spectrum disorders N = 162	4d edition of the Diagnostic and Statistical Manual of Mental Disorders (DSM-IV); Extended Version of the Brief Psychiatric Rating Scale (BPRS-E); Subjective Well-being under Neuroleptic Treatment scale (SWL); Index for Self-Esteem (ISE); Medical Outcomes Study Social Support Survey (MOS-SSS); Survey); RFS (Role Functioning Scale)	QoL and self-esteem added value to predicting suicidal ideation beyond clinical and demographic factors. Self-esteem mediates the relationship between QoL and suicidal ideation.
Yoo et al. (2015)	Associations between suicidality and self-esteem in patients with schizophrenia according to DSM-IV N = 87 (20 attempted suicide)	4d edition of the Diagnostic and Statistical Manual of Mental Disorders (DSM-IV); Positive and Negative Symptoms Scale (PANSS); Beck Depression Inventory (BDI); Beck Hopelessness Scale (BHS); Rosenberg Self-Esteem Scale (SES); Korean version of the Internalized Stigma of Mental Illness Scale (K-ISMI)	Patients with a history of suicide attempt had significantly higher scores on BDI ($p = 0.036$) and K-ISMI ($p = 0.009$) and significantly lower scores on SES ($p = 0.001$)

Five hundred and ten individuals with schizophrenia were studied by Ran et al. [52] with the aim of identifying clinical variables that could discern between patients with a history of suicide attempts and those without a history of suicide attempts. Of the 510 patients, 60.5% of patients that attempted suicide endorsed depressive symptoms and hopelessness. The suicide attempters also had more auditory hallucinations, delusions, and positive symptoms and presence of lifetime hopelessness.

3.2. Demoralization, Insight, and Stigma in Schizophrenia

How depression, demoralization, hopelessness, positive and negative symptoms, illness subtype, and suicidal tendency relate to one another in patients with schizophrenia is poorly understood but of great clinical relevance. Several studies have highlighted the link between high levels of insight, low self-esteem, and the quality of life [53,54] (Table 2). Patients with psychiatric illnesses experience discrimination, less life satisfaction, stigma, and feel demoralized and rejected by others [55]. Recent research has suggested that self-stigma results in reduced self-esteem, depression, and anxiety and hinders recovery [56,57]. In a cross-sectional study on 85 patients with schizophrenia receiving maintenance therapy, Birchwood et al. [58] investigated the relationship between depression, the acceptance or rejection of mental illness, the perceived controllability of illness and the acceptance of cultural stereotypes. Twenty-nine per cent of the patients with schizophrenia were considered 'depressed' using the cut-off point of 15 on the Beck Depression Inventory (BDI).

Table 2. Demoralization, insight, and stigma in schizophrenia.

Authors	Purpose	Measures	Results/Discussion
Birchwood et al. (1993)	Relationship between depression and acceptance or rejection of mental illness and perceived controllability of illness in chronic psychosis N = 84 (49 schizophrenia, 35 manic-depressive disorder)	Beck Depression Inventory (BDI); Personal Beliefs about Illness Questionnaire (PBIQ); Crown Self-Esteem Scale; degree of acceptance of two statements regarding acceptance or rejection of mental illness label	Patients' perception of controllability of their illness powerfully discriminated depressed from non-depressed psychotic patients. Label acceptance was not associated with depression, low self-esteem, or unemployment.
Aguilar et al. (1997)	Hopelessness in first-episode psychotic patients in 96 neuroleptic-naive psychotic patients (49 schizophrenic patients and 47 other non-affective psychotic patients)	Hopelessness Scale (HS)	High HS scores at baseline predicted poor short-term outcome in patients with schizophrenia, as evidenced by worse global functioning at the 12-month follow-up.
Carrol et al. (2004)	Explores the level of insight in patients with schizophrenia and its relationship to symptoms and history of violence. Relationship between the insight's dimensions of "compliance" and "awareness of illness" and hopelessness N = 28 (DSM-IV diagnosis of schizophrenia)	4d edition of the Diagnostic and Statistical Manual of Mental Disorders (DSM-IV); Beck Hopelessness Scale (BHS); Positive and Negative Symptoms Scale (PANSS);	Awareness of illness ($p = 0.028$), but not compliance with treatment, was positively correlated with level of hopelessness.
Lysaker et al. (2004)	Explores two aspects of hope (expectations of the future and motivation to persist), neurocognition, personality, symptoms, and social functioning in post-acute phase of schizophrenia N = 52 (39 DSM-IV diagnosis of schizophrenia; 13 DSM-IV diagnosis of schizoaffective disorder)	4d edition of the Diagnostic and Statistical Manual of Mental Disorders (DSM-IV); Positive and Negative Symptoms Scale (PANSS); Hopkins Verbal Learning Test (HVLT); Wisconsin Card Sorting Test (WCST); (NEO Five-Factor Inventory (NEO); Vocabulary; Beck Hopelessness Scale (BHS); Quality of Life Scale (QOL)	Neuroticism, verbal memory, and income were each related to expectations of the future. Neuroticism and social isolation were related to motivational hope. Positive and negative symptoms were unrelated to either form of hopelessness.

Table 2. *Cont.*

Authors	Purpose	Measures	Results/Discussion
White et al. (2007)	Relationship between psychiatric symptoms levels, beliefs about illness and hopelessness N = 100 (DSM-IV diagnosis of schizophrenia)	4d edition of the Diagnostic and Statistical Manual of Mental Disorders (DSM-IV); Personal Beliefs about Illness Questionnaire (PBIQ); Extended Version of the Brief Psychiatric Rating Scale (BPRS); Scale for the Assessment of Negative Symptoms (SANS); Beck Hopelessness Scale (BHS);	There were significant differences between the hopeless and non-hopeless participants on PBIQ, SANS, and BPRS. CDSS score, "humiliating need to be marginalized" PBIQ subscale and BPRS score contributed significantly (60% of the variance) to hopelessness scores.
Cavelti et al. (2012)	Mechanisms underlying the association of insight, depressive symptoms, and protective factors in patients with DSM-IV diagnosis of schizophrenic spectrum disorders N = 142	4d edition of the Diagnostic and Statistical Manual of Mental Disorders (DSM-IV); Scale to Assess Unawareness of Mental Disorder (SUMD); Beck Depression Inventory (BDI-II); Subjective Well-being under Neuroleptic Treatment scale (SWN); Illness Perception Questionnaire for Schizophrenia (IPQS);	Higher levels of insight and psychotic symptoms were associated with more depressive symptoms. Participants' perception of their illness as chronic and disabling mediates the relationship between insight and depressive symptoms. The association of insight and depressive symptoms was less pronounced in patients with positive recovery attitude
Cavelti et al. (2012)	Investigates self-stigma both as a moderator and as a mediator variable in the relationship between insight and demoralization in patients with DSM-IV diagnosis of schizophrenic spectrum disorder N = 145	4d edition of the Diagnostic and Statistical Manual of Mental Disorders (DSM-IV); Scale to Assess Unawareness of Mental Disorder (SUMD); Beck Depression Inventory (BDI); Subjective Well-being under Neuroleptic Treatment scale (SWN); Self-Stigma of Mental Illness Scale (SSMIS);	The association of insight and demoralization was stronger as self-stigma increased, confirming self-stigma as a moderator. Self-stigma also partially mediates the positive relationship between insight and demoralization. Demoralization fully mediates the adverse associations of self-stigma with psychotic symptoms and global functioning
Boursier et al. (2013)	Demoralization in psychotic patients N = 55 (schizophrenic disorder)	Positive and Negative Symptoms Scale (PANSS), Beck Hopelessness Scale (BHS), Poor quality of life (SqOL)	94% of the sample was found to be demoralized. Demoralization correlates with positive symptoms ($p = 0.016$), depression ($p < 0.001$), despair ($p = 0.015$), suicidality ($p < 0.01$), and poor quality of life ($p = 0.007$).

Table 2. *Cont.*

Authors	Purpose	Measures	Results/Discussion
Vass et al. (2015)	Impact of stigma on symptomatic and subjective recovery from psychosis (currently and longitudinally). Investigates whether self-esteem and hopelessness mediate the association between stigma and outcomes N = 80	International Classification of Diseases 10th Revision (ICD-10); Beck Hopelessness Scale (BHS); Questionnaire about the Process of Recovery (QPR); Positive and Negative Symptoms Scale (PANSS)	Stigma predicted both symptomatic and subjective recovery. Hopelessness and self-esteem mediated the effect of stigma on symptomatic and subjective recovery. At the follow-up, stigma predicted recovery and symptoms.
Wartelsteiner et al. (2016)	Examines the correlation of resilience, self-esteem, hopelessness, and psychopathology with quality of life N = 129 (52 DSM-IV diagnosis of schizophrenia; 77 healthy controls)	4d edition of the Diagnostic and Statistical Manual of Mental Disorders	Patients with schizophrenia had lower levels of QoL, resilience, self-esteem, and hope than healthy control subjects. In these patients, QoL correlated moderately with resilience, self-esteem, and hopelessness and weakly with symptoms (negative correlation with depression and positive symptoms)
Touriño et al. (2018)	Assesses prevalence of internalized stigma in patients with ICD-10 diagnosis of schizophrenia who attend psychosocial rehabilitation programs. Investigate the relationship between internalized stigma and sociodemographic, general clinical, psychopathologic, psychological, and suicidal behaviour variables in schizophrenic patients N = 71	ICD-10; ISMI; RSES; SUMD; BHS; CGI-SCH; CDS; SCS	Stigma was associated with higher prevalence of suicidal ideation, a higher number of suicide attempts, higher current suicidal risk, worse self-compassion, higher self-esteem, higher scores on depression, higher prevalence of depression, and higher hopelessness. Hopelessness and the existence of depression were independently associated with internalized stigma

The relationship between hopelessness and global functioning was investigated by Aguilar et al. [59] in first-episode psychosis patients. They found that patients with first-episode schizophrenia had higher levels of hopelessness than non-schizophrenia patients, and that higher hopelessness scores predicted worse global functioning at a one-year follow-up in patients with psychosis. In a cross-sectional study, Carroll et al. [60] explored the relationship between hopelessness and level of insight in 28 forensic patients with schizophrenia, testing the hypothesis that insight domains of 'compliance with treatment' and 'awareness of illness', as evaluated by the Schedule for Assessment of Insight (SAI), would be positively correlated with hopelessness. They showed that awareness of illness, but not compliance with the treatment, was positively correlated with level of hopelessness (i.e., patients who had a poor awareness of their illness generally had more hope for their future).

Lysaker et al. [61] investigated whether expectations about the future and motivation to persist (two aspects of hope) were correlated with neurocognitive patterns, personality, symptoms, and social functioning among 52 patients in a post-acute phase of schizophrenia. The authors suggested that both these aspects of hope were linked to lesser levels of stigma, fewer symptoms of schizophrenia, lesser anxiety, and lesser preference for avoidant forms of coping, emphasizing how different aspects of stigma are possibly linked to different domains of hope.

White et al. [62], in a study on 100 patients with schizophrenia, investigated the psychological features of non-hopeless patients (including personal beliefs about illness) and versus hopeless patients. Of the total sample, 25% of patients reported severe hopelessness, and hopelessness correlated significantly with "entrapment", "loss of autonomy", and "attribution: of self vs. illness" (the extent to which the individual believes that the origins of the illness lie in their personal psyche), using subscales of the Personal Beliefs about Illness Questionnaire (PBIQ). White et al. concluded that, although depression and hopelessness scores are highly correlated, the abovementioned aspects of a patient's personal belief about their illness were all independently associated with hopelessness after controlling for depression.

Cavelti et al. [63] demonstrated that the association between insight and demoralization is mediated by the participants' perception of their mental illness as being chronic, disabling, and out of control. The same authors [64] confirmed, in a study of 145 outpatients with schizophrenia, that the relationship between insight and demoralization was stronger as self-stigma increased, that is, patients with high insight tended to be more demoralized as a result, in part, of their increased likelihood of experiencing self-stigma in relation to their mental illness. In the same study, self-stigma also partially mediated the positive relationship between insight and demoralization, that is, the impact of insight on demoralization diminished after self-stigma was included in the regression equation. Moreover, demoralization fully mediated the adverse associations of self-stigma with psychotic symptoms and global functioning (i.e., higher levels of psychotic symptoms and lower levels of functioning were correlated with higher levels of demoralization).

Boursier et al. [65] investigated the presence of demoralization in 55 patients with schizophrenia, demonstrating that more than 94% of these patients experienced demoralization. The degree of demoralization was correlated with the intensity of positive symptoms, depression, despair, suicidality, poor quality of life, and low self-esteem.

A recent study by Wartelsteiner et al. [66] found that schizophrenia patients had significantly lower quality of life (QoL), resilience, self-esteem, and hope compared to healthy control subjects, highlighting the complex nature of QoL in patients suffering from schizophrenia and the importance of enhancing resilience and self-esteem and diminishing hopelessness and psychopathological features in patients with schizophrenia.

Recently Tourino et al. [67], in a sample of 71 outpatients with a diagnosis of schizophrenia, found that, in 21.1% of these patients, stigma was associated with suicidal ideation, a higher number of suicide attempts, higher current suicidal risk, worse self-compassion, higher scores for depression, a higher prevalence of depression, and higher levels of hopelessness.

4. Discussion

In this review, we have shown a clinical overlap between symptoms of demoralization and schizophrenia. Currently, it is estimated that the prevalence of depressive disorders in schizophrenia is around 40% [68,69] and the presence of depression is correlated with poorer outcomes in schizophrenia [70,71]. Bartels and Drake [27] suggested that depressive symptoms in schizophrenia included depressive symptoms secondary to organic factors, "nonorganic" depression intrinsic to the acute psychotic episode, and depressive symptoms that are not associated with the acute psychotic episode, such as symptoms associated with the prodromal, post-psychotic interval, as well as those symptoms that resemble depression that may represent negative symptoms of schizophrenia. Based on the results of this review, we suggest including the *Demoralization Syndrome* among the depressive syndromes in schizophrenia.

The demoralization syndrome can be differentiated from depression. In patients with chronic medical illness and in patients with psychiatric disorders, disability, bodily disfigurement, fear of loss of dignity, social isolation, feelings of greater dependency on others, and the perception of being a burden may predispose patients to develop symptoms of demoralization. Furthermore, patients with the demoralization syndrome, composed of the sense of impotence and helplessness, could progress to a desire to die by suicide. The research reviewed demonstrated clearly that suicide risk is associated with hopelessness and depression [21], and that suicidal intent in psychiatric inpatients correlates more strongly with hopelessness than with depression [72]. The results of this paper further support the argument for distinguishing demoralization syndrome and its constructs from clinical depression in patients affected by schizophrenia [9].

Previous research has shown that the patients with schizophrenia who are at a higher risk to die by suicide are those who are young, male, Caucasian, never married, with good premorbid function, post-psychotic depression, and with a history of substance abuse and suicide attempts. Furthermore, hopelessness, social isolation, hospitalization, deteriorating health with a high level of premorbid functioning, recent loss or rejection, limited external support, and family stress are considered important risk factors in patients with schizophrenia who die by suicide. How depression, demoralization, hopelessness, positive and negative symptoms, illness subtype, and suicidal tendency evolved in relation to each other in patients with schizophrenia is poorly understood but of clinical relevance. As shown above, several studies have highlighted the link between high levels of insight and low self-esteem and quality of life [52,53]. Patients with psychiatric illnesses experience discrimination, less life satisfaction, stigma, and feel demoralized and rejected by others [54].

The research review above shows how demoralization is frequently present in patients with schizophrenia and its significant association with suicide risk. Furthermore, hopelessness has been found to predict current and lifetime suicidality among patients with schizophrenia, independently of a diagnosis of major depression [43–71], emphasizing the importance of assessing demoralization symptoms in psychiatric patients to better evaluate suicide risk in clinical settings.

This review supports the hypothesis that the association between depression and suicide is moderated by hopelessness. Hopelessness may operate as a powerful potentiating variable, as demonstrated by the evidence showing that depression becomes a predictor of suicide only in the presence of hopelessness. Furthermore, the results of our review, which demonstrated the relationship between demoralization, insight, and stigma in patients affected by schizophrenia, suggest that demoralization may add valuable information about clinically relevant psychological distress in the context of psychiatric diseases. Self-insight may exert its effect on suicide risk through increasing demoralization, rather than through a direct impact on suicidal behavior. Studies in this field suggested that insight may represent a risk factor for suicide in patients with schizophrenia and this association appears to be mediated by other variables, such as depression and, above all, hopelessness. Further studies are required to analyze this issue in depth, given the crucial implications that it may have on the development of a model for suicide prevention in schizophrenia.

Limitations

When interpreting the results of this review, several limitations should be considered. First, all reviews of research are retrospective and, therefore, are subject to bias. Second, we selected only articles in English, omitting relevant articles in other languages from our review. Third, we did not examine the role of gender on suicide risk. Fourth, it was not always simple to apply the concept of "demoralization" retroactively to studies that did not specifically set out to study it, for example ones that look at "hopelessness" or "helplessness". Moreover, given this difficulty, the division of the two sub-chapters of the result section can sometimes seem confusing. Specifically, we included in the first section the studies that presented the main focus on suicidal risk and in the second chapter the studies that mainly considered demoralization, insight, stigma, and quality of life in patients affected by schizophrenia.

Finally, not all the studies reviewed in this paper distinguished completed suicide from attempted suicide. Suicide attempters and completers with schizophrenia appear to represent two overlapping but distinct groups, with different clinical and demographic profiles.

5. Conclusions

Despite increased screening for depression in clinical settings, demoralization symptoms in patients with schizophrenia are often either missed or dismissed by clinicians. This is at least in part because of the difficulty of distinguishing between symptoms of a concurrent mood disorder and those of the schizophrenia syndrome itself, in which disturbed affect and difficulty expressing emotions are central negative symptoms. Our results suggest that, in clinical practice, it is important to recognize the symptoms of demoralization, in particular hopelessness, using appropriate psychological tools in order to better approach the suffering of our patients and implement suicide prevention programs in patients with schizophrenia. Identifying specific subgroups of patients with schizophrenia with different suicide risk profiles, including the presence of demoralization symptoms, is an important goal for future research. Furthermore, in clinical practice, clinicians should definitely focus on the degree of insight in their clients in order to evaluate the suicidal risk, through a careful clinical evaluation and through the use of appropriate tools that evaluate and prevent suicidal risk.

Author Contributions: I.B. wrote the manuscript, S.S., E.R., M.H., G.C. and D.E. contributed to the collection of articles, D.L. corrected and reviewed the article. M.P. provided the original idea and the intellectual impetus.

Acknowledgments: No Acknowledgments.

References

1. Frank, J.D. Psychotherapy: The restoration of morale. *Am. J. Psychiatry* **1974**, *131*, 271–274. [CrossRef]
2. Robinson, S.; Kissane, D.W.; Brooker, J.; Burney, S. A Review of the construct of demoralization: History, definitions, and future direction for palliative care. *Am. J. Hos. Pall. Med.* **2014**, *33*, 93–101. [CrossRef]
3. Frank, J.D. *Persuasion and Healing: A Comparative Study of Psychotherapy*, 2nd ed.; JHU Press: Baltimore, MD, USA, 1993.
4. Frank, J.D. The role of hope in psychotherapy. *Int. J. Psychiatry* **1968**, *5*, 383–395. [PubMed]
5. Yalom, I.D. *The Yalom Reader: Selections from the Work of a Master Therapist and Storyteller*; Basic Books: New York, NY, USA, 1996.
6. De Figueiredo, J.M.; Frank, J.D. Subjective incompetence, the clinical hallmark of demoralization. *Compr. Psychiatry* **1982**, *23*, 353–363. [CrossRef]
7. Fava, G.A.; Freyberger, H.J.; Bech, P.; Christodoulou, G.; Sensky, T.; Theorell, T.; Wise, T.N. Diagnostic criteria for use in psychosomatic research. *Psychother. Psychosom.* **1995**, *63*, 1–8. [CrossRef]
8. Kissane, D.W.; Clarke, D.M.; Street, A.F. Demoralization syndrome: A relevant psychiatric diagnosis for palliative care. *J. Palliat. Care* **2001**, *17*, 12–21. [CrossRef]
9. Clarke, D.M.; Kissane, D.W. Demoralization: Its phenomenology and importance. *Aust. N. Z. J. Psychiatry* **2002**, *36*, 733–742. [CrossRef]
10. Sansone, R.A.; Sansone, L.A. Demoralization in patients with medical illness. *Psychiatry* **2010**, *7*, 42. [PubMed]
11. Slavney, P.R. Diagnosing demoralization in consultation psychiatry. *Psychosomatics* **1999**, *40*, 325–329. [CrossRef]
12. Angelino, A.F.; Treisman, G.J. Major depression and demoralization in cancer patients: Diagnostic and treatment considerations. *Support Care Cancer* **2001**, *9*, 344. [CrossRef] [PubMed]
13. Kissane, D.W. Distress, demoralization and depression in palliative care. *Curr Ther.* **2000**, *41*, 14–19.
14. Pasquini, M.; Berardelli, I.; Biondi, M. Ethiopathogenesis of depressive disorders. Clinical practice and epidemiology in mental health. *Clin. Pract. Epidemiol. Ment. Health* **2014**, *10*, 166–171. [CrossRef] [PubMed]

15. Tecuta, L.; Tomba, E.; Grandi, S.; Fava, G.A. Demoralization: A systematic review on its clinical characterization. *Psychol. Med.* **2015**, *45*, 673–691. [CrossRef] [PubMed]
16. Fava, G.A.; Cosci, F.; Sonino, N. Current psychosomatic practice. *Psychother. Psychosom.* **2017**, *86*, 13–30. [CrossRef]
17. Grassi, L.; Mangelli, L.; Fava, G.A.; Grandi, S.; Ottolini, F.; Porcelli, P.; Rafanelli, C.; Rigatelli, M.; Sonino, N. Psychosomatic characterization of adjustment disorders in the medical setting: Some suggestions for DSM-V. *J. Affect. Disord.* **2007**, *101*, 251–254. [CrossRef]
18. Nordentoft, M.; Wahlbeck, K.; Hallgren, J.; Westman, J.; Osby, U.; Alinaghizadeh, H.; Gissler, M.; Laursen, T.M. Excess mortality, causes of death and life expectancy in 270,770 patients with recent onset of mental disorders in Denmark, Finland and Sweden. *PLoS ONE* **2013**, *8*, e55176. [CrossRef]
19. Palmer, B.A.; Pankratz, V.S.; Bostwick, J.M. The lifetime risk of suicide in Schizophrenia: A reexamination. *Arch. Gen. Psychiatry* **2005**, *62*, 247–253. [CrossRef] [PubMed]
20. Bushe, C.J.; Taylor, M.; Haukka, J. Mortality in Schizophrenia: A measurable clinical endpoint. *J. Psychopharmacol.* **2010**, *24*, 17–25. [CrossRef]
21. Pompili, M.; Amador, X.F.; Girardi, P.; Harkavy-Friedman, J.; Harrow, M.; Kaplan, K.; Montross, L.P. Suicide risk in schizophrenia: Learning from the past to change the future. *Ann. Gen. Psychiatry* **2007**, *6*, 10. [CrossRef] [PubMed]
22. Pompili, M.; Serafini, G.; Innamorati, M.; Lester, D.; Shrivastava, A.; Girardi, P.; Nordentoft, M. Suicide risk in first episode psychosis: A selective review of the current literature. *Schizophr. Res.* **2011**, *129*, 1–11. [CrossRef]
23. Cassidy, R.M.; Yang, F.; Kapczinski, F.; Passos, I.C. Risk factors for suicidality in patients with schizophrenia: A systematic review, meta-analysis, and meta-regression of 96 studies. *Schizophr. Bull.* **2018**, *44*, 787–797. [CrossRef]
24. Vrbova, K.; Prasko, J.; Ociskova, M.; Latalova, K.; Holubova, M.; Grambal, A.; Slepecky, M. Insight in schizophrenia—A double-edged sword? *Neuro. Endocrinol. Lett.* **2017**, *38*, 457–464.
25. Drake, R.; Whitaker, A.; Gates, C.; Cotton, P. Suicide among schizophrenics: A review. *Compr. Psychiatry* **1985**, *26*, 90–100. [CrossRef]
26. Togay, B.; Noyan, H.; Tasdelen, R.; Ucok, A. Clinical variables associated with suicide attempts in schizophrenia before and after the first episode. *Psychiatry Res.* **2015**, *229*, 252–256. [CrossRef]
27. Bartels, S.J.; Drake, R.E. Depressive symptoms in schizophrenia: Comprehensive differential diagnosis. *Compr. Psychiatry* **1988**, *29*, 467–483. [CrossRef]
28. Hor, K.; Taylor, M. Suicide and schizophrenia: A systematic review of rates and risk factors. *J. Psychopharmacol.* **2010**, *24*, 81–90. [CrossRef] [PubMed]
29. Strauss, J.S. Chronicity: Causes, prevention, and treatment. *Psychiatr. Ann.* **1980**, *10*, 23–29. [CrossRef]
30. Regenold, M.; Sherman, M.F.; Fenzel, M. Getting back to work: Self-efficacy as a predictor of employment outcome. *Psychiatr. Rehabil. J.* **1999**, *22*, 361. [CrossRef]
31. Hoffmann, H.; Kupper, Z.; Kunz, B. Hopelessness and its impact on rehabilitation outcome in schizophrenia–an exploratory study. *Schizophr. Res.* **2000**, *43*, 147–158. [CrossRef]
32. Cohen, L.J.; Test, M.A.; Brown, R.L. Suicide and schizophrenia: Data from a prospective community treatment study. *Am. J. Psychiatry* **1990**, *147*, 602–607.
33. Ventura, J.; Neuchterlein, K.H.; Subotnik, K.L.; Gitlin, M.J.; Sharou, J. How are self-efficacy, neurocognition, and negative symptoms related to coping responses in schizophrenia? *Schizophr. Res.* **1999**, *36*, 186–187.
34. Lysaker, P.H.; Clements, C.A.; Wright, D.E.; Evans, J.; Marks, K.A. Neurocognitive correlates of helplessness, hopelessness, and well-being in schizophrenia. *J. Nerv. Ment. Dis.* **2001**, *189*, 457–462. [CrossRef]
35. Mechanic, D.; McAlpine, D.; Rosenfield, S.; Davis, D. Effects of illness attribution and depression on the quality of life among persons with serious mental illness. *Soc. Sci. Med.* **1994**, *39*, 155–164. [CrossRef]
36. Markowitz, F.E. The effects of stigma on the psychological well-being and life satisfaction of persons with mental illness. *J. Health Soc. Behav.* **1998**, *39*, 335–347. [CrossRef]
37. Wright, E.R.; Gronfein, W.P.; Owens, T.J. Deinstitutionalization, social rejection and the self-esteem of former mental patients. *J. Health Soc. Behav.* **2000**, *41*, 68–90. [CrossRef]
38. Cotton, P.G.; Drake, R.E.; Gates, C. Critical treatment issues in suicide among schizophrenics. *Hosp. Community Psychiatry* **1985**, *36*, 534–536. [CrossRef]
39. Drake, R.E.; Gates, C.; Cotton, P.G.; Whitaker, A. Suicide among schizophrenics. Who is at risk? *J. Nerv. Ment. Dis.* **1984**, *172*, 613–617. [CrossRef]

40. Drake, R.; Cotton, P.G. Depression, hopelessness and suicide in chronic schizophrenia. *Brit. J. Psychiat.* **1986**, *148*, 554–559. [CrossRef]
41. Fenton, W.S.; McGlashan, T.H.; Victor, B.J.; Blyler, C. Symptoms, subtype, and suicidality in patients with schizophrenia spectrum disorders. *Am. J. Psychiatry.* **1997**, *154*, 199–204.
42. Nordentoft, M.; Jeppesen, P.; Abel, M.; Kassow, P.; Petersen, L.; Thorup, A.; Krarup, G.; Hemmingsen, R.; Jørgensen, P. OPUS study: Suicidal behavior, suicidal ideation and hopelessness among patients with first-episode psychosis. *Br. J. Psychiatry* **2002**, *181*, 98–106. [CrossRef]
43. Kim, C.H.; Jayathilake, K.; Meltzer, H.Y. Hopelessness, neurocognitive function, and insight in schizophrenia: Relationship to suicidal behavior. *Schizophr. Res.* **2002**, *60*, 71–80. [CrossRef]
44. Montross, L.P.; Kasckow, J.; Golshan, S.; Solorzano, E.; Lehman, D.; Zisook, S. Suicidal ideation and suicide attempts among middle-aged and older patients with schizophrenia spectrum disorders and concurrent subsyndromal depression. *J. Nerv. Ment. Dis.* **2008**, *196*, 884–890. [CrossRef]
45. Restifo, K.; Harkavy-Friedman, J.M.; Shrout, P.E. Suicidal behavior in schizophrenia. *A test of the demoralization hypothesis. J. Nerv. Ment. Dis.* **2009**, *197*, 147–153. [CrossRef] [PubMed]
46. Pompili, M.; Lester, D.; Grispini, A.; Innamorati, M.; Calandro, F.; Iliceto, P.; De Pisa, E.; Tatarelli, R.; Girardi, P. Completed suicide in schizophrenia: Evidence from a case-control study. *Psychiatry Res.* **2009**, *167*, 251–257. [CrossRef] [PubMed]
47. David Klonsky, E.; Kotov, R.; Bakst, S.; Rabinowitz, J.; Bromet, E.J. Hopelessness as a predictor of attempted suicide among first admission patients with psychosis: A 10-year cohort study. *Suicide Life-Threat. Behav.* **2012**, *42*, 1–10. [CrossRef] [PubMed]
48. Fulginiti, A.; Brekke, J.S. Escape from discrepancy: Self-esteem and quality of life as predictors of current suicidal ideation among individuals with schizophrenia. *Community Ment. Health J.* **2015**, *51*, 654–662. [CrossRef] [PubMed]
49. Tarrier, N.; Barrowclough, C.; Andrews, B.; Gregg, L. Risk of non-fatal suicide ideation and behavior in recent onset schizophrenia—The influence of clinical, social, self-esteem and demographic factors. *Soc. Psych. Psych. Epid.* **2004**, *39*, 927–937. [CrossRef]
50. Acosta, F.J.; Aguilar, E.J.; Cejas, M.R.; Gracia, R. Beliefs about illness and their relationship with hopelessness, depression, insight and suicide attempts in schizophrenia. *Psychiatr. Danub.* **2013**, *25*, 0–54.
51. Yoo, T.; Kim, S.W.; Kim, S.Y.; Lee, J.Y.; Kang, H.J.; Bae, K.Y.; Yoon, J.S. Relationship between suicidality and low self-esteem in patients with schizophrenia. *Clin. Psychopharm. Neu.* **2015**, *13*, 296. [CrossRef] [PubMed]
52. Ran, M.S.; Xiang, M.Z.; Mao, W.J.; Hou, Z.J.; Tang, M.N.; Chen, E.Y.A.; Chan, C.L.W.; Yip, P.S.F.; Conwell, Y. Characteristics of suicide attempters and nonattempters with Schizophrenia in a rural community. *Suicide Life Threat Behav.* **2005**, *35*, 694–701. [CrossRef]
53. Drake, R.J.; Pickles, A.; Bentall, R.P.; Kinderman, P.; Haddock, G.; Tarrier, N.; Lewis, S.W. The evolution of insight, paranoia and depression during early schizophrenia. *Psychol. Med.* **2004**, *34*, 285–292. [CrossRef]
54. Hasson-Ohayon, I.; Kravetz, S.; Meir, T.; Rozencwaig, S. Insight into severe mental illness, hope, and quality of life of persons with schizophrenia and schizoaffective disorders. *Psychiatry Res.* **2009**, *167*, 231–238. [CrossRef]
55. Mansouri, L.; Dowell, D.A. Perceptions of stigma among the long-term mentally ill. *Psychosoc. Rehabil. J.* **1989**, *13*, 79. [CrossRef]
56. Schulze, B.; Angermeyer, M.C. Subjective experiences of stigma. A focus group study of schizophrenic patients, their relatives and mental health professionals. *Soc. Sci. Med.* **2003**, *56*, 299–312. [CrossRef]
57. Vass, V.; Morrison, A.P.; Law, H.; Dudley, J.; Taylor, P.; Bennett, K.M.; Bentall, R.P. How stigma impacts on people with psychosis: The mediating effect of self-esteem and hopelessness on subjective recovery and psychotic experiences. *Psychiatry Res.* **2015**, *230*, 487–495. [CrossRef]
58. Birchwood, M.; Mason, R.; MacMillan, F.; Healy, J. Depression, demoralization and control over psychotic illness: A comparison of depressed and non-depressed patients with a chronic psychosis. *Psychol. Med.* **1993**, *23*, 387–395. [CrossRef] [PubMed]
59. Aguilar, E.J.; Haas, G.; Manzanera, F.J.M.; Hernández, J.; Gracia, R.; Rodado, M.J.; Keshavan, M.S. Hopelessness and first-episode psychosis: A longitudinal study. *Acta Psychiatr. Scand.* **1997**, *96*, 25–30. [CrossRef]
60. Carroll, A.; Pantelis, C.; Harvey, C. Insight and hopelessness in forensic patients with schizophrenia. *Aust. N. Z. J. Psychiatry* **2004**, *38*, 169–173. [CrossRef] [PubMed]

61. Lysaker, P.H.; Davis, L.W.; Hunter, N.L. Neurocognitive, social and clinical correlates of two domains of hopelessness in schizophrenia. *Schizophr. Res.* **2004**, *70*, 277–285. [CrossRef] [PubMed]
62. White, R.G.; McCleery, M.; Gumley, A.I.; Mulholland, C. Hopelessness in schizophrenia: The impact of symptoms and beliefs about illness. *J. Nerv. Ment. Dis.* **2007**, *195*, 968–975. [CrossRef]
63. Cavelti, M.; Kvrgic, S.; Beck, E.M.; Kossowsky, J.; Vauth, R. The role of subjective illness beliefs and attitude toward recovery within the relationship of insight and demoralization among people with schizophrenia spectrum disorders. *J. Clin. Psychol.* **2012**, *68*, 462–476. [CrossRef]
64. Cavelti, M.; Kvrgic, S.; Beck, E.M.; Rüsch, N.; Vauth, R. Self-stigma and its relationship with insight, demoralization, and clinical outcome among people with schizophrenia spectrum disorders. *Compr. Psychiatry* **2012**, *53*, 468–479. [CrossRef]
65. Boursier, S.; Jover, F.; Pringuey, D. Relevance of the concept of demoralization in schizophrenic patients. *Eur. Psychiatry* **2013**, *28*, 1. [CrossRef]
66. Wartelsteiner, F.; Mizuno, Y.; Frajo-Apor, B.; Kemmler, G.; Pardeller, S.; Sondermann, C.; Hofer, A. Quality of life in stabilized patients with schizophrenia is mainly associated with resilience and self-esteem. *Acta Psychiatr. Scand.* **2016**, *134*, 360–367. [CrossRef]
67. Touriño, R.; Acosta, F.J.; Giráldez, A.; Álvarez, J.; González, J.M.; Abelleira, C.; Benítez, N.; Baena, E.; Fernández, J.A.; Rodriguez, C.J. Suicidal risk, hopelessness and depression in patients with schizophrenia and internalized stigma. *Actas Esp. Psiquiatr.* **2018**, *46*, 33–34.
68. Upthegrove, R.; Marwaha, S.; Birchwood, M. Depression and schizophrenia: Cause, consequence, or Trans-diagnostic issue? *Schizophr. Bull.* **2017**, *43*, 240–244. [CrossRef]
69. Conley, R.R.; Ascher-Svanum, H.; Zhu, B.; Faries, D.E.; Kinon, B.J. The burden of depressive symptoms in the long-term treatment of patients with schizophrenia. *Schizophr. Res.* **2007**, *90*, 186–197. [CrossRef]
70. Gardsjord, E.S.; Romm, K.L.; Friis, S.; Barder, H.E.; Evensen, J.; Haahr, U.; Ten Velden Hegelstad, W.; Joa, I.; Johannessen, J.O.; Langeveld, J.; et al. Subjective quality of life in first-episode psychosis. A ten year follow-up study. *Schizophr. Res.* **2016**, *172*, 23–28. [CrossRef]
71. Pompili, M.; Lester, D.; Innamorati, M.; Tatarelli, R.; Girardi, P. Assessment and treatment of suicide risk in schizophrenia. *Expert Rev. Neurother.* **2008**, *8*, 51–74. [CrossRef]
72. Wetzel, R.D.; Margulies, T.; Davis, R.; Karam, E. Hopelessness, depression, and suicide intent. *J. Clin. Psychiatry* **1980**, *41*, 159–160. [CrossRef]

12

Effects of Psychoactive Massage in Outpatients with Depressive Disorders: A Randomized Controlled Mixed-Methods Study

Michaela Maria Arnold [1,2,*], Bruno Müller-Oerlinghausen [3], Norbert Hemrich [2] and Dominikus Bönsch [1,4]

[1] Medizinische Fakultät, Julius-Maximilians-Universität Würzburg, 97070 Würzburg, Germany; dominikus.boensch@bezirkskrankenhaus-lohr.de
[2] Berufsfachschule für Massage am Universitätsklinikum Würzburg, 97080 Würzburg, Germany; Hemrich_N@ukw.de
[3] Charité, Universitätsmedizin Berlin, 10117 Berlin, Germany; bruno.mueller-oerlinghausen@web.de
[4] Bezirkskrankenhaus für Psychiatrie, Psychotherapie und Psychosomatische Medizin, 97816 Lohr am Main, Germany
* Correspondence: michaela-maria-arnold@web.de

Abstract: The clinical picture of depressive disorders is characterized by a plethora of somatic symptoms, psychomotor retardation, and, particularly, anhedonia. The number of patients with residual symptoms or treatment resistance is high. Touch is the basic communication among humans and animals. Its application professionally in the form of, e.g., psychoactive massage therapy, has been shown in the past to reduce the somatic and mental symptoms of depression and anxiety. Here, we investigated the effects of a specially developed affect-regulating massage therapy (ARMT) vs. individual treatment with a standardized relaxation procedure, progressive muscle relaxation (PMR), in 57 outpatients with depression. Patients were given one ARMT or PMR session weekly over 4 weeks. Changes in somatic and cognitive symptoms were assessed by standard psychiatric instruments (Hamilton Depression Scale (HAMD) and the Bech–Rafaelsen–Melancholia–Scale (BRMS)) as well as a visual analogue scale. Furthermore, oral statements from all participants were obtained in semi-structured interviews. The findings show clear and statistically significant superiority of ARMT over PMR. The results might be interpreted within various models. The concept of interoception, as well as the principles of body psychotherapy and phenomenological aspects, offers cues for understanding the mechanisms involved. Within a neurobiological context, the significance of C-tactile afferents activated by special touch techniques and humoral changes such as increased oxytocin levels open additional ways of interpreting our findings.

Keywords: massage therapy; psychoactive massage; affect-regulating massage therapy; affective touch; depression; pain; interoception; C-tactile fibers; body psychotherapy

---

1. Introduction

Depressive disorders are among the most common mental diseases in the western world [1]. In addition to the personal suffering of those affected and their environment, the disease represents a significant challenge for society as a whole. Lifetime prevalence has been found to range between 16% and 20%. The World Health Organization (WHO) has declared that it will become the leading cause of global disease burden in the future [2]. The course of the disorder in most patients is episodic and is characterized by a lowered, depressed mood lasting for at least 2 weeks, vital and cognitive retardation, negative thoughts, and the core symptom of anhedonia inflicting nearly all areas of normal life and making life dull and gray. Suicidal ideation and suicidal behavior occur frequently; 10–15% of patients with affective disorders who do not receive efficacious prophylactic long-term treatment (e.g., with lithium salts) will finally die from suicide. In addition, a plethora of somatic symptoms, including pain and physical fatigue affect quality of life, impair working function, increase healthcare utilization, worsen depression outcomes, and increase the risk of recurrence [3]. There is further evidence that depression is associated with substantially disturbed body awareness and desynchronization causing psychomotor retardation [4,5]. These aspects do not receive sufficient consideration if depression is simply called a "mood disorder" or "affective disorder" [6].

It is important to realize that the body ("Leib" in German language and philosophy) of a depressed individual is affected just as much as the mental state. Many facets of colloquial language illustrate the close connection of body and depression, e.g., talking about a person who is depressed or mortified, we may say "he/she is down in the mouth".

Although the diagnosis and treatment of depression has improved significantly in recent years, there are still deficits in the care and therapy of affected individuals. Optimal treatment success often cannot be achieved, so that in about 30% of cases residual symptoms can be observed. These include primarily, sleep disorders, chronic depressed and/or anxious mood, cognitive deficits, and somatic symptoms [7,8].

The main treatment modalities comprise different types of psychotherapy and/or treatment with antidepressants and other psychotropic agents. However, although prescriptions for antidepressants are rising from year to year in most European countries and in the US [9], their overall efficacy is far from satisfactory. In recent years critical voices based on meta-analyses and serious, independent studies have drawn the attention of a larger audience to the fact that in some patient cohorts the therapeutic efficacy of antidepressants was not found to be higher than that of placebo [10–12]. On the other side, increased awareness of patients, doctors, and the general public has been directed particularly to adverse reactions to these compounds, such as a worsened course of the illness, increased cardiovascular mortality, suicidal ideation, or persistent sexual disturbances even after withdrawal [13,14]. Furthermore, it also appears that the beneficial effects of psychotherapy on depression were overestimated in the past [15]. This might be the reason why patients with depression often seek help and relief from their symptoms with "alternative" or complementary therapies [16].

Treatment strategies such as body-oriented methods, including mindfulness-based approaches, have been discussed and explored recently, e.g., body psychotherapy for the management of chronic depression [17]. There is also sufficient evidence for the effectiveness of, e.g., physical training such as aerobic exercise for depression [18,19]. In addition, elements from yoga, tai chi, and qigong are increasingly being investigated and used to treat mental disorders, but evidence of their efficacy is preliminary [20,21].

Survey data suggest frequent utilization of massage therapy or other hands-on treatment among patients with depression [16]. Whether a passive treatment modality such as massage therapy would have a beneficial effect on symptoms of depression presents an intriguing question in view of the great number of patients with treatment-resistant depression [22] and the practical lack of side effects of most types of massage [23]. In medical practice, positive effects of massage therapy, such as relaxation or anxiety relief, and antidepressant effects have been observed. These clinical experiences are supported by a meta-analysis of available studies. On the basis of 10 randomized controlled trials (RCTs) comprising 249 participants, Moyer et al. (2004) found that treatment resulted in a lower post-treatment level of depression than in 73% of the control subjects. The authors considered this finding as persuasive evidence for an antidepressive effect in particular and concluded that the medium effect size equaled that of psychotherapy [24]. In addition, they also found strong evidence for reduced trait anxiety. An earlier meta-analysis by Peters (1999), however, had concluded that existing studies on the effectiveness of massage as a nursing intervention had only limited validity and that more rigorous research would be needed [25]. A meta-analysis of 17 RCTs was performed by Hou et al. in 2010, indicating significant effectiveness in the treatment vs. control groups in spite of only moderate quality of the included studies [26]. Baumgart et al. (2011) presented findings from a systematic survey of 22 carefully selected randomized studies published between 1996 and 2009, including seven studies on patients with depression, anxiety, or exhaustion/fatigue as the main diagnosis [27]. All seven studies, only two of them on hospitalized patients, showed a significant reduction in anxiety symptoms, and depression was significantly reduced in five studies. However, the authors also underlined that the heterogeneity of the diagnoses and the diversity of the controls and the assessment methods still limited valid general conclusions on the efficacy of massage therapy in the treatment of depression.

The website of the American Massage Therapy Association (www.amtamassage.org) clearly documents the still existing paucity of controlled studies in this area and the need for further studies recruiting patients with clinical depression. There is a great variety of massage methods, such as Swedish massage, Esalen massage, Thai massage, etc. [28–30]. Our research group has been concentrating for many years on studying the clinical effects of affective touch, also called soft or gentle touch or psychoactive massage, in patients and healthy volunteers. In a previous randomized controlled trial, the application of a specially developed one-hour psychoactive massage (Slow Stroke®Massage) showed antidepressive efficacy in hospitalized patients with depression [31]. Sufficient evidence could be provided that within the special setting of this study, gentle touch was the key element to produce the antidepressive/anxiolytic effect on the behavioral and somatic level. In the present study, we investigated the mental and subjective somatic effects of a special form of psychoactive massage, the affect-regulating massage therapy (ARMT) vs. progressive muscle relaxation (PMR) in outpatients with depression. (PMR has become an established relaxation method over the last decades and is already used regularly in the psychiatric and psychosomatic field [32,33]). A direct comparison of the effectiveness of psychoactive massage therapy and PMR in patients with depression has not been done so far. The present study, therefore, tested the following hypotheses:

Hypothesis 1. *It is expected that the application of ARMT will prove to be more effective in positively influencing the behavioral and somatic dimensions related to depression than a standardized relaxation method such as PMR. This difference will be reflected in the observer ratings using the assessment instruments described below.*

Hypothesis 2. *It is expected that a stronger effect in favor of ARMT will also be seen in patients' self-assessments. Significant results are expected in the pre-post differences of at least half of the items tested on a specially developed visual analogue scale.*

2. Materials and Methods

2.1. Study Design

The study was designed as a two-arm, monocentric, randomized controlled intervention study with a fixed number of cases. Every patient in the intervention group received four weekly treatments by means of a standardized massage technique (ARMT). Patients in the control group received four applications of PMR over the same time period. Before starting and immediately after completing the study, patients were assessed by an external rater blinded to the specific treatments the patients had been assigned to. A visual analogue scale was used for self-assessment, which was filled in by the patients before and after each treatment. The study center was the outpatient clinic of the vocational school for massage at the University Hospital of Würzburg (Würzburg, Germany), directed by N. Hemrich.

2.2. Instruments for Assessing Mental and Somatic Symptoms

2.2.1. HAMD

The Hamilton Depression Scale (HAMD) was used as the external assessment instrument [34,35]. A total of 17 items concerning the depressive symptoms of the previous seven days are checked. Each item is scored from 0 to 4. The severity of the depression is classified as follows [36]: 0–8 points:

no depression or clinically unremarkable or remitted; 9–16 points: mild depression; 17–24 points: moderate depression and ≥25 points: severe depression.

2.2.2. BRMS

The Bech–Rafaelsen Melancholia Scale (BRMS) was used as a further questionnaire for external assessment at multiple time points [37]. It comprises a total of 11 items, which refer to the depressive symptoms of the previous three days. Each item is scored between 0 and 4. The interrater reliability of the German version has been found to be $r = 0.80$ and higher [38]; it has also generally been found to be $r = 0.80$ and higher. The severity of depression is classified according to the sum of all scores as follows: 0–5 points: no depression; 6–14 points: mild depression; 15–25 points: moderate depression and 26–44 points: severe depression.

2.2.3. VAS

A specially designed 100 mm visual analogue scale (VAS) was used for subjective assessment of depressive symptoms consisting of 8 items for self-assessment of the current mood [39]. It was completed by the patients immediately before and after each intervention in order to document changes that occurred during the intervention. Only the symptom of sleep disorder could not be recorded due to the given time frame. In addition, patients could write down free-form personal comments. The following items, indicating the negative poles (zero points) of the scale, were assessed:

VAS 1: Stress/tension
"I'm very tense"/"I'm completely relaxed"

VAS 2: Hopelessness
"I feel hopeless"/"I'm full of hope"

VAS 3: Internal unrest
"I am very restless"/"I am full of inner peace"

VAS 4: Pain sensations
"I'm feeling pain"/"I'm not feeling any pain"

VAS 5: Psychomotor retardation
"I feel rigid and immobile"/"I feel light and lively"

VAS 6: Tendency to brood
"Negative thoughts are circulating in my head"/"I'm thinking positive and optimistic"

VAS 7: Loss of drive
"I feel limp and listless"/"I feel full of energy and drive"

VAS 8: Unpleasant physical sensations
"I'm not comfortable in my body"/"I'm comfortable in my body"

2.2.4. Assessment on Clinical Interview

The initial examination included an assessment of the patient's general history as well as a detailed disease-focused interview. After the end of the treatment series, a final consultation was held. During this semi-structured interview, the patient's subjective experiences and attitudes toward the study were questioned and documented. All interviews were conducted by the principal investigator (first author) and recorded in writing.

2.3. Conducting the Study

2.3.1. Sample Size Calculation

The study by Müller-Oerlinghausen et al. served as the basis for the sample size calculation [31,40]. The mean values and mean differences between pre- and post-assessments and the standard deviation could be derived with regard to VAS. Differences of about 20 scale points with a standard deviation of

25 had been described for several VAS variables. Against this empirical background and assuming a significance level of 5% for two-sided tests, we calculated an optimal sample size of 58.75 cases, which was rounded up to 60. No potential attrition rate was taken into consideration.

2.3.2. Ethical Approval

The study was approved by the Ethics Committee of the Medical Faculty of the Julius Maximilian University of Würzburg. Performance of the study, including informed consent of the patients, followed the Declaration of Helsinki.

2.3.3. Recruitment and Randomization

The patients were recruited in cooperating psychiatric or psychotherapeutic practices in Würzburg. Advertisements were placed in the press and leaflets were distributed at the University Hospital of Würzburg.

Inclusion criteria were as follows:

- Patients of both sexes between the ages of 18 and 65;
- The presence of a mild to moderate depressive episode diagnosed by a general practitioner or specialist, including the following ICD-10 diagnoses: F32.0, F32.1, F32.2, F32.8, F32.9, F33.0, F33.1, F33.2, F33.8, F33.9.

Exclusion criteria:

- Acute comorbid medical condition.
- Eczematous skin disease;
- Marked varicose veins or venous thrombosis;
- Pregnancy;
- Simultaneous participation in another clinical trial.

The first contact of potential study participants was usually made by phone or email. Suitability for participation in the study was checked on the basis of the inclusion and exclusion criteria. If there was agreement, the patient's written consent to participate in the study was then obtained. Within two months, 60 patients were recruited. Randomization took place in the order of admission to the study. A randomization list was used, which was based on numbers from the random number generator of the SPSS® statistical program package. After being notified of the randomization result, three participants in the control group terminated their participation in the study prematurely because they did not agree with the assigned group. This resulted in 30 participants in the intervention group and 27 participants in the control group. The initial rating was carried out by an external observer blinded with regard to the randomization result. The threshold for inclusion in the study was set before as 9 points on the HAMD 17 and 6 points on the BRMS. No financial or other compensation was offered to the study participants. The process is shown in Figure 1.

2.4. Description of Interventions (ARMT and PMR)

2.4.1. Massage Group (ARMT)

The study was performed in cooperation with the vocational school for massage at the University Hospital of Würzburg. A working group was formed consisting of nine masseurs under training, the principal of the vocational school, and the principal investigator/first author, who is also a certified massage therapist. Through intensive training and communication, a standardized treatment procedure was developed, which was carried out by all therapists equally. Techniques for psychoactive massage described in the literature, e.g., Slow Stroke© Massage [28,31], were taken as the matrix for developing our own massage technique, described in detail below. (To get an idea of these special touch techniques ref. also to some video material under www.bruno-mueller-oerlinghausen.de or www.affective-touch.com).

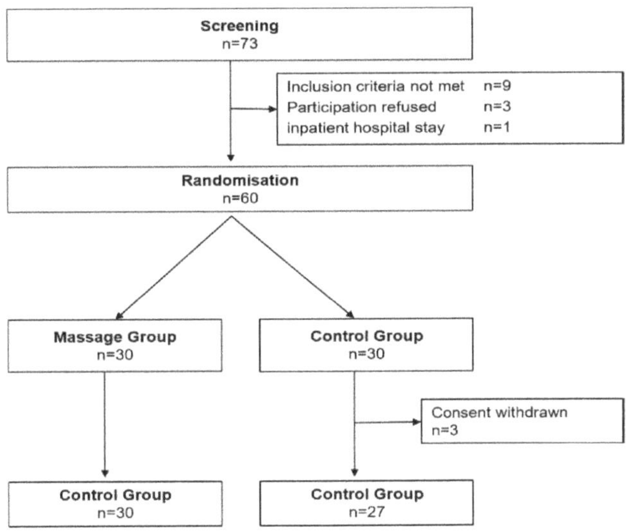

Figure 1. Recruitment and randomization.

Any massage session lasted 60 min including rest. It took place in a quiet room. A constant room temperature of at least 25 °C was ensured. The massage oil was preheated to 35 °C. Massage always began with the undressed patient in a supine position. The genital area was covered by a towel. At the beginning, the preheated massage oil was distributed on the ventral body surface to the abdomen, legs, and arms to ensure continuous treatment without interruption. Afterwards, the therapist's hands rested on the palmar side of the patient's feet to achieve conscious contact. Subsequently, extensive whole-body strokes were performed. Both hands were used to massage from the legs over the flanks up to the arms and over the pelvis and legs, and back to the starting point. This was followed by treatment of the lower extremities with superficial, partially stretching strokes and soft kneading. The sequence was continued by strokes from the middle of the body cranially and caudally as a diagonal whole-body stroke. After classical abdominal, thoracic, and arm treatment, as well as symmetrical whole-body strokes, the patient changed to the prone position. The treatment then began analogous to the ventral side, starting from the heel bone and continuing over the legs, back, and arms. This was followed by a sequence of diagonal and symmetrical whole-body strokes and soft kneading of the dorsal body. Finally, to mark the end of the treatment, the hands rested on the plantar sides of the feet. The patient was then allowed to rest for another 10–15 min. During this time, he or she was covered with sheets and a woolen blanket. Overall, the treatment was carried out very calmly and evenly. Possible muscular tension was not addressed in order to not interrupt the massage flow by any painful perceptions. No conversations were held during the treatment and no background music was played. Care was taken to ensure that patients were always treated by the same therapist within a treatment series.

2.4.2. Control Group (PMR)

In the control group, progressive muscle relaxation (PMR) according to Jacobson, a widely recognized relaxation method, was used [32,33]. In order to make the general conditions as equivalent as possible to those of the massage group, PMR was not performed in the group, but as an individual 45-min treatment. The instructions were given by the same therapists who were also active in the massage group. At the beginning of PMR, the patient was asked to get into in a comfortable supine position, using a massage table or gymnastics mat as a base. Care was taken to ensure a comfortable position through appropriate room temperature and the use of pillows and blankets. The patient was then individually guided through a PMR whole-body schedule. The standardized instructions were presented in a calm and pleasant tone. Afterwards, the patient could rest for 10–15 min. During the treatment, no conversations were held and no background music was played. Care was taken to ensure that the patients were always treated by the same therapist within one series.

2.5. Accompanying Therapy

Any existing therapy with psychotropic drugs and/or psychotherapy could be continued. Changes in this respect were documented at the end of the trial period.

2.6. Statistical Evaluation

Absolute and relative frequencies, as well as mean and standard deviation, were used to present personal data such as age, gender, marital status, etc. All data collected manually by the questionnaire were first transferred to an Excel spreadsheet. Data were then analyzed using IBM SPSS Statistics (version 25). Since normal distribution of the parameters could not be assumed, the Mann–Whitney U-test, a nonparametric test, was chosen to calculate statistical significance. The level of statistical significance was set as $p < 0.05$ (two-sided). Pearson's correlation coefficient r was calculated for estimation of effect size.

3. Results

3.1. Description of Sample

3.1.1. Sociodemographic Data

The ARMT group consisted of 30 participants. The mean age was 45.2 years; the youngest patient was 24, the oldest, 60 years old; 76.7% were female. About half of the participants were married or in a stable partnership (53.3%). The majority of participants (76.7%) had an intermediate or high school diploma and had qualified employment.

The PMR group consisted of 27 participants. The mean age was 45.0 years; the youngest patient was 19, the oldest, 64 years old; 81.5% of were female. About half of the participants were married or living in a stable partnership (55.6%). Almost all participants (96.3%) had an intermediate or high school diploma and had qualified employment; in this respect they were somewhat different from the subjects of the ARMT group. The sociodemographic data is shown in Table 1.

Table 1. Sociodemographic variables of the two patient groups.

	ARMT	$n = 30$	**PMR**	$n = 27$
	M	*SD*	*M*	*SD*
Age (years)	45.2	9.43	44.9	12.29
Sex	*n*	%	*n*	%
female (n)	22	73.33	22	81.48
male (n)	8	26.67	5	18.52
Civil status				
single	9	30.00	9	33.33
married/partnership	16	53.33	15	55.55
divorced/widowed	5	16.67	3	11.11
Children				
childless	11	36.67	15	55.55
one or two children	13	43.33	6	22.22
three or more children	6	20.00	6	22.22
Education				
primary school	7	23.33	1	3.7
secondary school	13	43.33	25	92.6
high school	10	33.33	1	3.7
Employment				
vocational training	23	76.67	22	81.48
academic career	7	23.33	5	18.52
unemployed	6	20.00	7	25.92

ARMT = affect regulating massage therapy; PMR = progressive muscle relaxation; M = Mean; SD = Standard Deviation.

3.1.2. Depression-Related Data

In the ARMT group, the severity of depression was rated as moderately severe, corresponding to 18.2 points on average on the HAMD at the beginning of the study. Assessment by means of the BRMS (mean value 16.1 points) also confirmed moderately severe depression. Psychopharmacological treatment as mono- or combination therapy was reported by 56.7% of the participants. There was no change in dosage for 83.3% of the patients over the duration of the study. About half (53.33%) of the participants were under psychotherapeutic treatment during participation in the study.

In the PMR group, the severity of depression rated by means of the HAMD averaged 19.2 points at the beginning of the study, also indicating a moderately severe depressive episode. The BRMS scores suggested an identical classification, with an average of 17.4 points. Psychopharmacological treatment as mono or combination therapy accounted for 55.5% of the participants. There was no change in dosage for 85.2% of the participants during participation in the study. Almost half (48.2%) of the participants were under psychotherapeutic treatment during the study.

3.2. Effects of ARMT and PMR Assessed by HAMD and BRMS

The averaged differences between the HAMD assessment at time TA, before the first treatment, and time TB, after the fourth treatment, were calculated. The reduction in symptom burden over 4 weeks was significantly more pronounced in the ARMT group than in the control group ($p = 0.034$, $r = 0.28$). The results are shown in Figure 2.

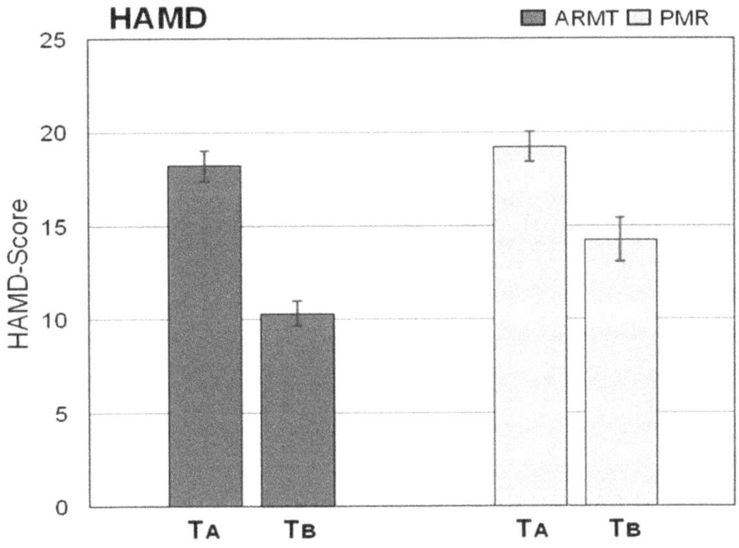

Figure 2. Summed up Hamilton Depression Scale (HAMD) scores in ARMT and PMR groups before (TA) and after (TB) completing the full series of treatments (mean ± SEM).

Focusing on individual items of the HAMD, changes in the following items proved to be highly statistically significant with a moderate effect size:

- HAMD 1: Depressive mood ($p = 0.004$, $r = 0.39$)
- HAMD 13: Somatic symptoms ($p = 0.021$, $r = 0.30$)

Although statistical significance was not reached, we consider the numerical change of item five (sleep disorders) to be particularly noteworthy ($p = 0.059$, $r = 0.25$). The course of the BRMS scores is depicted in Figure 3. The reduction in symptom burden during 4 weeks was significantly more pronounced in the massage group than in the control group ($p = 0.04$, $r = 0.27$). Focusing on individual items, the difference of the following single BRMS dimensions over time proved to be statistically significant:

- BRMS 8: Emotional retardation ($p = 0.037$, $r = 0.28$)
- BRMS 9: Sleep disorders ($p = 0.038$, $r = 0.28$)

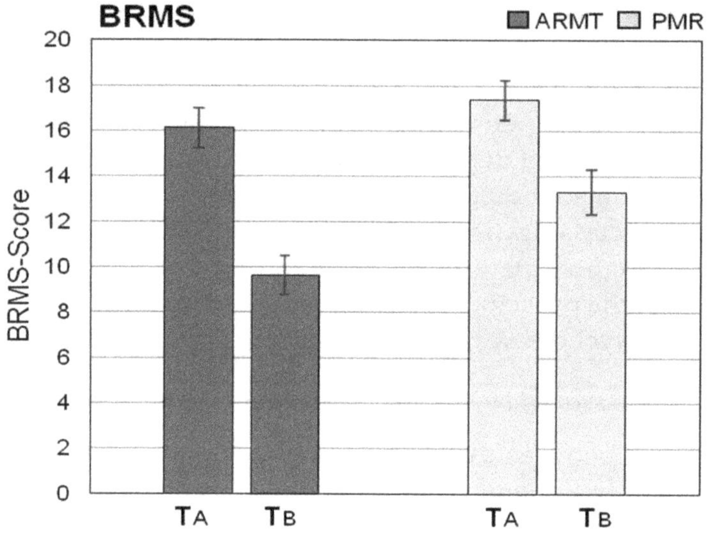

Figure 3. Summed up Bech–Rafaelsen Melancholia Scale (BRMS) scores in ARMT and PMR groups before (*T*A) and after (*T*B) completing the full series of treatments (mean ± SEM).

Although statistical significance was not achieved, special attention might be given to the change in item one, motor activity ($p = 0.063$, $r = 0.25$).

In summary, the findings so far are in accordance with Hypothesis 1 (see above).

3.3. Results of Participant's Self-Assessment (VAS)

For each VAS item (one to eight), the pre-post differences related to each treatment session were averaged over time points *T*1–*T*4. Figure 4 shows that the treatment effects were markedly and significantly more pronounced in the ARMT group as compared to the PMR group. Statistical significance of this difference existed for six of the eight items. (Descriptions of single items can be found in Section 2.2.3).

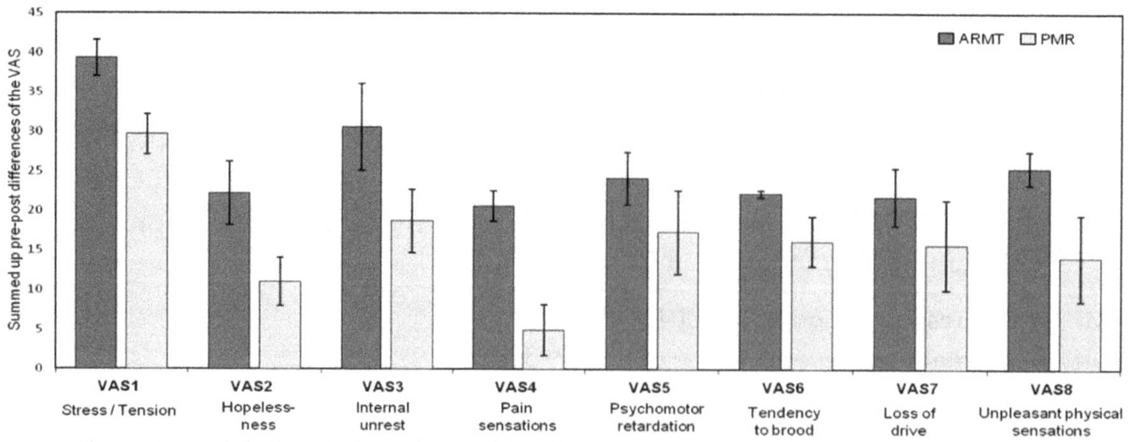

Figure 4. Averaged differences (± SD) of individual pre-/post-treatment visual analogue scale (VAS) values over total study period (*T*1–*T*4).

Please note that a value of 100 on, e.g., VAS 1 ("tension") would signify that the proband felt completely relaxed. (A score of 100 is always the positive pole and zero the negative pole of each

VAS item.) In detail, the following individual VAS items show (highly) significant changes in favor of the massage treatment, i.e., greater pre-post differences of particularly those variables closely associated with depression:

VAS 1: Stress/tension ($p = 0.035$, $r = 0.28$)
VAS 2: Hopelessness ($p = 0.032$, $r = 0.28$)
VAS 3: Internal unrest ($p = 0.009$, $r = 0.35$)
VAS 4: Pain sensations ($p = 0.003$, $r = 0.39$)
VAS 5: Psychomotor retardation ($p = 0.012$, $r = 0.33$)
VAS 8: Unpleasant physical sensations ($p = 0.011$, $r = 0.34$)

A moderate effect size was observed for most of the changes. The pre-post differences in VAS 6 (tendency to brood/negative thoughts, $p = 0.075$, $r = 0.24$) and VAS 7 (lack of drive, $p = 0.070$, $r = 0.24$) were not different between the two treatment groups. To illustrate the therapeutic process, Figure 5, as an example, presents the time course of VAS 5, psychomotor retardation (pre- and post-treatment scores) over the four treatment sessions. Obviously, the treatment effects are more marked in the ARMT group.

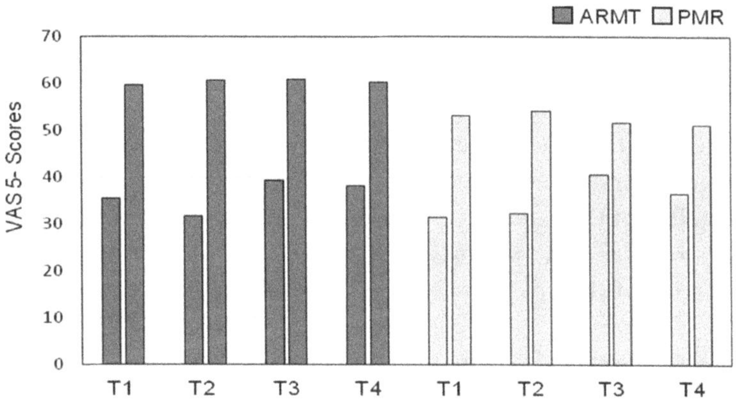

Figure 5. Time course of VAS 5 (psychomotor retardation) scores over time points *T1*–*T4* in ARMT vs. PMR groups. Arithmetic means before and after treatment (right and left columns, respectively). Note: A score of 100 signifies that the proband agrees fully with the statement "My body feels light and mobile".

Consequently, Hypothesis 2 could be confirmed, i.e., it is expected that a stronger effect will also be seen in the patients' self-assessment. Significant results are assumed in at least half of the VAS items.

3.4. Statements of Study Participants in Clinical Interviews

The statistical results are underlined by the personal statements of the study participants. Particularly frequent positive comments were made by patients assigned to the massage group:

- Better body awareness and deep relaxation;
- Interruption of brooding and negative thoughts;
- Increased motivation for everyday life activities.

As points of criticism, some patients mentioned a feeling of coldness and a sense of shame about taking off their clothes before the massage.

Additionally, patients in the control group described positive effects of PMR:

- Useful in everyday life and as a sleeping aid;
- Easy relaxation and better body awareness.

The lack of background music was occasionally mentioned as a point of criticism. Patients in both groups indicated that they had particularly benefited from the morning sessions. The early treatment appointment significantly reduced the burden of a matutinal depressive mood and had a positive effect for the rest of the day. Some participants also experienced a continuous increase in the perceived positive effects during the course of the study. As a point of criticism, study participants from both groups mentioned particular unfavorable external conditions, such as noise from the adjacent construction site.

4. Discussion

As outlined above, somatic symptoms such as psychomotor retardation, sleep disorders, or general fatigue are prominent features of the clinical picture of depression. Thomas Fuchs perceives depression as a physical illness existing not only against the background of functional disorders of the entire organism, such as dysregulation of the hormone system and biorhythmics, metabolic and immunological changes. Rather, as a phenomenologist, he describes a disorder of the basic physical constitution that presents itself as a "corporisation of the body" (ref. [41] the contrasting significance of "corpse" and "body" in English). Like an objectification, the patient experiences himself distanced from his body-self and no longer "at home in his body", as the sociologist Hartmut Rosa illustrates it in general terms. The depressed person does not feel "comfortable in his skin", where the skin in Rosa's terminology constitutes an organ of resonance [42]. This disturbed bodily feeling manifests itself in different regions, such as tightness in the chest, heaviness of the limbs, or chronic fatigue. The body loses drive and spontaneity. Everything feels heavy. This is also reflected in the subject's exchange with the environment: breathing is flattened, facial expressions are reduced, libido is often tuned down. The "feeling of numbness" overshadows every perception, so that even crying is no longer possible. It is not mourning that is felt, but the feeling of emptiness and lifelessness that is expressed primarily in the body. "Being a body is replaced by having a body" [43]. Would it not be possible that the cognitive and emotional characteristics of depression are secondary reactions to the perception of the primary bodily changes [44,45]?

Hartmut Rosa tries to separate the depressive experience from grief: "Grief is an element of a relationship to the world that is, on the whole, quite resonant. [...] Depression, on the other hand, is characterized by the fact that there are no more tears: the relationship to the world can no longer be liquefied, it is petrified" [42]. The patient feels unable to counteract this weighing feeling of heaviness, and this fundamental phenomenon might induce speculation on a potential bridge to the concept of "learned helplessness" [46].

Against this background, it seems a rational approach to use body-oriented therapies in the treatment of depression. Our findings indicate antidepressive, anxiolytic, and analgesic effects, which were significantly more pronounced among the participants in the massage therapy group as compared to those in the PRM group. How can these remarkable therapeutic effects of a professional, empathetic, affective touch technique be explained? We shall discuss some options on various explanatory levels.

One of the most obvious effects of massage therapy, according to the patients' self-assessment, is the pronounced psychomotor relaxation, which is also reflected in the reduction in inner restlessness. However, it was not only general tension that was released by the treatment. Rather, feelings of hopelessness and inner restlessness were also significantly reduced. The therapeutic touch technique also had a positive effect on the existing obsessive brooding tendency. In the final open talks with the patients, we often heard statements such as that the massage finally allowed the individual to "turn off my thoughts" or "to break loose". One patient made a written comment after the third massage session: "Never before did I experience such a deep relaxation. None of the usual relaxing (mind–body) exercises had this strong effect".

However, even if this feeling of relaxation is a significant part of the overall effect, there must be other factors involved, otherwise the superiority of massage over a standardized relaxation method would hardly make sense. In modern theories of depression, the concept of interoception has been given increasing attention [47,48]. Interoception, i.e., the perception of the processes of the body's interior, distinguishes between proprioception (perception of body position and movement in space) and visceroception (perception of the inner organs' activity). In contrast to exteroception, the signals making up interoception are sent from the entire inner milieu of the individual to the brain. Interoception can likewise be understood as a skill that can be trained through regular practice (e.g., in mindfulness methods), thus contributing to a more conscious body perception and better emotional self-regulation.

In order to explain the effects of the body-oriented interventions examined in this study, we may refer to this concept. The external conditions per se that were more or less concordant in both groups provided a framework for increased body perception. A calm atmosphere without distractions was created to enable the patients to experience consciously their bodily condition, in the sense of an "inner view". The special feature of affective touch is the calm, mindful approach enabling patients to consciously experience their body. This procedure can thus be described as an intensive training of interoception. The patients' oral statements underline this assumption.

Recently a hypothesis was put forward that the antidepressive effect of affective touch can be explained by a normalization of disturbed interoception [49]. Another special factor that could explain the significant superiority of affect-regulating massage based on its basic element, affective touch, is the factor of touch itself. A gentle, empathetic touch is generally experienced as pleasant. It can soothe feelings of social exclusion and facilitate interpersonal binding [50,51]. The neurophysiological correlates of this type of touch have been intensively investigated during the last two decades. The specific feeling of well-being that humans and hairy mammals experience with this type of touch is based neurophysiologically on the activation of so-called C-actile afferents. In particular, Swedish researchers were able to show that a neuronal network of slowly conducting, non-myelinated C-fibers reacts to special receptors of the hairy skin (located, e.g., on the back of the hand, but not on the palm). For these receptors, gentle, slow, and rhythmic touch at a speed of about 3 cm/sec is the appropriate stimulus, projected directly and predominantly into the insular area. The stimulation of such C tactile fibers seems to have as its only "purpose" creating a feeling of well-being [52]. This might also have evolutionary biological significance, e.g., by promoting the feeling of kinship within a group. Other afferent projections via A-beta or A-alpha fibers as well as signals from mechanoreceptors in the hairy skin most likely will also contribute to the overall interoceptive signaling taking place in various limbic structures.

Switching to the level of experience and behavior, it should be kept in mind that touch is the basal medium of communication among humans and animals [53,54]. Against the background of anhedonia, described as the most common feature of depressive experience and behavior, our findings are in some way "paradoxical". How can patients with depression feel and express bodily and verbally affective touch as a positive experience? Obviously empathic, professional touch can slip into this basic communication disorder, i.e., can enter the disturbed emotional world of the patient. It fits into this concept that participants in the massage group often expressed feelings of having been "accepted" in the final talks with the first author. The following English translation of a patient's original final statement might help us in understanding some essentials of the therapeutic process:

"I cried a lot the first time. For the first time I was able to feel my legs and my feet. Tears of joy during the treatment. From the second session onwards, even better with a warming pad. Meeting of the hands on my belly—very touching. I never experienced such a loving touch before. With further treatments I was loosening up completely. Already during the second session I perceived more than the first time. Even my hands were treated! Because of the depression I couldn't allow touching me otherwise.... My shell has become softer, my heart is opened. The massage therapist was totally super gentle, helped me to become a "whole person" again".

Even though the patient quoted above was in all probability not familiar with the work of Wilhelm Reich [55], in her description she nevertheless takes up an essential aspect that plays an important role in modern body psychotherapy [56]. In Reichian terminology, one can speak of an armoring of the emotions [55], which can be influenced, if not eliminated, by massage therapy. According to our observations, patients often are taken by surprise that after a massage session their body feels "less heavy". A trusting therapist–patient relationship in the field of physiotherapy seems to be just as important as is already recognized in psychotherapy. The therapeutic relationship thrives on appropriate empathy and the right balance between affectionate empathy and professional demarcation. In contrast to psychotherapy, however, in the physiotherapeutic context it is specifically the body of the patient that is perceived and accepted and thus enters into resonance with the therapist. This leads to new, possibly corrective (body) experiences, which can be of decisive importance for the therapeutic process. To quote the clinical psychologist C.A. Moyer from his meta-analysis of studies on the effects of massage therapy in depression: "The finding that massage therapy has an effect on trait anxiety and depression that is similar in magnitude to what would be expected to result from psychotherapy suggests the possibility that these different treatments may be more similar than previously considered" [24].

However, coming back to the mechanism involved, a decisive difference exists in healing touch: according to Changaris, we offer the patient direct affect-regulating "bottom-up" therapy in contrast or addition to the "top-down" technique of cognitive psychotherapy [57]. Finally, humoral effects such as increased oxytocin levels and reduced cortisol, e.g., in saliva might add to the interpretation of the antidepressive effects of psychoactive massage within a neurobiological context [58,59]. Oxytocin has been attributed with significant effects on social interaction, as well as feelings of trust and connectedness [60]. Thus, it does not seem unlikely that depressive patients suffering from social withdrawal and isolation could profit from increased oxytocin release, possibly facilitating contact and communication [61]. Additionally, the analgesic effects of massage therapy might be related to increased oxytocin release [62]. Tiffany Field [58], against the background of various experimental studies, has often emphasized the importance of markedly reduced cortisol levels in urine or saliva of various diagnostic groups of depressed or stressed patients having been given massage therapy. The strong relaxing effect observed also in our patients might well be related to this hormonal change. Tiffany Field, however, has often argued that the lowered cortisol levels are related to increased vagal activity [63].

4.1. Strengths of the Study

4.1.1. Control Group

It was already pointed out that the choice of an adequate control group, besides the impossibility of blinding, is one of the biggest methodical problems in developing a meaningful design in massage studies. Often the control conditions are chosen in such a way that only a standard therapy, waiting list, or general relaxation (quiet sitting/lying, relaxing music or movies) is used. In our study, a more adequate procedure was chosen instead, which led to the most equal conditions possible for all study participants, with the essential difference that therapeutic touch occurred only in the massage group. This allowed us to strengthen the evidence that it is not a bunch of mostly unknown unspecific effects such as personal devotion, but the affective touch as such that is responsible for the greater effectiveness of massage therapy. "Adequate control conditions" signifies that participants in both the massage and control groups always received individual treatments. PMR is typically performed as group therapy. It can be assumed that performing PMR as an individual treatment increased its effectiveness. In other words, we selected a rather conservative approach, which resulted in moderate effect sizes. Use of a "placebo" control would most likely produce much greater effect sizes. In addition, an identical group of therapists were involved in both groups in order to avoid distorting personal influence. Furthermore, the same premises were used for both the massage and control groups. All treatments took place in comparable periods within four months and in a constant environment.

4.1.2. Study Participants

Relatively few studies on the efficacy of massage therapy have been conducted so far in patients with mental illness. The present study provides further evidence of the positive effects of massage therapy in depression. In selecting the study participants, we focused on patients with mild to moderate depression whose clinical picture and disease severity reflected a broad section of the general population. In this way we were able to create largely realistic conditions as they are encountered daily in practices of both GPs and psychiatrists, but also physiotherapists.

4.1.3. Assessments

Standardized and widely used psychiatric scales for assessing and quantifying depressive symptoms were employed in validated German translation.

4.1.4. Conducting the Study

In both groups, care was taken to ensure the consistency of therapists in individual treatment series. In addition to reducing variance, this also served to maximize the effects, as other studies have shown the importance of therapist consistency [64]. Furthermore, all therapists were equally prepared for the study owing to intensive training. This ensured a standardized and comparable execution of individual therapies.

4.2. Limitation

One important criterion for the quality of studies contributing to the bulk of evidence-based medicine, besides randomization and active control, is the blinding of study participants and directly involved investigators. For obvious methodological reasons, this requirement could not be met in the present study, as in many comparable studies. However, according to a recent meta-analysis, the absolute postulate of blinding when carrying out a sound study might be somewhat questioned in the future [65]. Furthermore, the self-assessment questionnaires (before and after each treatment) were handed out to the patients by the treating therapists themselves. In retrospect, the critical question came up as to whether this circumstance may have led to distortion. One may speculate whether it would have been important for some patients to leave a positive impression or not to "disappoint" the therapist by filling out a questionnaire in a neutral or negative way. However, since the same questionnaire handling was used in both groups, this possible bias was not further discussed, which might have caused a greater overall effect, but probably did not distort the difference between the two groups

4.3. Outlook

Due to the limited effectiveness of the currently available and widely used treatments in depression, it seems reasonable to expand the therapeutic spectrum for inpatients and outpatients with body-oriented procedures. In this context, affect-regulating or comparable psychoactive massage therapies represent a noteworthy opportunity to open up new access routes for acute treatment. They can be used as low-threshold offerings in the outpatient setting in order to achieve a rapid antidepressive effect. Their use in an inpatient setting is also conceivable according to the findings of a previous controlled study [31]. Very good adherence can be expected, as the present study was also able to prove. Body-oriented therapeutic approaches should be given higher value within the spectrum of antidepressive treatments. They also deserve a special place beside much propagated mind–body techniques [66,67]. A severely depressed patient will often be unable to participate in special psychological training sessions aimed at stress reduction.

5. Conclusions

This randomized controlled intervention study examined the psychophysical effects of body-oriented treatment methods on patients suffering from mild to moderate depression in an outpatient setting. We tested the hypothesis that a one-hour massage based on a special gentle touch technique (affect regulating massage therapy = ARMT) is superior in its positive effects to a relaxation method that has long been established in the clinical field, progressive muscle relaxation according to Jacobson. Our results confirm this assumption. In both the observer ratings and self-assessments of patients using a visual analogue scale, statistically significant superiority of massage therapy was shown. When focusing on individual dimensions of the HAMD, the superior effects were particularly evident in the items "depressive mood" and "general somatic symptoms". Assessment using the BRMS showed statistically significant superiority of massage therapy particularly in the items "emotional retardation" and "sleep disorders". As for the sleep disorders so often encountered in patients with depression, it should be noted that massage had a positive effect, especially on difficulty remaining asleep, while difficulty getting to sleep responded better to PMR. This observation also coincides with the free-form statements of some study participants who used the PMR technique outside of the study, independently as an aid to fall asleep. Especially in the self-assessment (VAS) of patients, massage therapy proved to be superior. This became obvious for the vast majority of items questioned. When inspecting the pre-post differences of individual VAS items, the stronger impact of massage therapy on the dimensions stress/tension, internal unrest, unpleasant physical sensation, psychomotor retardation, and hopelessness is particularly impressive. Changes were also marked for pain sensations. Overall, we were able to document the doubtless superiority of ARMT for core symptoms of depressive experience and behavior.

Author Contributions: M.M.A.: conceptualization, investigation, writing—review and editing; B.M.-O.: methodology, supervision, writing—original draft; N.H.: resources; D.B.: supervision. All authors have read and agreed to the published version of the manuscript.

Acknowledgments: Thanks are due to Ulrich Stefenelli for his advice and help in statistical matters and to Michael Eggart for methodical input. Thanks are also due the Karl and Veronica Carstens Foundation (Essen, Germany) for scientific advice during M.M.A.'s work on her doctoral thesis.

References

1. Jacobi, F.; Höfler, M.; Strehle, J.; Mack, S.; Gerschler, A.; Scholl, L.; Busch, M.A.; Maske, U.; Hapke, U.; Gaebel, W.; et al. Psychische Störungen in der Allgemeinbevölkerung: Studie zur Gesundheit Erwachsener in Deutschland und ihr Zusatzmodul Psychische Gesundheit (DEGS1-MH). *Nervenarzt* **2014**, *85*, 77–87. [CrossRef] [PubMed]
2. *Depression and Other Common Mental Disorders: Global Health Estimates*; World Health Organization: Geneva, Switzerland, 2017.
3. Kapfhammer, H.P. Somatic symptoms in depression. *Dial. Clin. Neurosci.* **2006**, *8*, 227–239.
4. Fuchs, T.; Schlimme, J.E. Embodiment and psychopathology: A phenomenological perspective. *Curr. Opin. Psychiatry* **2009**, *22*, 570–575. [CrossRef] [PubMed]
5. Fuchs, T. Melancholia as a desynchronization. Towards a psychopathology of interpersonal time. *Psychopathology* **2001**, *34*, 179–186. [CrossRef]
6. Danielsson, L.; Rosberg, S. Depression embodied: An ambigous striving against fading. *Nord. Coll. Caring Sci.* **2014**, *29*, 501–509. [CrossRef]
7. Paykel, E.S.; Ramana, R.; Cooper, Z.; Hayhurst, H.; Kerr, J.; Barocka, A. Residual symptoms after partial remission: An important outcome in depression. *Psychol. Med.* **1995**, *25*, 1171–1180. [CrossRef]
8. Nierenberg, A.A. Residual symptoms in depression: Prevalence and impact. *J. Clin. Psychiatry* **2015**, *76*, e1480. [CrossRef]
9. Lohse, M.; Müller-Oerlinghausen, B. Psychopharmaka. In *Arzneiverodnungsreport 2019*; Schwabe, U., Paffrath, D., Ludwig, W.-D., Klauber, J., Eds.; Springer: Berlin, Germany, 2019; pp. 927–959.
10. Cuiipers, P.; Cristea, A. What if a placebo effect explained all the activity of depression treatments? *World Psychiatry* **2015**, *14*, 310–311. [CrossRef]

11. Munkholm, K.; Paludan-Müller, A.S.; Boesen, K. Considering the methodological limitations in the evidence base of antidepressants for depression: A reanalysis of a network meta-analysis. *BMJ Open* **2019**, *9*, e024886. [CrossRef]
12. Pigott, H.E.; Leventhal, A.M.; Alter, G.S.; Boven, J.J. Efficacy and effectiveness of antidepressants: Current status of research. *Psychother. Psychosom.* **2010**, *79*, 267–279. [CrossRef]
13. Fava, G.A.; Tomba, E.; Grandi, S. The road to recovery from depression. Don't drive today with yesterday's map. *Psychother. Psychosom.* **2007**, *6*, 260–265. [CrossRef] [PubMed]
14. Andrews, P.W.; Thomson, J.A.; Amstadter, A.; Neale, M.C. Primum nil nocere: An evolutionary analysis of whether antidepressants do more harm than good. *Front. Psychol.* **2012**, *3*, 117. [CrossRef] [PubMed]
15. Cuiipers, P.; van Straten, A.; Bohlmeijer, E. The effects of psychotherapy for adult depression are overestimated: A meta-analysis of study quality and effect size. *Psychol. Med.* **2010**, *40*, 211–223. [CrossRef] [PubMed]
16. Wu, P.; Fuller, C.; Liu, X.; Lee, H.; Fan, B.; Hoven, C.W.; Mandell, D.; Wade, C.; Kronenberg, F. Use of complementary and alternative medicine among women with depression: Results of a national survey. *Psychiatr. Serv.* **2007**, *58*, 349–356. [CrossRef]
17. Röhricht, F.; Papadopoulos, N.; Priebe, S. An exploratory randomized controlled trial of body psychotherapy for patients with chronic depression. *J. Affect. Dis.* **2013**, *151*, 85–91. [CrossRef]
18. Cooney, G.M.; Dwan, K.; Greig, C.A.; Lawlor, D.A.; Rimer, J.; Waugh, F.R.; McMurdo, M.; Mead, G.E. Exercise for depression. *Cochrane Database Syst. Rev.* **2013**, CD004366. [CrossRef]
19. Kvam, S.; Kleppe, C.L.; Nordhus, I.H.; Hovland, A. Exercise as a treatment for depression: A meta-analysis. *J. Affect. Disord.* **2016**, *202*, 67–86. [CrossRef]
20. Cramer, H.; Lauche, R.; Langhorst, J.; Dobos, G. Yoga for depression: A systematic review and meta-analysis. *Depress Anxiety* **2013**, *30*, 1068–1083. [CrossRef]
21. Oh, B.; Choi, S.M.; Inamori, A.; Rosenthal, D.; Yeung, A. Effects of qigong on depression: A systemic review. *Evid. Based Complement. Alternat. Med.* **2013**, *2013*, 134737. [CrossRef]
22. Jaffe, D.H.; Rive, B.; Denee, T.R. The humanistic and economic burden of treatment-resistant depression in Europe: A cross-sectional study. *BMC Psychiatry* **2019**, *19*, 247. [CrossRef]
23. Ernst, E. The safety of massage therapy. *Rheumatology* **2003**, *42*, 1101–1106. Available online: https://academic.oup.com/rheumatology/article/42/9/1101/1772218 (accessed on 2 May 2020). [CrossRef] [PubMed]
24. Moyer, C.A.; Rounds, J.; Hannum, J.W. A meta-analysis of massage therapy research. *Psychol. Bull.* **2004**, *130*, 3–18. [CrossRef] [PubMed]
25. Peters, R.H. The effectiveness of therapeutic touch: A meta-analytic view. *Nurs. Sci. Q.* **1999**, *12*, 52–61. [CrossRef] [PubMed]
26. Hou, W.H.; Chiang, P.T.; Hsu, Y.T.; Chiu, S.; Yen, Y.C. Treatment effects of massage therapy in depressed p 2eople: A meta-analysis. *J. Clin. Psychiatry* **2010**, *71*, 894–901. [CrossRef] [PubMed]
27. Baumgart, S.; Müller-Oerlinghausen, B.; Schendera, C.F.G. Efficacy of massage therapy on depression and anxious disorders as well as on depressiveness and anxiety as comorbidity. A systematic overview of controlled studies. (Article in German with English abstract). *Phys. Rehab. Kur. Med.* **2011**, *21*, 167–182. [CrossRef]
28. Reichert, B. (Ed.) *Massage-Therapie*; Georg Thieme: Stuttgart, Germany, 2015.
29. Hoyme, R.J. *The Complete Guide to Modern Massage: Step-by-Step Massage Basis and Techniques from Around the World*; Althea Press: New York, NY, USA, 2018.
30. Müller-Oerlinghausen, B.; Kiebgis, G.M. *Berührung- Warum Wir Sie Brauchen und Wie Sie Uns Heilt*, 2nd ed.; Ullstein: München, Germany, 2018.
31. Müller-Oerlinghausen, B.; Berg, C.; Scherer, P.; Mackert, A.; Moestl, H.P.; Wolf, J. Effects of slow-stroke massage as complimentary treatment of depressed hospitalized patients: Results of a controlled study (SeSeTra). (Article in German with English abstract). *Dtsch. Med. Wochenschr.* **2004**, *129*, 1363–1368.
32. Jacobson, E. *Entspannung als Therapie: Progressive Relaxation in Theorie und Praxis*, 7th ed.; Klett-Cotta: Stuttgart, Germany, 2011.
33. Petermann, F. *Entspannungsverfahren: Das Praxishandbuch. Mit E-Book Inside*; Neuausgabe, 6., überarbeitete Auflage; Julius Beltz GmbH & Co: Weinheim, Germany, 2020.
34. Hamilton, M. A rating scale for depression. *J. Neurol. Neurosurg. Psychiatry* **1960**, *23*, 56–62. [CrossRef]
35. Weyer, G.; Koeppen, D. *Internationale Skalen für Psychiatrie 6*; überarb. und erw. Aufl; Beltz-Test: Göttingen, Germany, 2015.

36. Zimmerman, M.; Martinez, J.H.; Young, D.; Chelminski, I.; Dalrymple, K. Severity classification on the Hamilton Depression Rating Scale. *J. Affect. Disord.* **2013**, *150*, 384–388. [CrossRef]
37. Stieglitz, R.D. *Bech-Rafaelsen-Melancholie-Skala*; Hogrefe: Göttingen, Germany, 1998.
38. Maier, W.; Philipp, W. Comparative analysis of observer rating scales. *Acta Psychiatr. Scand.* **1985**, *72*, 239–245. [CrossRef]
39. Schomacher, J. Gütekriterien der visuellen Analogskala zur Schmerzbewertung. *Physioscience* **2008**, *4*, 125–133. [CrossRef]
40. Müller-Oerlinghausen, B.; Berg, C.; Droll, W. Die Slow Stroke Massage als ein körpertherapeutischer Ansatz bei Depression. *Psychiatr. Prax.* **2007**, *34*, S305–S308. [CrossRef] [PubMed]
41. Fuchs, T. Corporealized and disembodied minds. A phenomenological view of the body in melancholia and schizophrenia. *Psychiatry Psychol.* **2005**, *12*, 95–107.
42. Rosa, H. *Resonanz: Eine Soziologie der Weltbeziehung*, 1st ed.; Suhrkamp: Berlin, Germany, 2016.
43. Faller, H. *Depression: Klinik, Ursachen, Therapie*; Königshausen & Neumann: Würzburg, Germany, 2011.
44. Röhricht, F. Leibgedächtnis und Körper-Ich: Zwei zentrale Bezugspunkte in der störungsspezifischen körperorientierten Psychotherapie. *Psychol. Österreich.* **2011**, *4*, 239–248.
45. Gallagher, S. *How the Body Shapes the Mind*; Oxford University Press: New York, NY, USA, 2005.
46. Seligman, M.E.P. Learned helpnessless. *Ann. Rev. Med.* **1972**, *23*, 407–412. [CrossRef] [PubMed]
47. Eggart, M.; Lange, A.; Binser, M.J.; Queri, S.; Müller-Oerlinghausen, B. Major Depressive disorder is associated with Impaired interoceptive accuracy: A systematic review. *Brain Sci.* **2019**, *9*, 131. [CrossRef] [PubMed]
48. Arikha, N. The Interoceptive Turn. The Science of How We Sense Ourselves from within, Including Our Bodily States, is Creating a Radical Picture of Selfhood. 2019. Available online: https://aeon.co/essays/the-interoceptive-turn-is-maturing-as-a-rich-science-of-selfhood (accessed on 9 June 2020).
49. Eggart, M.; Queri, S.; Müller-Oerlinghausen, B. Are the antidepressive effects of massage therapy mediated by restoration of impaired interoceptive functioning? A novel hypothetical mechanism. *Med. Hypotheses* **2019**, *128*, 28–32. [CrossRef]
50. Von Mohr, M.; Kirsch, L.P.; Fotopoulou, A. The soothing function of touch: Affective touch reduces feelings of social exclusion. *NeuroImage* **2018**, *169*, 162–171. [CrossRef]
51. Takeuchi, M.S.; Miyaoka, H.; Tomoda, A.; Suzuki, M.; Liu, Q.; Kitamura, T. The effect of interpersonal touch during childhood on adult attachment and depression: A neglected area of family and developmental psychology? *J. Child Fam. Stud.* **2010**, *19*, 109–117. [CrossRef]
52. Olausson, H.; Wessberg, J.; Morrison, I.; McGlone, F. *Affective Touch and the Neurophysiology of CT Afferents*; Springer: New York, NY, USA, 2016.
53. Montagu, A. *Touching: The Human Significance of the Skin*; Columbia University Press: New York, NY, USA; London, UK, 1971.
54. Field, T. Massage therapy research review. *Complement. Ther. Clin. Pract.* **2016**, *24*, 19–31. [CrossRef]
55. Reich, W. *Character Analysis*, 3rd ed.; Farrar, Straus, Giroux: New York, NY, USA, 1972.
56. Röhricht, F. Body oriented psychotherapy—The state of the art in empirical research and evidence based practice: A clinical perspective. *Body Mov. Dance* **2009**, *4*, 135–156. [CrossRef]
57. Changaris, M. *Touch: The Neurobiology of Health, Healing, and Human Connection*; LifeRhythm: Mendocino, CA, USA, 2015.
58. Field, T.; Hernandez-Reif, M.; Diego, M.; Schanberg, S.; Kuhn, C. Cortisol decreases and serotonin and dopamine increase following massage therapy. *Int. J. Neurosci.* **2005**, *115*, 1397–1413. Available online: https://www.tandfonline.com/doi/pdf/10.1080/00207450590956459?needAccess=true (accessed on 2 May 2020). [CrossRef] [PubMed]
59. Kosfeld, M.; Heinrichs, M.; Zak, P.J.; Fischbacher, U.; Fehr, E. Oxytocin increases trust in humans. *Nature* **2005**, *435*, 673–676. [CrossRef] [PubMed]
60. Uvnäs-Moberg, K. *The Hormone of Closeness: The Role of Oxytocin in Relationships1. Aufl*; Springer Spektrum: Berlin/Heidelberg, Germany, 2016.
61. Wang, J.; Lloyd-Evans, B.; Giacco, D.; Forsyth, R.; Nebo, C.; Mann, F.; Johnson, S. Social isolation in mental health: A conceptual and methodological review. *Soc. Psychiatry Psychiatr. Epidemiol.* **2017**, *52*, 1451–1461. [CrossRef] [PubMed]

62. Paloyelis, Y.; Krahé, C.; Maltezos, S.; Williams, S.C.; Howard, M.A.; Fotopoulou, A. The Analgesic Effect of Oxytocin in Humans: A Double-Blind, Placebo-Controlled Cross-Over Study Using Laser-Evoked Potentials. *J. Neuroendocrinol.* **2016**, *28*. [CrossRef] [PubMed]
63. Diego, M.A.; Field, T.; Hernandez-Reif, M. Vagal Activity, Gastric Motility, and Weight Gain in Massaged Preterm Neonates. *J. Pediatrics* **2005**, *147*, 50–55. [CrossRef] [PubMed]
64. Listing, M.; Reißhauer, A.; Krohn, M.; Voigt, B.; Tjahono, G.; Becker, J.; Klapp, B.F.; Rauchfuß, M. Massage therapy reduces physical discomfort and improves mood disturbances in women with breast cancer. *Psycho-Oncology* **2009**, *18*, 1290–1299. [CrossRef]
65. Moustgard, H.; Clayton, G.L.; Jones, H.E.; Boutron, I. Impact of blinding on estimated treatment effects in randomized clinical trials: Meta-epidemiological study. *BMJ* **2020**, *368*, 6802. [CrossRef]
66. Dorsett, M.D.; Friccione, G.L.; Benson, H. A new era for mind-body medicine. *N. Engl. J. Med.* **2020**, *382*, 1390–1391. [CrossRef]
67. Michalak, J.; Burg, J.; Heidenreich, T. Don't forget your body: Mindfulness embodiment and the treatment of depression. *Mindfulness* **2012**, *3*, 190–199. [CrossRef]

13

Affective Temperaments and Clinical Course of Bipolar Disorder: An Exploratory Study of Differences among Patients with and without a History of Violent Suicide Attempts

Giovanna Fico [1,*], Vito Caivano [1], Francesca Zinno [1], Marco Carfagno [1], Luca Steardo Jr. [2], Gaia Sampogna [1], Mario Luciano [1] and Andrea Fiorillo [1]

1 Department of Psychiatry, University of Campania "L. Vanvitelli", Largo Madonna Delle Grazie, 80139 Naples, Italy
2 Department of Health Sciences, Psychiatric Unit, University Magna Graecia of Catanzaro, Viale Europa, 88100 Catanzaro CZ, Italy
* Correspondence: giov.fico@gmail.com;

Abstract: *Background and Objectives:* Suicide is the leading cause of death in patients with Bipolar Disorder (BD). In particular, the high mortality rate is due to violent suicide attempts. Several risk factors associated with suicide attempts in patients with BD have been identified. Affective temperaments are associated with suicidal risk, but their predictive role is still understudied. The aim of this study is to assess the relationship between affective temperaments and personal history of violent suicide attempts. *Materials and Methods*: 74 patients with Bipolar Disorder type I (BD-I) or II (BD-II) were included. All patients filled in the short version of Munster Temperament Evaluation of the Memphis, Pisa, Paris and San Diego (short TEMPS-M) and the Temperament and Character Inventory, revised version (TCI-R). The sample was divided into two groups on the basis of a positive history for suicidal attempts and the suicidal group was further divided into two subgroups according to violent suicide attempts. *Results*: Violent suicide attempts were positively associated with the cyclothymic temperament and inversely to the hyperthymic one. BD-I patients and patients with a clinical history of rapid cycling were significantly more represented in the group of patients with a history of violent suicide attempts. *Conclusions*: Our study highlights that several clinical and temperamental characteristics are associated with violent suicide attempts, suggesting the importance of affective temperaments in the clinical management of patients with BPI.

Keywords: bipolar; suicide; affective temperament; violent suicide; aggressive behaviors

---

1. Introduction

According to the World Health Organization (WHO), suicide is one of the leading causes of death worldwide accounting for nearly 800,000 deaths every year [1]. Psychiatric disorders are an important contributing factor to suicide attempts [2] and bipolar disorders (BDs) are associated with the highest suicide risk [3], which is 15–30 times higher than the general population. Up to one-half of patients with BDs attempt suicide in their lifetime [4].

Suicide is a complex and multivariate phenomenon, defined as "death caused by self-directed injurious behavior with intent to die" [5] which can be performed by several means, including violent and non-violent methods. Suicide methods are noteworthy to be characterized, since they can contribute defining a suicidal subpopulation more vulnerable to suicide completion. In fact, violent suicide attempters have been proved to have an elevated risk of future suicide attempts [6], as well as a higher immediate lethality of an attempt [7] with a fatality rate over 70% [8]. Although a violent suicide attempt is usually defined by the method, there is no clear consensus about its definition. Asberg [9] identifies a few violent attempts (i.e., hanging, gas poisoning and drowning), whereas drug overdoses are considered to be non-violent suicide attempts. Subsequently, Giner (2014) [10] and Penas-Lledo (2015) [11] adopted and extended Asberg's criteria by including in the definition of "violent attempts" the use of firearms, jumping from heights, several deep cuts, car crash, burning, electrocution, and jumping under a train. Likewise, Dumais (2005) [12] enlarges the list of non-violent suicide attempts by adding drowning and gas poisoning. The identification of a subpopulation, such as the violent suicide attempters, of patients with mental disorders at higher risk to commit suicide and the identification of the risk factors of suicide attempts is a stepping stone in the development of a better suicide prevention strategy.

Several risk factors linked to suicide attempts in patients with BD have been identified in previous studies, including a long duration of illness, untreated BD, female sex, positive history for suicide attempts, comorbidity with substance abuse or personality disorders, anxiety, depressive polarity [13], recent affective episodes, and recent psychiatric inpatient care [14]. Personality and temperamental traits have also been considered, and anger, impulsivity, aggression, anxiety and two factors (i.e., "harm avoidance" and "novelty seeking") of the Temperament and Character Inventory (TCI) have been identified to be associated with suicide attempts [15]. Only recently temperament and, in particular, affective temperaments have been considered as possible factors linked to suicide attempts [16]. Temperament represents the "temporally stable biological core of personality" affecting several aspects of an individual's life (activity level, rhythms, moods and related cognitions) while personality, a broader phenotype, also refers to "acquired characterological determinants and interpersonal operations" [16]. Akiskal et al. conceptualized a *spectrum* of *affective* conditions ranging from *temperament* to clinical episodes [17] and proposed criteria defining five temperaments: (1) Cyclothymic temperament, characterized by chronic cycling between mood polarities and unstable self-esteem and energy; (2) hyperthymic temperament, characterized by increased energy and optimism [17]; (3) irritable temperament, characterized by irritable and angry behavior; (4) anxious temperament, characterized by a tendency to worry; (5) depressive temperament, characterized by low levels of energy, introversion and worrying [18]. Affective temperaments, conceptualized as stable, subclinical forms of the manic-depressive illness by Akiskal (1983), have a role in the clinical evolution of the mood disorders and the outcome, including the risk of suicide attempts [19]. In particular, hyperthymic temperament has been shown to be associated with a reduced risk of suicide attempts [20,21], whereas cyclothymic, irritable, depressive and anxious temperaments are more present in patients with a positive history of suicide attempts [22,23]. Besides, cyclothymic and irritable temperaments are highly connected with both aggression [24] and impulsivity [25], which play a role in suicidal behavior. A widely used questionnaire to evaluate affective temperaments is the Temperament Evaluation of Memphis, Pisa, Paris and San Diego (TEMPS) [18,26] which has been developed in different formats and used in clinical and research settings [27]. It has been documented that affective temperaments individually considered, have reduced predictive power if used to anticipate suicidal risk [28], while composite TEMPS-A score yields stronger associations with suicidal risk and better identify subjects at risk for suicide attempts [20]. A few data on the clinical characteristics of violent attempters with BDs are available. Existing data suggest that violent attempters are more likely to be men [29], have the first episode of manic/hypomanic type [30] and carry the serotonin transporter gene S allele [31].

To our knowledge, there are no previous studies that specifically addressed the issue of the association between affective temperament subtypes and a history of violent suicide attempts in BDs. Thus, the aim of our study is to investigate the relationship between affective temperaments and personal history of violent suicide attempts, defined according to Asberg's criteria, in a clinical sample of bipolar patients.

2. Materials and Methods

The exploratory study was carried out in the bipolar outpatient unit of the Department of Psychiatry of the University of Campania "Luigi Vanvitelli", in Naples between January and June 2018. The only inclusion criterion was a diagnosis of bipolar disorder type I or II according to the DSM 5 criteria. Patients were excluded if they have presented affective illness as a consequence of alcohol/substance abuse or dependence, medical illness, an organic brain disorder or medication, and if not able to provide written informed consent (i.e., dementia, cognitive impairment or delirium). The study was approved by the local ethical review board (N001567/28.01.2018).

All patients filled in the short version of the Munster Temperament Evaluation of the Memphis, Pisa, Paris and San Diego (short TEMPS-M) [32,33], a 35 items questionnaire used to assess affective temperaments described by Akiskal (depressive, anxious, hyperthymic, cyclothymic and irritable) using a dimensional approach with a five-point Likert type scale ranging from 1 to 5 (1 = "not at all"; 2 = "a little"; 3 = "moderately"; 4 = "much"; 5 "very much") [34] and the Temperament and Character Inventory, revised version (TCI-R) [35]. The TCI was developed by Cloninger, with the goal of assessing factors underlying the psychobiological aspect of personality. The revised version (TCI-R) is a questionnaire consisting of 240 items, with a 5-point Likert-type scale, grouped into four temperament dimensions, novelty seeking (NS), harm avoidance (HA), reward dependence (RD) and persistence (PS), and three character dimensions, self-directiveness (SD), cooperativeness (CO) and self-transcendence (ST) samples [36].

Patients' and clinicians' socio-demographic and clinical characteristics were analyzed using descriptive and frequency counts, as appropriate. The sample was divided into two groups on the basis of a positive history for a suicidal attempt. Differences among groups were evaluated using χ^2 or Bonferroni-adjusted T-test, as appropriate. Suicidal patients were further divided into two subgroups according to the history of violent suicide attempts, in line with Asberg's criteria (1976). A logistic multivariable regression model was performed in order to identify factors associated with a positive history of suicidal behavior. All possible confounders were entered in the model. Statistical analyses were performed using SPSS version 18, the level of statistical significance was set at the level of $p < 0.05$.

3. Results

The sample consists of 74 patients. Patients' sociodemographic characteristics, as well as patients' clinical features, are reported in Table 1. The sample is composed by 36 men (48.7%) and 38 women (51.3%), with a mean age of 48.92 years (SD = 12.38), the most frequent diagnosis was bipolar II disorder (59.5%). The samples grouped according to a positive history of suicide attempts (Table 2). Forty patients have a positive history of suicide attempts (45.9%). Psychotic symptoms are more frequent in patients with a history of suicide attempts compared to patients without a history of suicide attempts ($p < 0.019$), and particularly during mixed episodes ($p < 0.008$). Furthermore, suicidal attempters show a higher rate of aggressive behaviors, but no differences were found between the two groups in terms of the clinical course of the disease, number of psychiatric admissions, number of affective episodes and seasonality. Depressive, anxious and cyclothymic temperaments are more represented in suicidal attempters, while hyperthymic in non-suicidal ones. Suicidal attempters have been further divided into two subgroups according to violent suicide attempts in line with Asberg's criteria (Table 3). Twenty-four patients report a history of violent suicide attempts, 54.2% being females and 45.8% males with a mean age of 49.46 (SD = 13.02); the most frequent diagnosis is BDI (75%); 41.7% of violent attempters and 45.83% of non-violent attempters were on lithium therapy. A clinical course of rapid cycling (4 or more affective episodes during a year) is significantly more represented in the group of patients with a history of violent suicide attempts. Furthermore, violent attempters show a higher rate of cyclothymic temperament and lower rates of hyperthymic temperament. At the multivariate logistic regression, we found that the hyperthymic temperament reduces the likelihood to have a positive history of suicidal attempts ($p < 0.01$) (Table 4).

Table 1. Socio-demographic and clinical characteristics of the sample (N = 74).

Gender, male (N; %)	(36; 48.6)
Diagnosis, Bipolar disorder type I (N; %)	(30; 40.5%)
Age (mean ± SD)	(48.92 ± 12.38)
Age at illness onset (mean ± SD)	(27.71 ± 9.8)
Duration of illness (mean ± SD)	(16.07 ± 9.46)
Number of depressive episodes (mean ± SD)	(7.1 ± 5.22)
Number of manic episodes (mean ± SD)	(3.79 ± 2.06)
Number of hypomanic episodes (mean ± SD)	(6.48 ± 4.5)
Number of mixed episodes (mean ± SD)	(2.53 ± 1.16)
Lifetime number of affective episodes (mean ± SD)	(14.17 ± 9.59)
Number of affective episodes during last year (mean ± SD)	(2.04 ± 2.28)
Lifetime number of psychiatric admissions (mean ± SD)	(0.493 ± 0.92)
Duration of psychiatric admissions (mean ± SD)	(0.7 ± 1.44)
Clinical Course (N; %)	
Mania–Depression–Interval (MDI)	(11; 14.9)
Depression–Mania–Interval (DMI)	(10; 13.5)
Mania–Interval–Depression (MID)	(8; 10.8)
Depression–Interval–Mania (DIM)	(3; 4.1)
Rapid cycling	(8; 10.8)
Irregular cycling	(25; 33.8)
History of suicide attempts (N; %)	(40; 54.1)
Presence of psychotic symptoms, yes (N; %)	(36; 49.3)
during depressive episodes	(13; 9.5)
during manic episodes	(7; 17.6)
during mixed episodes	(15; 20.3)
Aggressive behaviours (N; %)	(32; 43.2)
brief TEMPS-M subscores (mean ± SD)	
Depressive (dep)	(23.58 ± 5.93)
Cyclothymic (cyc)	(23.76 ± 7.1)
Irritable (irr)	(18.96 ± 7.59)
Anxious (anx)	(19.82 ± 6.3)
Hyperthymic (hyp)	(19.97 ± 6.3)

Table 2. Socio-demographic and clinical characteristics of the sample divided by history of suicide attempts.

Factors	Suicidal	Non-Suicidal
Cases (N; %)	40; 45.9%	34; 54.1%
Gender, male (N; %)	19; 47.5	17; 50
Diagnosis, Bipolar disorder type I, (N; %)	18; 45%	12; 30%
Age (mean ± SD)	49.53 ± 13.16	48.21 ± 11.56
Age at illness onset (mean ± SD)	26.76 ± 9.230	28.67 ± 10.45
Duration of illness (mean ± SD)	16.69 ± 8.92	15.34 ± 10.14
Number of depressive episodes (mean ± SD)	6.49 ± 3.55	7.82 ± 6.67
Number of manic episodes (mean ± SD)	3.93 ± 1.92	3.62 ± 2.24
Number of hypomanic episodes (mean ± SD)	5.61 ± 2.48	7.50 ± 5.96
Number of mixed episodes (mean ± SD)	2.55 ± 0.86	2.51 ± 1.45
Lifetime number of affective episodes (mean ± SD)	12.97 ± 5.92	15.59 ± 12.57
Number of affective episodes during last year (mean ± SD)	1.74 ± 0.68	2.39 ± 3.28
Lifetime number of psychiatric admissions (mean ± SD)	0.58 ± 1.07	0.38 ± 0.69
Duration of psychiatric admissions (mean ± SD)	0.800 ± 1.63	0.588 ± 1.2090

Table 2. *Cont.*

Factors	Suicidal	Non-Suicidal
Clinical Course (N; %)		
Mania–Depression–Interval (MDI)	6; 15	5; 14.7
Depression–Mania–Interval (DMI)	6; 15	4; 11.8
Mania–Interval–Depression (MID)	3; 7.5	5; 14.7
Depression–Interval–Mania (DIM)	2; 5	1; 2.9
Rapid cycling	2; 5	6; 17.6
Irregular cycling	12; 30	13; 38.2
Presence of psychotic symptoms, yes (N; %)	25; 62.5 *	11; 32.4
during depressive episodes	4; 10	3; 8.8
during manic episodes	8; 20	5; 14.7
during mixed episodes	13; 32.5 *	2; 5.9
Seasonality (N; %)	16; 40.0	15; 32.4
Aggressive behaviours (N; %)	21; 52.5 *	11; 32.3
brief TEMPS-M subscores (mean ± SD)		
Depressive (dep)	25 ± 5.54	21.91 ± 6.01
Cyclothymic (cyc)	25.7 ± 6.38	21.47 ± 7.3
Irritable (irr)	19.68 ± 7.86	18.12 ± 7.29
Anxious (anx)	21.33 ± 6.31	18.06 ± 5.9
Hyperthymic (hyp)	18.13 ± 6.38 *	22.15 ± 5.53
TCI-R subscores (mean ± SD)		
NS total score	107.04 ± 18.19	106.34 ± 17.20
HA total score	113.85 ± 23.03	107.44 ± 23.87
RD total score	99.61 ± 16.54	99.04 ± 16.54
PS total score	100.09 ± 26.47	109.6 ± 24.85
SD total score	115.4 ± 22.16	123.2 ± 21.72
C total score	122.8 ± 16.14	124.3 ± 20.93
ST total score	73.13 ± 17.75	71.27 ± 13.25

Abbreviations: novelty seeking (NS), harm avoidance (HA), reward dependence (RD) and persistence (PS), self-directiveness (SD), cooperativeness (CO) and self-transcendence (ST). * $p < 0.002$ (Bonferroni).

Table 3. Socio-demographic and clinical characteristics of patients with a history of violent suicide attempts (N = 24).

Gender, male (N; %)	11; 45.8
Diagnosis, Bipolar disorder type I, (N; %)	18; 75%
Age (mean ± SD)	49.46 ± 13.02
Age at illness onset (mean ± SD)	27. 09 ± 8.73
Duration of illness (mean ± SD)	15.94 ± 10.42
Number of depressive episodes (mean ± SD)	7.57 ± 5.89
Number of manic episodes (mean ± SD)	3.76 ± 1.94
Number of hypomanic episodes (mean ± SD)	7.01 ± 5.20
Number of mixed episodes (mean ± SD)	2.52 ± 1.19
Lifetime number of affective episodes (mean ± SD)	14.88 ± 11.01
Number of affective episodes during last year (mean ± SD)	2.23 ± 11.01
Lifetime number of psychiatric admissions (mean ± SD)	0.380 ± 0 .69
Duration of psychiatric admissions (mean ± SD)	0.56 ± 1.12
Clinical Course (N; %)	
Mania–Depression–Interval (MDI)	4; 16.7
Depression–Mania–Interval (DMI)	5; 20.8
Mania–Interval–Depression (MID)	3; 12.5
Depression–Interval–Mania (DIM)	1; 4.2
Rapid cycling	8; 33.3 *
Irregular cycling	7; 29.2

Table 3. *Cont.*

Presence of psychotic symptoms, yes (N; %)	13; 54.2
during depressive episodes during manic episodes during mixed episodes	3; 12.5 6; 25 4; 16.7
Aggressive behaviours (N; %)	17; 70.8
Lithium Therapy (N; %)	10; 41.7%
brief TEMPS-M subscores	
Depressive (dep) Cyclothymic (cyc) Irritable (irr) Anxious (anx) Hyperthymic (hyp)	24.04 ± 6.29 27.6 ± 5.39 * 18.58 ± 7.64 20.54 ± 5.71 17.25 ± 5.60 *
TCI-R subscores (mean ± SD)	
NS total score HA total score RD total score PS total score SD total score C total score ST total score	103.91 ± 18.59 112.70 ± 26 99.31 ± 13.9 101.6 ± 27.45 119.25 ± 21.79 124.02 ± 16.06 71.3 ± 18.75

Abbreviations: novelty seeking (NS), harm avoidance (HA), reward dependence (RD) and persistence (PS), self-directiveness (SD), cooperativeness (CO) and self-transcendence (ST). * $p < 0.002$ (Bonferroni).

Table 4. Multivariate logistic regression, dependent variable: suicidal behavior vs. non-suicidal behavior.

Number of subjects included on the analysis	46		
F (df)	4.816 (1)		
P	0.000		
Adjusted R square	0.443		
Constant	1.572 (−2.037 to 2.493)		
	O.R.	**C.I. 95%**	*p*
Lithium therapy	0.185	0–9.628	0.149
Age	1.005	0.76–1.146	0.944
Gender	0.415	0.008–3.64	0.407
Presence of psychotic symptoms	0.692	0.003–7.39	0.726
Aggressive behavior	0.130	0.003–5.236	0.103
Seasonality	1.172	0.002–4.764	0.870
Duration of illness	1.026	0.862–1.215	0.668
Lifetime number of affective episodes (1–10)	-	0.852–1.356	0.229
Lifetime number of affective episodes (11–21)	11.233	0.523–1.112	0.098
Lifetime number of affective episodes (>22)	12.099	0.654–1.288	0.139
Lifetime number of psychiatric admissions	0.702	0.123–1.789	0.598
brief TEMPS-M subscores			
Depressive	0.875	0.448–1.096	0.294
Hyperthymic	0.800	0.526–1021	0.018
Anxious	1.098	0.681–1.428	0.461
Cyclothymic	1.127	0.974–2.015	0.271
Irritable	1.064	0.719–1.147	0.414

F-test; df, degree of freedom; C.I., confidence interval; O.R., Odds Ratio.

4. Discussion

The impact of affective temperaments on the risk of suicidal behavior is an emerging theme in the field of mental health [18,37,38]. Our sample is mainly composed of BD-II patients, considered at the highest risk of suicide attempts among patients with the bipolar spectrum [39]. Recent research showed that suicide attempts are 1.5 times more frequent among women than men and that the risk of suicide attempts decreases from BDII to major depression, BDI, other psychiatric disorders and to psychotic disorders, which carry the lowest risk [40]. This can be explained by the evidence that BDII patients experience more chronicity [41], higher rates of rapid cycling [42], greater disabling depressive symptoms [39], a higher probability of misdiagnosis [41], more anxiety disorders in comorbidity [43], agitated depression and residual symptoms [44]. Our study confirms that hyperthymic temperament is associated with a reduced risk of suicide attempts in BD patients, while depressive, cyclothymic and anxious temperaments have a strong association with suicide attempts [45]. These findings are in line with previous reports [16,22,46]. Hyperthymic temperament may exert protective effects in different ways, such as better drive, greater energy, more ambition, as well as better coping and decrease the risk of suicidal behavior [19,46]. On the other hand, the low rating of hyperthymic temperament has been associated with increased hopelessness, an important predictor of suicide attempts [47]. Contrary to previous studies [28], our data do not confirm the role of irritable temperament on suicide risk, probably due to the small sample size. In our study emerged that psychotic symptoms are more represented in patients with a history of suicide attempts particularly during mixed episodes [45]. Several studies have suggested that individuals who experience psychotic symptoms have an increased sensitivity to stress, in terms of affective reactions to life events [48], as well as poorer coping skills [49], which may contribute to a greater risk of suicidal behavior when faced with acute life stressors. Other potential mechanisms may be the presence of shared risk factors for suicidal behavior and psychotic symptoms, including traumatic early life experiences, especially physical and sexual abuse [45], as reported by a recent meta-analysis by Ng et al. [50]. Therefore, mixed states, both with or without psychotic symptoms, are associated with an elevated risk of suicidal behavior, due to a greater proportion of time spent being depressed than patients without mixed episodes [51]. Furthermore, our study has outlined several clinical characteristics of violent suicide attempters. Rapid cycling patients were more likely to be violent attempters, as well as patients with BD-I and with cyclothymic temperament. Increased impulsivity, which is often a characteristic of cyclothymic temperament, is associated with a worse prognosis of BD [52,53], and with a more severe clinical course of the disease with history of rapid cycling, mixed episodes and substance abuse [54]. Our findings are in line with other studies showing that cyclothymic temperament is associated with a behavioral instability, increased sensitivity to a stressful event and higher levels of impulsivity [22,55–57], and a risk factor for suicide attempts [21]. Therefore, identifying those conditions such as cyclothymic temperament, a rapid cycling course or mixed episodes, more related to an impulsive dimension in patients with BD, could help to more easily typify a subpopulation of patients at risk of committing violent suicide attempts.

The higher rates of cyclothymic dominant temperament among patients with BD have been widely shown in several studies [38,57]. There is still an open debate whether cyclothymic temperaments and cyclothymia as a psychiatric disorder have overlapping characteristics. In particular, cyclothymia has been conceptualized as the extreme of a cyclothymic temperament, characterized by high rates of impulsivity, emotional lability and mood swings [55]; it is estimated that up to one third of patients with cyclothymia have more possibilities to develop BD, particularly the type II [58]. A great number of patients are misclassified as bipolar, depressed or with a personality disorder instead of receiving a diagnosis of cyclothymia by the use of DSM-5 diagnostic criteria [55,59,60]; thus, is it possible that patients with a diagnosis of cyclothymia with BDs have been included in the study. A broader approach, considering not only a categorical diagnosis based on strict DSM-5 criteria but including temperamental dimension also, could help to better identify patients with cyclothymia and plan individualized treatments [50].

Underdiagnosis or misdiagnosis are relatively common in BD [61,62], and they are linked with the presence of milder symptoms not fitting a BD diagnosis, but falling into the "soft bipolar spectrum" definition [63]. In particular, Akiskal and Pinto (1999) [63] described two subtypes of bipolar spectrum not associated with manic or hypomanic state: bipolar II1/2 (depression superimposed on cyclothymic temperament) and bipolar IV (depression superimposed on hyperthymic temperament). A recent work by Goto and colleagues [64] proved that depression in those who have cyclothymic (bipolar II1/2) and hyperthymic temperament (bipolar IV) may predict bipolarity, giving validity to the bipolar II 1/2 and bipolar IV concepts; this is in line with our results on cyclothymic temperament which is highly represented in the total sample and significantly higher in violent attempters.

It is important to emphasize that this was an exploratory study with several potential limitations. The small sample size reduces the statistical power of our findings, especially in the sub-analysis made in the population of violent suicide attempters. Furthermore, we could not assess some socio-demographical characteristics and levels of education. Moreover, we only collected data on lithium treatment, but we have no data on other psychiatric medications. The time during which the study was conducted was relatively short; this can affect, for example, data on seasonality. Finally, data on aggression, as well as on clinical course, number or duration of admissions, presence of psychotic symptoms, were not assessed with objective measures, but they were referred by patients. The paper has also several strengths, such as the naturalistic setting and the fact that it is one of the first clinical studies on the possible role of affective temperaments in patients with BD. Moreover, in this study we evaluated the subpopulation of violent suicide attempters of BD patients, which can be considered an early detection target and can be taken into account for personalized treatments for BD.

5. Conclusions

Our study outlined several clinical and temperamental characteristics of violent suicide attempters. Temperaments, in particular the affective ones, should be routinely assessed in clinical settings in order to identify people at higher risk of suicide attempts and to develop preventive programs, although it would be reductive to build a "suicide attempter profile" only on the basis of temperaments. A wider clinical evaluation, including also different clinical aspects such as current affective episodes and severity of the disease, pharmacological treatments, and the use of coping strategies in stressful situations should be taken into consideration in order to have effective early interventions.

Author Contributions: Conceptualization, A.F., M.L. and G.F. and Y.Y.; methodology, G.S., L.J.S., V.C., F.Z., M.C.; formal analysis, G.S., M.L. and G.F.; writing—original draft preparation, G.F., M.L., V.C., F.Z., M.C.; writing—review and editing, A.F., M.L., F.Z.; supervision, A.F.

References

1. WHO. *Suicide Data*; WHO: Geneva, Switzerland, 2018.
2. Bachmann, S. Epidemiology of Suicide and the Psychiatric Perspective. *Int. J. Environ. Res. Public Health* **2018**, *15*, 1425. [CrossRef] [PubMed]
3. Gonda, X.; Pompili, M.; Serafini, G.; Montebovi, F.; Campi, S.; Dome, P.; Duleba, T.; Girardi, P.; Rihmer, Z. Suicidal behavior in bipolar disorder: Epidemiology, characteristics and major risk factors. *J. Affect. Disord.* **2012**, *143*, 16–26. [CrossRef] [PubMed]
4. Schaffer, A.; Isometsa, E.T.; Tondo, L.; H Moreno, D.; Turecki, G.; Reis, C.; Cassidy, F.; Sinyor, M.; Azorin, J.-M.; Kessing, L.V.; et al. International Society for Bipolar Disorders Task Force on Suicide: Meta-analyses and meta-regression of correlates of suicide attempts and suicide deaths in bipolar disorder. *Bipolar Disord.* **2015**, *17*, 1–16. [CrossRef] [PubMed]

5. Vijayakumar, L.; Phillips, M.R.; Silverman, M.M.; Gunnell, D.; Carli, V. Suicide. In *Mental, Neurological, and Substance Use Disorders: Disease Control Priorities*; Patel, V., Chisholm, D., Dua, T., Laxminarayan, R., Medina-Mora, M.E., Eds.; The International Bank for Reconstruction and Development/The World Bank: Washington, DC, USA, 2016; ISBN 9781464804267.
6. Runeson, B.; Tidemalm, D.; Dahlin, M.; Lichtenstein, P.; Langstrom, N. Method of attempted suicide as predictor of subsequent successful suicide: National long term cohort study. *BMJ* **2010**, *341*, c3222. [CrossRef] [PubMed]
7. Stenbacka, M.; Jokinen, J. Violent and non-violent methods of attempted and completed suicide in Swedish young men: The role of early risk factors. *BMC Psychiatry* **2015**, *15*, 196. [CrossRef]
8. Gunnell, D.; Bennewith, O.; Hawton, K.; Simkin, S.; Kapur, N. The epidemiology and prevention of suicide by hanging: A systematic review. *Int. J. Epidemiol.* **2005**, *34*, 433–442. [CrossRef]
9. Asberg, M.; Traskman, L.; Thoren, P. 5-HIAA in the cerebrospinal fluid. A biochemical suicide predictor? *Arch. Gen. Psychiatry* **1976**, *33*, 1193–1197. [CrossRef]
10. Giner, L.; Jaussent, I.; Olié, E.; Béziat, S.; Guillaume, S.; Baca-Garcia, E.; Lopez-Castroman, J.; Courtet, P. Violent and serious suicide attempters: One step closer to suicide? *J. Clin. Psychiatry* **2014**, *75*, e191–e197. [CrossRef]
11. Penas-Lledo, E.; Guillaume, S.; Delgado, A.; Naranjo, M.E.G.; Jaussent, I.; LLerena, A.; Courtet, P. ABCB1 gene polymorphisms and violent suicide attempt among survivors. *J. Psychiatry Res.* **2015**, *61*, 52–56. [CrossRef]
12. Dumais, A.; Lesage, A.D.; Lalovic, A.; Seguin, M.; Tousignant, M.; Chawky, N.; Turecki, G. Is violent method of suicide a behavioral marker of lifetime aggression? *Am. J. Psychiatry* **2005**, *162*, 1375–1378. [CrossRef]
13. Costa Lda, S.; Alencar, Á.P.; Nascimento Neto, P.J.; dos Santos Mdo, S.; da Silva, C.G.; Pinheiro Sde, F.; Silveira, R.T.; Bianco, B.A.; Pinheiro, R.F., Jr.; de Lima, M.A.; et al. Risk factors for suicide in bipolar disorder: A systematic review. *J. Affect. Disord.* **2015**, *170*, 237–254. [CrossRef]
14. Hansson, C.; Joas, E.; Palsson, E.; Hawton, K.; Runeson, B.; Landen, M. Risk factors for suicide in bipolar disorder: A cohort study of 12 850 patients. *Acta Psychiatr. Scand.* **2018**, *138*, 456–463. [CrossRef] [PubMed]
15. Perroud, N.; Baud, P.; Ardu, S.; Krejci, I.; Mouthon, D.; Vessaz, M.; Guillaume, S.; Jaussent, I.; Olie, E.; Malafosse, A.; et al. Temperament personality profiles in suicidal behaviour: An investigation of associated demographic, clinical and genetic factors. *J. Affect. Disord.* **2013**, *146*, 246–253. [CrossRef] [PubMed]
16. Rihmer, Z.; Akiskal, K.K.; Rihmer, A.; Akiskal, H.S. Current research on affective temperaments. *Curr. Opin. Psychiatry* **2010**, *23*, 12–18. [CrossRef] [PubMed]
17. Akiskal, H.S.; Akiskal, K. Cyclothymic, hyperthymic, and depressive temperaments as subaffective variants of mood disorders. In *Annual Review, Vol. II*; Tasman, A., Riba, M.B., Eds.; American Psychiatric Press: Washington, DC, USA, 1992; pp. 43–62.
18. Akiskal, H.S.; Akiskal, K.K.; Haykal, R.F.; Manning, J.S.; Connor, P.D. TEMPS-A: Progress towards validation of a self-rated clinical version of the Temperament Evaluation of the Memphis, Pisa, Paris, and San Diego Autoquestionnaire. *J. Affect. Disord.* **2005**, *85*, 3–16. [CrossRef] [PubMed]
19. Pompili, M.; Innamorati, M.; Gonda, X.; Serafini, G.; Sarno, S.; Erbuto, D.; Palermo, M.; Elena Seretti, M.; Stefani, H.; Lester, D.; et al. Affective temperaments and hopelessness as predictors of health and social functioning in mood disorder patients: A prospective follow-up study. *J. Affect. Disord.* **2013**, *150*, 216–222. [CrossRef]
20. Tondo, L.; Vazquez, G.H.; Sani, G.; Pinna, M.; Baldessarini, R.J. Association of suicidal risk with ratings of affective temperaments. *J. Affect. Disord.* **2018**, *229*, 322–327. [CrossRef] [PubMed]
21. Baldessarini, R.J.; Vazquez, G.H.; Tondo, L. Affective temperaments and suicidal ideation and behavior in mood and anxiety disorder patients. *J. Affect. Disord.* **2016**, *198*, 78–82. [CrossRef]
22. Pompili, M.; Rihmer, Z.; Akiskal, H.S.; Innamorati, M.; Iliceto, P.; Akiskal, K.K.; Lester, D.; Narciso, V.; Ferracuti, S.; Tatarelli, R.; et al. Temperament and personality dimensions in suicidal and nonsuicidal psychiatric inpatients. *Psychopathology* **2008**, *41*, 313–321. [CrossRef]
23. Rihmer, A.; Rozsa, S.; Rihmer, Z.; Gonda, X.; Akiskal, K.K.; Akiskal, H.S. Affective temperaments, as measured by TEMPS-A, among nonviolent suicide attempters. *J. Affect. Disord.* **2009**, *116*, 18–22. [CrossRef]
24. Dolenc, B.; Dernovšek, M.Z.; Sprah, L.; Tavcar, R.; Perugi, G.; Akiskal, H.S. Relationship between affective temperaments and aggression in euthymic patients with bipolar mood disorder and major depressive disorder. *J. Affect. Disord.* **2015**, *174*, 13–18. [CrossRef] [PubMed]

25. Walsh, M.A.; Royal, A.M.; Barrantes-Vidal, N.; Kwapil, T.R. The association of affective temperaments with impairment and psychopathology in a young adult sample. *J. Affect. Disord.* **2012**, *141*, 373–381. [CrossRef] [PubMed]
26. Akiskal, H.S.; Placidi, G.F.; Maremmani, I.; Signoretta, S.; Liguori, A.; Gervasi, R.; Mallya, G.; Puzantian, V.R. TEMPS-I: Delineating the most discriminant traits of the cyclothymic, depressive, hyperthymic and irritable temperaments in a nonpatient population. *J. Affect. Disord.* **1998**, *51*, 7–19. [CrossRef]
27. Elias, L.R.; Kohler, C.A.; Stubbs, B.; Maciel, B.R.; Cavalcante, L.M.; Vale, A.M.O.; Gonda, X.; Quevedo, J.; Hyphantis, T.N.; Soares, J.C.; et al. Measuring affective temperaments: A systematic review of validation studies of the Temperament Evaluation in Memphis Pisa and San Diego (TEMPS) instruments. *J. Affect. Disord.* **2017**, *212*, 25–37. [CrossRef]
28. Vazquez, G.H.; Gonda, X.; Lolich, M.; Tondo, L.; Baldessarini, R.J. Suicidal Risk and Affective Temperaments, Evaluated with the TEMPS-A Scale: A Systematic Review. *Harv. Rev. Psychiatry* **2018**, *26*, 8–18. [CrossRef] [PubMed]
29. Nivoli, A.M.A.; Pacchiarotti, I.; Rosa, A.R.; Popovic, D.; Murru, A.; Valenti, M.; Bonnin, C.M.; Grande, I.; Sanchez-Moreno, J.; Vieta, E.; et al. Gender differences in a cohort study of 604 bipolar patients: The role of predominant polarity. *J. Affect. Disord.* **2011**, *133*, 443–449. [CrossRef]
30. Neves, F.S.; Malloy-Diniz, L.F.; Correa, H. Suicidal behavior in bipolar disorder: What is the influence of psychiatric comorbidities? *J. Clin. Psychiatry* **2009**, *70*, 13–18. [CrossRef]
31. Gonda, X.; Fountoulakis, K.N.; Harro, J.; Pompili, M.; Akiskal, H.S.; Bagdy, G.; Rihmer, Z. The possible contributory role of the S allele of 5-HTTLPR in the emergence of suicidality. *J. Psychopharmacol.* **2011**, *25*, 857–866. [CrossRef]
32. Erfurth, A.; Gerlach, A.L.; Hellweg, I.; Boenigk, I.; Michael, N.; Akiskal, H.S. Studies on a German (Munster) version of the temperament auto-questionnaire TEMPS-A: Construction and validation of the briefTEMPS-M. *J. Affect. Disord.* **2005**, *85*, 53–69. [CrossRef]
33. Naderer, A.; Keller, F.; Plener, P.; Unseld, M.; Lesch, O.M.; Walter, H.; Erfurth, A.; Kapusta, N.D. The brief TEMPS-M temperament questionnaire: A psychometric evaluation in an Austrian sample. *J. Affect. Disord.* **2015**, *188*, 43–46. [CrossRef]
34. Fico, G.; Luciano, M.; Sampogna, G.; Zinno, F.; Steardo, L., Jr.; Perugi, G.; Pompili, M.; Tortorella, A.; Volpe, U.; Fiorillo, A.; et al. Validation of the brief TEMPS-M temperament questionnaire in a clinical Italian sample of bipolar and cyclothymic patients. *J. Affect. Disord* **2019**, in press.
35. Tor, E.N.; Cloninger, R.; Przybeck, T.R.; Svrakic, D.; Wetzel, R.D. *TCI-Guide to Its Development and Use*; Center for Psychobiology of Personality Washington University: St. Louis, MO, USA, 2014.
36. Fossati, A.; Cloninger, C.R.; Villa, D.; Borroni, S.; Grazioli, F.; Giarolli, L.; Battaglia, M.; Maffei, C. Reliability and validity of the Italian version of the Temperament and Character Inventory-Revised in an outpatient sample. *Compr. Psychiatry* **2007**, *48*, 380–387. [CrossRef] [PubMed]
37. Karam, E.G.; Salamoun, M.M.; Yeretzian, J.S.; Mneimneh, Z.N.; Karam, A.N.; Fayyad, J.; Hantouche, E.; Akiskal, K.; Akiskal, H.S. The role of anxious and hyperthymic temperaments in mental disorders: A national epidemiologic study. *World Psychiatry* **2010**, *9*, 103–110. [CrossRef] [PubMed]
38. Kochman, F.J.; Hantouche, E.G.; Ferrari, P.; Lancrenon, S.; Bayart, D.; Akiskal, H.S. Cyclothymic temperament as a prospective predictor of bipolarity and suicidality in children and adolescents with major depressive disorder. *J. Affect. Disord.* **2005**, *85*, 181–189. [CrossRef] [PubMed]
39. Rihmer, Z.; Kiss, K. Bipolar disorders and suicidal behaviour. *Bipolar Disord.* **2002**, *4*, 21–25. [CrossRef] [PubMed]
40. Pompili, M.; Baldessarini, R.J.; Innamorati, M.; Vazquez, G.H.; Rihmer, Z.; Gonda, X.; Forte, A.; Lamis, D.A.; Erbuto, D.; Serafini, G.; et al. Temperaments in psychotic and major affective disorders. *J. Affect. Disord.* **2018**, *225*, 195–200. [CrossRef] [PubMed]
41. Vieta, E.; Benabarre, A.; Colom, F.; Gasto, C.; Nieto, E.; Otero, A.; Vallejo, J. Suicidal behavior in bipolar I and bipolar II disorder. *J. Nerv. Ment. Dis.* **1997**, *185*, 407–409. [CrossRef] [PubMed]
42. Maj, M.; Pirozzi, R.; Formicola, A.M.; Tortorella, A. Reliability and validity of four alternative definitions of rapid-cycling bipolar disorder. *Am. J. Psychiatry* **1999**, *156*, 1421–1424.
43. Henry, C.; Van den Bulke, D.; Bellivier, F.; Etain, B.; Rouillon, F.; Leboyer, M. Anxiety disorders in 318 bipolar patients: Prevalence and impact on illness severity and response to mood stabilizer. *J. Clin. Psychiatry* **2003**, *64*, 331–335. [CrossRef]

44. Benazzi, F. Prevalence and clinical correlates of residual depressive symptoms in bipolar II disorder. *Psychother. Psychosom.* **2001**, *70*, 232–238. [CrossRef]
45. Kelleher, I.; Corcoran, P.; Keeley, H.; Wigman, J.T.W.; Devlin, N.; Ramsay, H.; Wasserman, C.; Carli, V.; Sarchiapone, M.; Hoven, C.; et al. Psychotic symptoms and population risk for suicide attempt: A prospective cohort study. *JAMA Psychiatry* **2013**, *70*, 940–948. [CrossRef] [PubMed]
46. Vazquez, G.H.; Gonda, X.; Zaratiegui, R.; Lorenzo, L.S.; Akiskal, K.; Akiskal, H.S. Hyperthymic temperament may protect against suicidal ideation. *J. Affect. Disord.* **2010**, *127*, 38–42. [CrossRef] [PubMed]
47. Gonda, X.; Fountoulakis, K.N.; Kaprinis, G.; Rihmer, Z. Prediction and prevention of suicide in patients with unipolar depression and anxiety. *Ann. Gen. Psychiatry* **2007**, *6*, 23. [CrossRef] [PubMed]
48. Lataster, T.; Wichers, M.; Jacobs, N.; Mengelers, R.; Derom, C.; Thiery, E.; Van Os, J.; Myin-Germeys, I. Does reactivity to stress cosegregate with subclinical psychosis? A general population twin study. *Acta Psychiatr. Scand.* **2009**, *119*, 45–53. [CrossRef] [PubMed]
49. Wigman, J.T.W.; Devlin, N.; Kelleher, I.; Murtagh, A.; Harley, M.; Kehoe, A.; Fitzpatrick, C.; Cannon, M. Psychotic symptoms, functioning and coping in adolescents with mental illness. *BMC Psychiatry* **2014**, *14*, 97. [CrossRef] [PubMed]
50. Perugi, G.; Hantouche, E.; Vannucchi, G. Diagnosis and Treatment of Cyclothymia: The "Primacy" of Temperament. *Curr. Neuropharmacol.* **2017**, *15*, 372–379. [CrossRef] [PubMed]
51. Persons, J.E.; Coryell, W.H.; Solomon, D.A.; Keller, M.B.; Endicott, J.; Fiedorowicz, J.G. Mixed state and suicide: Is the effect of mixed state on suicidal behavior more than the sum of its parts? *Bipolar Disord.* **2018**, *20*, 35–41. [CrossRef]
52. Moeller, F.G.; Barratt, E.S.; Dougherty, D.M.; Schmitz, J.M.; Swann, A.C. Psychiatric aspects of impulsivity. *Am. J. Psychiatry* **2001**, *158*, 1783–1793. [CrossRef]
53. Swann, A.C.; Anderson, J.C.; Dougherty, D.M.; Moeller, F.G. Measurement of inter-episode impulsivity in bipolar disorder. *Psychiatry Res.* **2001**, *101*, 195–197. [CrossRef]
54. Etain, B.; Mathieu, F.; Liquet, S.; Raust, A.; Cochet, B.; Richard, J.R.; Gard, S.; Zanouy, L.; Kahn, J.P.; Cohen, R.F.; et al. Clinical features associated with trait-impulsiveness in euthymic bipolar disorder patients. *J. Affect. Disord.* **2013**, *144*, 240–247. [CrossRef]
55. Perugi, G.; Hantouche, E.; Vannucchi, G.; Pinto, O. Cyclothymia reloaded: A reappraisal of the most misconceived affective disorder. *J. Affect. Disord.* **2015**, *183*, 119–133. [CrossRef] [PubMed]
56. Popovic, D.; Vieta, E.; Azorin, J.-M.; Angst, J.; Bowden, C.L.; Mosolov, S.; Young, A.H.; Perugi, G. Suicide attempts in major depressive episode: Evidence from the BRIDGE-II-Mix study. *Bipolar Disord.* **2015**, *17*, 795–803. [CrossRef] [PubMed]
57. Jiménez, E.; Bonnín, C.D.M.; Solé, B.; Sánchez-Moreno, J.; Reinares, M.; Torrent, C.; Torres, I.; Salagre, E.; Varo, C.; Ruíz, V.; et al. Spanish validation of the Barcelona TEMPS-A questionnaire in patients with bipolar disorder and general population. *J. Affect. Disord.* **2019**, *249*, 199–207. [CrossRef] [PubMed]
58. Vieta, E.; Berk, M.; Schulze, T.G.; Carvalho, A.F.; Suppes, T.; Calabrese, J.R.; Gao, K.; Miskowiak, K.W.; Grande, I. Bipolar disorders. *Nat. Rev. Dis. Prim.* **2018**, *4*, 18008. [CrossRef] [PubMed]
59. Utsumi, T.; Sasaki, T.; Shimada, I.; Mabuchi, M.; Motonaga, T.; Ohtani, T.; Tochigi, M.; Kato, N.; Nanko, S. Clinical features of soft bipolarity in major depressive inpatients. *Psychiatry Clin. Neurosci.* **2006**, *60*, 611–615. [CrossRef]
60. Perugi, G.; Toni, C.; Travierso, M.C.; Akiskal, H.S. The role of cyclothymia in atypical depression: Toward a data-based reconceptualization of the borderline-bipolar II connection. *J. Affect. Disord.* **2003**, *73*, 87–98. [CrossRef]
61. Katzow, J.J.; Hsu, D.J.; Ghaemi, S.N. The bipolar spectrum: A clinical perspective. *Bipolar Disord.* **2003**, *5*, 436–442. [CrossRef]
62. De Fruyt, J.; Demyttenaere, K. Bipolar (spectrum) disorder and mood stabilization: Standing at the crossroads? *Psychother. Psychosom.* **2007**, *76*, 77–88. [CrossRef]
63. Akiskal, H.S.; Pinto, O. The evolving bipolar spectrum. Prototypes, I., II, III, and IV. *Psychiatr. Clin. N. Am.* **1999**, *22*, 517–534. [CrossRef]
64. Goto, S.; Terao, T.; Hoaki, N.; Wang, Y. Cyclothymic and hyperthymic temperaments may predict bipolarity in major depressive disorder: A supportive evidence for bipolar II1/2 and IV. *J. Affect. Disord.* **2011**, *129*, 34–38. [CrossRef]

14

Suicidality in Borderline Personality Disorder

Joel Paris *

Institute of Community and Family Psychiatry, McGill University, 4333 chemin de la cote ste. Catherine, Montreal, QC H3T1E4, Canada

Abstract: Borderline personality disorder (BPD) is associated with suicidal behaviors and self-harm. Up to 10% of BPD patients will die by suicide. However, no research data support the effectiveness of suicide prevention in this disorder, and hospitalization has not been shown to be useful. The most evidence-based treatment methods for BPD are specifically designed psychotherapies.

Keywords: suicide suicidality personality disorder; borderline personality disorder; self-harm

---

1. Introduction

This review is based on a search with the key words "borderline personality disorder" and "suicide or suicidality" in MEDLINE and PsycINFO of all articles since 2000 (along with some important older articles). This review focuses on articles that are most relevant to the following questions:

(1) What suicidal behaviors are seen in patients with borderline personality disorder (BPD), and what is their motivation?

(2) What is the risk for death by suicide in BPD?

(3) Is there evidence for the value of hospitalizing suicidal BPD patients?

(4) What are the most evidence-based treatments for suicidal BPD patients?

2. Suicidal Behaviors in BPD

As defined by the DSM-5 [1] and by the ICD-11 [2], personality disorders (PDs) are characterized by abnormal patterns of inner experience and behavior. These affect cognition, emotion, interpersonal functioning, impulse control, are inflexible and pervasive, lead to clinically significant distress or impairment, are stable and of long duration, and have an onset in adolescence or early adulthood. Personality disorders are common in practice, and can be found, above and beyond other diagnoses, in up to 45% of all outpatients [3]. Of these, BPD is by far the most researched category due to the clinical challenges it presents.

BPD is associated with a wide range of psychopathology, including unstable mood, impulsive behaviors, as well as unstable interpersonal relationships [1]. BPD patients have a mean of three lifetime suicide attempts, mostly by overdose [4].

Self-harm behaviors (i.e., non-suicidal self-injury) (NSSI) [5], are also common in BPD. NSSI usually presents as superficial cuts to the wrists and arms. However, NSSI is not suicidal in intent; BPD patients have problems with emotional regulation and cut themselves addictively to reduce painful inner states [6]. Cutting relieves emotional tension, but does not reflect a wish to die [7].

While drug overdoses can sometimes be life threatening, these behaviors vary greatly in nature and intent. They usually occur following stressful life events, and patients describe their motivation as a wish to escape [7]. Most incidents reflect ambivalent motivation, involving small quantities of medication and/or calling significant others for help. Even when potentially fatal overdoses occur, patients often contact people who are in a position to intervene.

It has long been established that suicide attempters and completers are separate but overlapping populations [8]. In a large-scale follow-up of attempters seen in an emergency room (ER), only about

3% eventually died by suicide [9]. Most repetitive attempts occur in young women, and decrease with time [10].

3. Death by Suicide in BPD Patients

Follow-back research has found that suicide occurs in up to 10% of BPD cases [11,12]. However, lower rates (3%–6%) have been reported in prospectively followed cohorts [13–15]. These discrepancies could reflect less-severe suicidality in patients who agree to be followed in research studies.

By and large, suicides in BPD occur later in the course of the illness and follow long courses of unsuccessful treatment [16]. A 15-year follow-back study found that the mean age at suicide to be 30 [12], while a 27-year follow-up reported a mean age of 37, with a standard deviation of 10 [11]. Thus, patients are not at their highest risk of suicide when they are young and frequent visitors to the ER.

Even so, patients with BPD do kill themselves. Psychological autopsy methods, which involve post-mortem interviews with families, have examined the frequency of this diagnosis in death by suicide [17–19]. In these studies, PDs were present in about half of the cases under the age of 35, with BPD being the most common category.

A meta-analysis by Pompili et al. [20] noted that suicidality is "more alarming" in young people, with a high level of suicidal behaviors. Yet the great majority of BPD patients eventually improve over time [16], and those who die by suicide tend to be those who fail to recover.

Males with BPD have a different pattern. Nearly a third of youth suicides, most of whom are male, can be diagnosed with BPD by psychological autopsy [17]. Other studies of BPD patients who died by suicide also show a preponderance of males [21]. Few of these patients were in treatment at the time of their death.

4. Hospitalization for Suicidality in BPD Patients

Many BPD patients have courses of treatment marked by multiple failed suicide attempts. These treatments are associated with multiple trials of psychotherapy, multiple prescriptions, repeated emergency room visits, and hospitalization for suicide attempts and threats [22]. Yet the research literature on the management of suicidality in BPD does not provide evidence-based guidelines for the prevention of death by suicide [23].

It has long been known that clinicians lack algorithms that can predict a fatal outcome in major mental disorders with any accuracy. As summarized in an article in The Lancet [24], in spite of a large body of research on suicide prediction, there is still no effective algorithm that can be used in practice to predict suicide. At best, clinicians are left with guidelines that may be commonsensical, but that lack empirical support.

However, the absence of evidence for prevention has not changed practice in managing BPD. Specifically, many patients are admitted to hospital when they attempt or threaten suicide. It is understandable that clinicians want to err on the safe side, but the absence of controlled data prevents us from concluding that hospital stays offer an effective method of suicide prevention. Admission for suicidal threats was recommended by the American Psychiatric Association guidelines for the treatment of BPD [25]. However, these guidelines, which have never been updated, were based on clinical opinion, and not on data showing that hospital admission has a preventive effect.

Repeated hospitalization for suicidal threats and attempts can also be counter-productive, since it interferes with out-patient treatment, and makes it impossible for patients to remain in the workplace [26–28]. It can also lead to a kind of "regression", with an increase of symptoms based on the behavioral reinforcement of suicidal behavior. Linehan [6] recommends not admitting patients for suicidality beyond an overnight hold in a crisis.

5. Evidence-Based Treatments for BPD

We now know that well-structured ambulatory treatment, using methods specifically developed for BPD, is an effective intervention for most BPD patients. The most extensively investigated treatment is dialectical behavior therapy (DBT) [6], whose efficacy has been confirmed by randomized clinical trials [29,30]. The main outcomes are reductions in overdoses, in emergency room visits for suicidality, reduced frequency of self-harm, and reduced hospital admissions. DBT specifically aims to modify the regulation of emotion, teaching patients how to regulate negative emotions in ways other than cutting or overdosing [6].

Several other psychotherapy methods have also been tested in randomized clinical trials: mentalization-based therapy [31,32]; transference-focused psychotherapy [33]; schema-focused therapy [34]; and standard cognitive therapy [35].

All these methods target the affective instability (emotion dysregulation) that characterizes BPD [6,36], as well as impulsivity [37]. Emotion dysregulation accompanied by a lack of control over impulses makes patients more likely to turn to suicidal actions, and the frequency of suicide attempts is strongly related to these traits [10]. Thus, all methods of psychotherapy attempt to teach patients to stand outside their emotions, to self-reflect before acting on them, and to develop a better understanding of interpersonal conflict.

By and large, all psychological treatments that are well-structured and specifically designed for BPD patients are superior to standard clinical management. A Cochrane report [38] as well as a systematic meta-analysis [39] have summarized this evidence, supporting the conclusion that specific forms of psychotherapy for BPD are efficacious. These methods are usually provided in out-patient settings, and do not require hospital admission. As noted by Zanarini [40], BPD patients need to "get a life", which means therapists must work actively to involve them with life goals, such as career and social networks.

In contrast, the efficacy of pharmacological agents in BPD is not well established. No clinical trials have documented remission of the disorder with successful drug treatment, and a Cochrane report did not find sufficient evidence to prescribe *any* drug for patients with BPD [41]. Recent research has also shown that anticonvulsant mood stabilizers are not efficacious [42]. There is some evidence for the use of antipsychotics for short periods [43]. A similar conclusion has been reached by the UK National Institute on Clinical Excellence [44]. Unfortunately, it has long been observed that most BPD patients are often on multiple medications, including antidepressants, mood stabilizers, and/or neuroleptics [22], and this practice does not seem to have changed. These interventions do not require hospital admission. There is also no evidence that pharmacological regimes are effective for suicide prevention.

6. Implications for Practice

One of the most unique aspects of BPD is chronic suicidal ideation [27]. Patients with mood disorders can be suicidal when depressed, but usually put these ideas aside when they go into remission. In contrast, BPD patients may consider suicide on a daily basis for months to years, and only go into remission much later. Suicidal ideas will vary in intensity over time, waxing when life events are stressful, and waning when they are not.

Yet by themselves, suicidal thoughts are too common to be useful in predicting suicidal actions. But while patients with suicidal behaviors have a statistically higher risk, one cannot predict who is most likely to die by suicide. Deaths by suicide are rare events relative to attempts, which is why large-scale follow-up studies have found that algorithms based on risk factors fail to predict who will die by suicide [45,46]. The problem is false positives (patients who fit a profile but never kill themselves).

Most patients with BPD, despite having suicidal thoughts for long periods of time and multiple suicide attempts, never kill themselves. Thus, the level of alarm created by patients with BPD who present in clinics and ERs with suicidal ideas is not necessarily justified, even when threats are dramatic or blood-curdling. Clinicians need to work on making these patents more functional, and should not be distracted from these therapeutic tasks by suicidality.

Needless to say, chronic suicidality can be draining for therapists, and no one wants to lose a patient in this way. Yet in BPD, suicidality "goes with the territory" [47], and most patients cannot be treated without accepting a calculated risk [48]. Moreover, recommending ER visits and hospitalization reinforces the very behaviors they are designed to treat [6].

Hospitalization has not been supported by evidence, and when suicidality is chronic, admission to hospital provides only temporary relief; most patients continue to have suicidal ideas after discharge. While some research describes intensive treatment in hospital [49], similar programs could be offered on an out-patient basis. To avoid the harm of repetitive admissions, one might prefer day treatment, which offers the advantages of admission (intensive treatment by an experienced team) without its disadvantages, and has some supporting evidence for its efficacy [31]. Unfortunately, day programs usually have waiting lists and are not useful in a crisis.

In practice, BPD patients are commonly held in ERs (or admitted to wards) when they threaten suicide, cut themselves, or overdose. These choices are partly determined by a fear of litigation. However, to minimize the risk of lawsuits, clinicians can ensure careful record keeping, consult frequently with colleagues, and get families involved early on in treatment [50].

Based on current evidence, it is reasonable to conclude that we should treat suicidal patients with BPD on an out-patient basis using specialized forms of psychotherapy. Psychopharmacology remains adjunctive and optional. Hospital admission can be justified by either a near-fatal attempt (requiring a re-evaluation), or a micro-psychotic episode (requiring pharmacological intervention) [27]. Since we have no firm evidence that death by suicide in BPD can be prevented, we should focus on providing existing evidence-based psychological treatments designed for this challenging population.

References

1. American Psychiatric Association. *Diagnostic and Statistical Manual of Mental Disorders*, 5th ed.; Text Revision; American Psychiatric Press: Washington DC, USA, 2013.
2. World Health Organization. *International Classification of Diseases*, 11th ed.; World Health Organization: Geneva, Switzerland, 2018.
3. Zimmerman, M.; Rothschild, L.; Chelminski, I. The prevalence of DSM-IV personality disorders in psychiatric outpatients. *Am. J. Psychiatry* **2005**, *162*, 1911–1918. [CrossRef]
4. Soloff, P.H.; Lynch, K.G.; Kelly, T.M.; Malone, K.M.; Mann, J.J. Characteristics of suicide attempts of patients with major depressive episode and borderline personality disorder: A comparative study. *Am. J. Psychiatry* **2000**, *157*, 601–608. [CrossRef] [PubMed]
5. Nock, M.K.; Favazza, A. Nonsuicidal self-injury: Definition and classification. In *Understanding Nonsuicidal Self- Injury: Origins, Assessment, and Treatment*; Nock, M.K., Ed.; American Psychological Association: Washington, DC, USA, 2009; pp. 9–18.
6. Linehan, M.M. *Cognitive Behavioral Therapy of Borderline Personality Disorder*; Guilford: New York, NY, USA, 1993.
7. Brown, M.Z.; Comtois, K.A.; Linehan, M.M. Reasons for suicide attempts and nonsuicidal self-injury in women with borderline personality disorder. *J. Abnorm. Psychol.* **2002**, *111*, 198–202. [CrossRef]
8. Beautrais, A.L. Suicides and serious suicide attempts: Two populations or one? *Psychol. Med.* **2001**, *31*, 837–845. [CrossRef] [PubMed]
9. Hawton, K.; Zahl, D.; Weatherall, R. Suicide following deliberate self-harm: Long-term follow-up of patients who presented to a general hospital. *Br. J. Psychiatry* **2003**, *182*, 537–542. [CrossRef] [PubMed]
10. Paris, J. *The Treatment of Borderline Personality Disorder*, 2nd ed.; Guilford: New York, NY, USA, 2019.
11. Paris, J.; Zweig-Frank, H. A twenty-seven year follow-up of borderline patients. *Compr. Psychiatry* **2001**, *42*, 482–487. [CrossRef]
12. Stone, M.H. *The Fate of Borderline Patients*; Guilford: New York, NY, USA, 1990.

13. Gunderson, J.G.; Stout, R.L.; McGlashan, T.H.; Shea, T.; Morey, L.C.; Grilo, C.M.; Zanarini, M.C.; Yen, S.; Markowitz, J.C.; Sanislow, C.; et al. Ten-year course of Borderline Personality Disorder: Psychopathology and function from the Collaborative Longitudinal Personality Disorders Study. *Arch. Gen. Psychiatry* **2011**, *68*, 827–837. [CrossRef] [PubMed]
14. Zanarini, M.C.; Frankenburg, F.; Reich, B.; Fitzmaurice, G. Attainment and stability of sustained symptomatic remission and recovery among borderline patients and Axis II comparison subjects: A 16-year prospective followup study. *Am. J. Psychiatry* **2012**, *169*, 476–483. [CrossRef]
15. Temes, C.M.; Frankenburg, F.; Fitzmaurice, G.; Zanarini, M.C. Deaths by suicide and other causes among patients with borderline personality disorder and personality-disordered comparison subjects over 24 years of prospective follow-up. *J. Clin. Psychiatry* **2019**, in press. [CrossRef]
16. Paris, J. *Personality Disorders Over Time*; American Psychiatric Press: Washington, DC, USA, 2003.
17. Lesage, A.D.; Boyer, R.; Grunberg, F.; Morisette, R.; Vanier, C.; Morrisette, R.; Ménard-Buteau, C.; Loyer, M. Suicide and mental disorders: A case control study of young men. *Am. J. Psychiatry* **1994**, *151*, 1063–1068.
18. Hunt, I.M.; Kapur, N.; Robinson, J.; Shaw, J.; Flynn, S.; Bailey, H.; Meehan, J.; Bickley, H.; Burns, J.; Appleby, L.; et al. Suicide within 12 months of mental health service contact in different age and diagnostic groups: National clinical survey. *Br. J. Psychiatry* **2006**, *188*, 135–142. [CrossRef] [PubMed]
19. Tidemalm, D.; Elofsson, S.; Stefansson, C.-G.; Waern, M.; Runeson, B. Predictors of suicide in a community-based cohort of individuals with severe mental disorder. *Soc. Psychiatry Psychiatry Epidemiol.* **2005**, *40*, 595–600. [CrossRef] [PubMed]
20. Pompili, M.; Girardi, P.; Ruberto, A.; Tatarelli, R. Suicide in borderline personality disorder: A meta-analysis. *Nord. J. Psychiatry* **2005**, *59*, 319–324. [CrossRef] [PubMed]
21. McGirr, A.; Paris, J.; Lesage, A.; Renaud, J.; Turecki, G. Risk factors for suicide completion in borderline personality disorder: A case-control study of cluster B comorbidity and impulsive aggression. *J. Clin. Psychiatry* **2007**, *68*, 721–729. [CrossRef]
22. Zanarini, M.C.; Frankenburg, F.R.; Khera, G.S.; Bleichmar, J. Treatment histories of borderline inpatients. *Compr. Psychiatry* **2001**, *42*, 144–150. [CrossRef]
23. Goodman, M.; Roiff, T.; Oakes, A.H.; Paris, J. Suicidal risk and management in Borderline Personality Disorder. *Curr. Psychiatry Rep.* **2012**, *14*, 79–85. [CrossRef] [PubMed]
24. Turecki, G.; Brent, D. Suicide and suicidal behavior. *Lancet* **2016**, *387*, 19–25. [CrossRef]
25. Oldham, J.M.; Gabbard, G.O.; Goin, M.K.; Gunderson, J.; Soloff, P.; Spiegel, D.; Stone, M.; Phillips, K.A. Practice guideline for the treatment of Borderline Personality Disorder. *Am. J. Psychiatry* **2001**, *158*, 1–52.
26. Gunderson, J.G. *Borderline Personality Disorder: A Clinical Guide*, 2nd ed.; American Psychiatric Press: Washington, DC, USA, 2008.
27. Paris, J. *Half in Love with Death: The Meaning of Chronic Suicidality*; Laurence Erlbaum: Mahwah, NJ, USA, 2006.
28. Paris, J. *Stepped Care for Borderline Personality Disorder*; Academic Press: New York, NY, USA, 2017.
29. Linehan, M.M.; Armstrong, H.E.; Suarez, A.; Allmon, D.; Heard, H. Cognitive behavioral treatment of chronically parasuicidal borderline patients. *Arch. Gen. Psychiatry* **1991**, *48*, 1060–1064. [CrossRef] [PubMed]
30. Linehan, M.M.; Comtois, K.A.; Murray, A.M.; Brown, M.Z.; Gallop, R.J.; Heard, H.L.; Korslund, K.E.; Tutek, D.A.; Reyonolds, S.K.; Lindenboim, N. Two-year randomized controlled trial and follow-up of dialectical behavior therapy vs therapy by experts for suicidal behaviors and borderline personality disorder. *Arch. Gen. Psychiatry* **2006**, *63*, 757–766. [CrossRef] [PubMed]
31. Bateman, A.; Fonagy, P. Effectiveness of partial hospitalization in the treatment of borderline personality disorder: A randomized controlled trial. *Am. J. Psychiatry* **1999**, *156*, 1563–1569. [CrossRef] [PubMed]
32. Bateman, A.; Fonagy, P. Randomized controlled trial of out-patient mentalization-based treatment versus structured clinical management for borderline personality disorder. *Am. J. Psychiatry* **2009**, *166*, 1355–1364. [CrossRef] [PubMed]
33. Clarkin, J.F.; Levy, K.N.; Lenzenweger, M.F.; Kernberg, O.F. Evaluating three treatments for borderline personality disorder: A multiwave study. *Am. J. Psychiatry* **2007**, *164*, 1–8. [CrossRef]
34. Giesen-Bloo, J.; Van Dyck, R.; Spinhoven, P.; Van Tilburg, W.; Dirksen, C.; Van Asselt, T.; Kremers, I.; Nadort, M.; Arntz, A. Outpatient psychotherapy for borderline personality disorder: Randomized trial of schema-focused therapy vs. transference-focused psychotherapy. *Arch. Gen. Psychiatry* **2006**, *63*, 649–658. [CrossRef]

35. Davidson, K.; Norrie, J.; Tyrer, P.; Gumley, A.; Tata, P.; Murray, H. The effectiveness of cognitive behavior therapy for borderline personality disorder: Results from the borderline personality disorder study of cognitive therapy [BOSCOT] trial. *J. Personal. Disord.* **2006**, *20*, 450–465. [CrossRef]
36. Koenigsberg, H.W.; Harvey, P.D.; Mitropoulou, V.; Schmeidler, J.; New, A.S.; Goodman, M.; Silverman, J.M.; Serby, M.; Schopick, F.; Siever, L. Characterizing affective instability in borderline personality disorder. *Am. J. Psychiatry* **2002**, *159*, 784–788. [CrossRef]
37. Crowell, S.E.; Beauchaine, T.P.; Linehan, M.M. A biosocial developmental model of borderline personality: Elaborating and extending Linehan's theory. *Psychol. Bull.* **2009**, *135*, 495–510. [CrossRef]
38. Stoffers-Winterling, J.M.; Völlm, B.A.; Rücker, G.; Timmer, A.; Huband, N.; Lieb, K. Psychological interventions for borderline personality disorder. *Cochrane Library* **2012**. [CrossRef]
39. Cristea, I.A.; Gentilla, C.; Cotet, C.D.; Palomba, D.; Barbui, C.; Cuijpers, P. Efficacy of psychotherapies for Borderline Personality Disorder: A systematic review and meta-analysis. *JAMA Psychiatry* **2017**, *74*, 319–328. [CrossRef] [PubMed]
40. Zanarini, M.C. Psychotherapy of borderline personality disorder. *Acta Psychiatry Scand.* **2009**, *120*, 373–377. [CrossRef] [PubMed]
41. Binks, C.A.; Fenton, M.; McCarthy, L.; Lee, T.; Adams, C.E.; Duggan, C. Pharmacological interventions for people with borderline personality disorder. *Cochrane Database Syst. Rev.* **2012**, *1*, CD005653.
42. Crawford, M.; Sanatinia, R.; Barrett, B.M.; Cunningham, G. The clinical effectiveness and cost-effectiveness of lamotrigine in borderline personality disorder: A randomized placebo-controlled trial. *Am. J. Psychiatry* **2018**, *175*, 576–580. [CrossRef]
43. Black, D.W.; Zanarini, M.C.; Ronine, A.; Shaw, M.; Allen, J.; Schulz, S.C. Comparison of low and moderate dosages of extended-release quetiapine in Borderline Personality Disorder: A randomized, double-blind, placebo-controlled trial. *Am. J. Psychiatry* **2014**, *171*, 1174–1182. [CrossRef] [PubMed]
44. National Institutes of Clinical Excellence. Guidelines for the Treatment of Borderline Personality Disorder. 2009. Available online: http://www.nice.org.uk/guidance/index.jsp?action=byID&o=11651 (accessed on 10 May 2018).
45. Goldstein, R.B.; Black, D.W.; Nasrallah, A.; Winokur, G. The prediction of suicide. *Arch. Gen. Psychiatry* **1991**, *48*, 418–422. [CrossRef]
46. Pokorny, A.D. Prediction of suicide in psychiatric patients: Report of a prospective study. *Arch. Gen. Psychiatry* **1982**, *40*, 249–257. [CrossRef]
47. Schwartz, D.A.; Flinn, D.E.; Slawson, P.F. Treatment of the suicidal character. *Am. J. Psychiatry* **1974**, *28*, 194–207. [CrossRef]
48. Maltsberger, J.T. Calculated risk taking in the treatment of suicidal patients: Ethical and legal problems. *Death Stud.* **1994**, *18*, 439–452. [CrossRef]
49. Fowler, J.C.; Clapp, J.D.; Madan, A.; Allen, J.G.; Frueh, C.; Fonagy, P.; Oldham, J.M. A naturalistic longitudinal study of extended inpatient treatment for adults with borderline personality disorder: An examination of treatment response, remission and deterioration. *J. Affect. Disord.* **2018**, *235*, 323–331. [CrossRef] [PubMed]
50. Gutheil, T.G. Suicide and suit: Liability after self-destruction. In *Suicide and Clinical Practice*; Jacobs, D., Ed.; American Psychiatric Press: Washington, DC, USA, 1992; pp. 147–167.

15

Transcranial Direct Current Stimulation for Obsessive-Compulsive Disorder

Jérôme Brunelin [1,2,3,4,*], Marine Mondino [1,2,3,4], Rémy Bation [1,2,3,4,5], Ulrich Palm [6], Mohamed Saoud [1,2,3,4,5] and Emmanuel Poulet [1,2,3,4,7]

1 INSERM, U1028, Lyon Neuroscience Research Center, PSY-R2 team, F-69000 Lyon, France; marine.mondino@ch-le-vinatier.fr (M.M.); remy.bation@chu-lyon.fr (R.B.); mohamed.saoud@chu-lyon.fr (M.S.); emmanuel.poulet@chu-lyon.fr (E.P.)
2 CNRS, UMR5292, Lyon Neuroscience Research Center, PSY-R2 Team, F-69000 Lyon, France
3 University Lyon, F-69000 Lyon, France
4 Centre Hospitalier le Vinatier, F-69678 Bron, France
5 Psychiatry Unit, Wertheimer Hospital, CHU Lyon, F-69500 Bron, France
6 Department of Psychiatry and Psychotherapy, Klinikum der Universität München, D-80336 Munich, Germany; Ulrich.Palm@med.uni-muenchen.de
7 Psychiatry Emergency Unit, Edouard Herriot Hospital, CHU, F-69000 Lyon, France
* Correspondence: jerome.brunelin@ch-le-vinatier.fr;

Abstract: Despite the advances in psychopharmacology and established psychotherapeutic interventions, more than 40% of patients with obsessive-compulsive disorder (OCD) do not respond to conventional treatment approaches. Transcranial direct current stimulation (tDCS) has been recently proposed as a therapeutic tool to alleviate treatment-resistant symptoms in patients with OCD. The aim of this review was to provide a comprehensive overview of the current state of the art and future clinical applications of tDCS in patients with OCD. A literature search conducted on the PubMed database following PRISMA guidelines and completed by a manual search yielded 12 results: eight case reports, three open-label studies (with 5, 8, and 42 participants), and one randomized trial with two active conditions (12 patients). There was no sham-controlled study. A total of 77 patients received active tDCS with a large diversity of electrode montages mainly targeting the dorsolateral prefrontal cortex, the orbitofrontal cortex or the (pre-) supplementary motor area. Despite methodological limitations and the heterogeneity of stimulation parameters, tDCS appears to be a promising tool to decrease obsessive-compulsive symptoms as well as comorbid depression and anxiety in patients with treatment-resistant OCD. Further sham-controlled studies are needed to confirm these preliminary results.

Keywords: OCD; tDCS; brain stimulation; neuromodulation; obsession; compulsion

---

1. Introduction

Obsessive-compulsive disorder (OCD) is a frequent and debilitating psychiatric condition that occurs in 2–3% of the population [1]. Symptoms consist of unwanted intrusive thoughts and compulsive behaviours, leading to the inability to maintain social and occupational functioning [2].

Established treatments consist of a combination of psychopharmacology (especially selective serotonin reuptake inhibitor—SSRI) and psychotherapeutic interventions, such as cognitive behavioral therapy—CBT [3]. Despite augmentation strategies with other psychotropic drugs and advances in psychopharmacology [4], it is assumed that nearly 40% of patients do not show a sufficient response to conventional treatments [3]. Therefore, the development of new therapeutic approaches is warranted.

Among the recently developed therapeutic approaches, non-invasive brain stimulation techniques (NIBS), such as transcranial direct current stimulation (tDCS) hold promises to alleviate symptoms and improve cognitive functioning in various psychiatric conditions [5,6]. tDCS consists of applying a weak direct current (1–2 mA) between two electrodes placed on the scalp of a subject. Neurophysiological studies have reported that depending on the electrode polarity and current intensity, tDCS may increase cortical excitability in the vicinity of the anode whereas cathodal tDCS may decrease it [7]. The effects of tDCS are not restricted to the area beneath the electrodes and could reach a widespread network of cortical and subcortical regions that are connected to the targeted region [8]. The ability of tDCS to modulate a network is of particular interest since abnormal activity and connectivity within the orbitofronto-striato-pallido-thalamic network is described in patients with OCD. Indeed, imaging studies in patients with OCD showed abnormalities, which can be either hyper- or hypo activities, within numerous brain regions along a widespread network including the orbitofrontal cortex (OFC), the (pre-) supplementary motor area (SMA), the cingulate gyrus, the caudate, the thalamus, the right and left cerebellum, and the parietal cortex [9]. These abnormalities, which can be either trait- or state-dependent, have been revealed in resting conditions as well as by symptom provocation paradigms, depending on the studies. Moreover, it has been reported that some of these abnormalities were reverted after successful treatment [10,11]. It has thus been hypothesized that applying tDCS over these abnormal brain regions would lead to a decrease in obsessive-compulsive (OC) symptoms by modulating the underlying abnormal brain network. For instance, the use of anodal tDCS over the pre-SMA is based on imaging studies revealing an interaction between pre-SMA hypoactivity and deficient response inhibition with reciprocal striatal hyperactivity in patients with OCD [12]. The use of cathodal tDCS over the OFC is based on imaging studies reporting hyperactivity at rest and during symptom provocation paradigms of the OFC in patients with OCD [9,13]. Targeting the dorsolateral prefrontal cortex (DLPFC) is based on NIBS studies reporting beneficial clinical effects when stimulating this specific brain region in numerous psychiatric conditions [5,6], and on imaging studies reporting abnormalities in the cortico-striato-thalamo-cortical pathways, especially the 'DLPFC-caudate nucleus-thalamus' loop that is implicated in the pathophysiology of OCD [13]. This review aimed to provide a comprehensive overview of existing literature on the effects of tDCS applied as a therapeutic tool to reduce OC symptoms in patients with treatment-resistant OCD and to discuss future applications of tDCS in OCD.

2. Materials and Methods

Search Strategy

A systematic review was conducted following the recommendations of the PRISMA guidelines. A primary search on the PubMed database until December 2017 with the keywords (tDCS AND OCD) yielded 21 results. This primary search was completed by a manual search on articles cited by retrieved articles and on Google allowing for adding five articles (see Figure 1—PRISMA diagram).

The inclusion criteria were: (i) full length original articles published in English language in peer-reviewed journals, (ii) patients with OCD according to DSM or ICD-10 criteria, (iii) detailed description of the stimulation method, and (iv) the use of repeated sessions of tDCS. Among the 26 articles from the primary search, 11 articles were excluded for the following reasons: six were review articles not specifically dealing with tDCS in OCD, four did not concern OCD, and one offered a modelling of the electrical field induced by tDCS in patients with OCD. One of the articles issued by the manual search showed no data on OC symptoms [14], as well as a study investigating the clinical interest of transcranial alternating current stimulation (tACS) and not tDCS [15] were excluded from the qualitative analysis. Another article investigating the effect of a single session of tDCS (anode, cathode, sham) over the medial prefrontal cortex (PFC) on anxiety symptoms after exposure in 12 patients with treatment resistant OCD was also excluded [16].

A total of 12 articles was included in the qualitative analysis, nine from the primary search and three from the manual search [17–19].

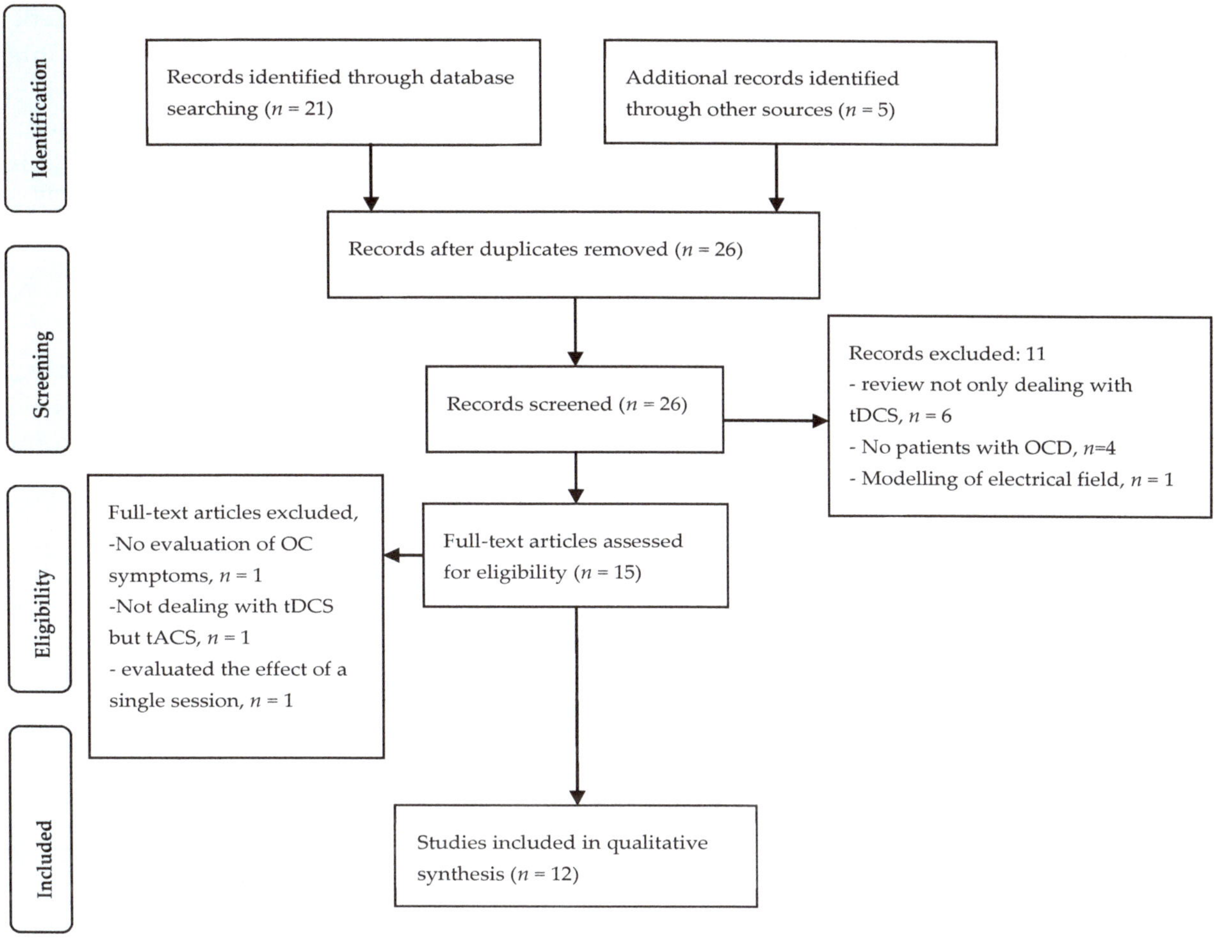

Figure 1. PRISMA flow diagram of selected studies in the qualitative analysis.

3. Results

Amongst the 12 included studies investigating the clinical effects of tDCS in patients with OCD, eight were case reports [17,19–25], three were open-label studies, including 5, 8, and 42 patients [18,26,27] and one was a randomized-controlled study including 12 patients with OCD [28]. Remarkably, none of the studies was sham-controlled (Table 1).

In the first case report, Volpato and colleagues [20] observed no significant effects of 10 sessions of tDCS (20 min, 2 mA) on OC symptoms when the cathode was placed over the left dorsolateral prefrontal cortex (DLPFC; over F3, according to the 10/20 international electroencephalography EEG system) and the anode extra-cephalically (on the neck). Interestingly, the authors reported a significant decrease of depression and anxiety symptoms. Other studies have tried different electrode montages and have shown beneficial outcomes on OC symptoms (see Figure 2 for an illustration of the electrode montages). Namely, two studies targeted the left DLPFC by placing the anode over the left DLPFC (F3) and the cathode either over the right DLPFC (F4) [25] or the right orbitofrontal cortex (OFC) /supraorbital area (Fp2) [18]. Three studies used an electrode montage positioning the cathode over the left OFC (Fp2) and the anode over the occipital region (O2) or the cerebellum [19,22,26]. One study targeted the right OFC (Fp2) with the cathode and the left parieto-temporo-occipital region with the anode (midway between P1, C3, and T7) [27]. Finally, five studies targeted the pre-supplementary motor area (SMA). Among them, two placed the anode over the pre-SMA (Fz/FCz) and the cathode over the right orbitofrontal cortex (Fp2) [17,21], one placed the cathode over the pre-SMA and the anode extra-cephalically over the right deltoid [24], and two compared two different montages with either the anode or the cathode over the pre-SMA and the other electrode extra cephalically over the right deltoid [23,28]. In the included studies, different sizes of electrodes were used: 25 cm^2 [19,23,24,28], 35 cm^2 [18,20–22,25,26] and 5.5 cm^2 [27]. The intensity of stimulation was set at 2 mA in all of the tDCS studies (2–3 mA in [27]) and tDCS duration varied from 20 min [17–20,22,23,26,28] to 30 min [24,25,27]. The number of tDCS sessions also varied; most of the studies delivered 10 [19,20,22,23,26,28] or 20 sessions [17,21,24,25] and one study delivered 15 sessions [18]. tDCS sessions were delivered daily [18,19,23,24,27,28] or twice daily [17,21,22,25,26]. All of the studies used the Yale–Brown Obsessive and Compulsive Scale score (Y-BOCS) [29] to assess OC symptoms.

In summary, a total of 77 patients with OCD received active tDCS with different electrode montages. Most of the studies reported a significant effect of tDCS on OC symptoms, more specifically, a decrease of the YBOCS score. Several studies also reported beneficial effects of tDCS on other symptoms that are often observed in patients with OCD, such as depression and anxiety [18–20,24,25].

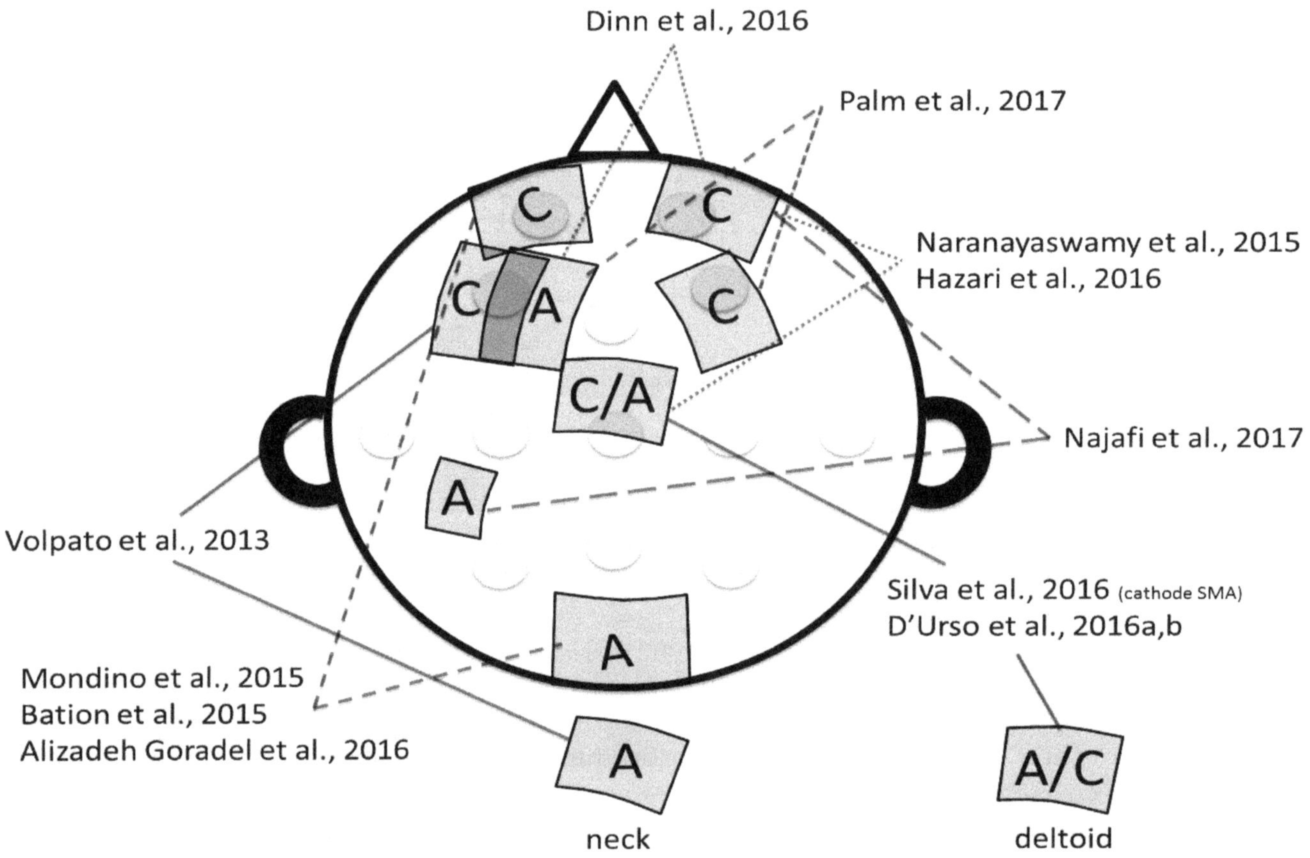

Figure 2. Illustration of the diversity in electrodes montage observed in transcranial direct current stimulation (tDCS) studies aiming to alleviate obsessive-compulsive symptoms in patients with treatment-resistant obsessive-compulsive disorder. A: Anode; C: Cathode. Hazari et al., 2016 [17]; Dinn et al., 2016 [18]; Alizadeh Goradel et al., 2016 [19]; Volpato et al., 2013 [20]; Narayanaswamy et al., 2015 [21]; Mondino et al., 2015 [22]; D'Urso et al., 2016a [23]; Silva et al., 2016 [24]; Palm et al., 2017 [25]; Bation et al., 2015 [26]; Najafi et al., 2017 [27]; D'Urso et al., 2016b [28].

Table 1. Main findings of studies investigating the clinical interest of transcranial direct current stimulation (tDCS) to decrease symptoms in patients with obsessive-compulsive disorder (OCD).

Articles	N	Patients Characteristics	Target	Intensity Electrode Size	Duration and Number of Sessions	Main Results
Volpato et al., 2013 [20]	1	Age: 35, male Type*: 2,3,4 Previous TTT: SSRI, SNRI, CBT	Anode: posterior neck-base Cathode: left DLPFC	2 mA, 35 cm^2	20 min, 10 sessions (1/day)	No effect on OC symptoms. Depression score decreased (−34% HDRS); anxiety score decreased (−17%).
Mondino et al., 2015 [22]	1	Age: 52, female Type*: 3,4 Previous TTT: tricyclic, SSRI, SNRI, AP, Lithium, CBT	Anode: right cerebello-occipital (100 cm^2) Cathode: left OFC	2 mA, 35 cm^2	20 min, 10 sessions (2/day; 2 h between 2 sessions)	YBOCS score decreased (−26%)
Hazari et al., 2016 [17]	1	Age: 24, male Type*: 1,2 Previous TTT: SSRI, ECT	Anode: SMA Cathode: right OFC	2 mA, ND	20 min, 20 sessions (2/day, at least 3 h between 2 sessions)	YBOCS decreased (−80%) during 7 months
D'Urso et al., 2016 [23]	1	Age: 33, female Type*: 3 Previous TTT: SSRI, BZD, tricyclic, CBT	Anode: Pre-SMA Cathode: right deltoid And then, Reverse montage	2 mA, 25 cm^2	20 min, 10 sessions (1/day)	Worsening of symptoms after anodal tDCS. YBOCS score decreased (−30%) after cathodal tDCS,
Alizadeh Goradel et al., 2016 [19]	1	Age: 23, female Type*: 1 Previous TTT: SSRI	Anode: right occipital Cathode: left OFC	2 mA, 25 cm^2	20 min, 10 sessions (1/day)	YBOCS score decreased (−64%); Depression score decreased (−87%); −100% anxiety
Palm et al., 2017 [25]	1	Age: 31, male Type*: 1,3 Previous TTT: tricyclic, SSRI, AP, CBT	Anode: left DLPFC Cathode: Right DLPFC	2 mA, 35 cm^2	30 min, 20 sessions (2/day, 3 h between 2 sessions)	Combined with Sertraline, YBOCS score (−22%), depression (−10%) and anxiety (−21%) decreased
Narayanaswamy et al., 2015 [21]	2	Age: 39, female Type*: 1 Previous TTT: SSRI, exposure	Anode: left pre-SMA Cathode: right OFC	2 mA, 35 cm^2	20 min, 20 sessions (2/day, at least 3 h between 2 sessions)	Patient 1: YBOCS score decreased (−40%), −52% at day 17
		Age: 24, male Type*: 1 Previous TTT: tricyclic, SSRI				Patient 2: YBOCS score decreased (−46.7%)
Silva et al., 2016 [24]	2	Age: 37, male Type*: 2 Previous TTT: tricyclic, SSRI, CBT	Anode: right deltoid Cathode: bilateral SMA	2 mA, 25 cm^2	30 min, 20 sessions (1/day)	Patient 1: no effect at Week 4, YBOCS score decreased at week 12 (−18%). No changes in anxiety nor depression
		Age: 31, male Type*: 1,3 Previous TTT: tricyclic, SSRI				Patient 2: YBOCS score decreased, (−17%) at Week 4; −55% at week 12). 50% improvement in anxiety and depression

Table 1. *Cont.*

Dinn et al., 2016 [18]	5	Age: 40.4 (8.4), 4 females, 1 male Type*: ND Previous TTT: SSRI, SNRI, AP	Anode: left DLPFC Cathode: right OFC	2 mA, 35 cm^2	20 min, 15 sessions (1/day)	Open Label Study OC symptoms decreased (−23%); depression decreased (−30%)
Bation et al., 2015 [26]	8	Age: 44.2 (13.8), 6 females, 2 males Type*: 1 (n = 5), 3 (n = 3) Previous TTT: tricyclic, 3 SSRI, AP, CBT	Anode: right cerebellum Cathode: left OFC	2 mA, 35 cm^2	20 min, 10 sessions (2/day, at least 3 h between 2 sessions)	Open Label Study YBOCS score decreased (−24.6%)
D'Urso et al., 2016 [28]	12	Age: 39.0 (13.1), 7 females, 5 males Type*: 1 (n = 4), 2 (n = 2), 3 (n = 6) Previous TTT: at least SSRI, CBT	Anode midline pre SMA Cathode: right deltoid (n = 6) OR reverse montage	2 mA, 25 cm^2	20 min, 10 sessions (1/day)	RCT—10 patients completed the study Cathodal tDCS was significantly more effective than anodal tDCS. In cathodal arm, YBOCS score decreased (−17.5%) after 10 sessions, −20.1% after 20 sessions
Najafi et al., 2017 [27]	42	Age: 29.1 (10.1), 23 females, 19 males Type*: ND Previous TTT: at least 2 SSRI, CBT	Anode: parieto-temporo-occipital areas Cathode: right OFC	2–3 mA, 5.5 cm^2	30 min, 15 sessions (1/day)	Open Label Study YBOCS score decreased (−63.4%) Maintenance of the effect at 3 months follow up (−77.6%)

DLPFC: dorsolateral prefrontal cortex; HDRS: Hamilton Depression Rating Scale; ND: Not Done; OFC: orbitofrontal cortex; (pre) SMA: (pre) supplementary motor area; Y-BOCS: Yale-Brown Obsessive Compulsive Scale. Age: mean (standard deviation) years, TTT: treatment, AP: antipsychotic, SSRI: selective serotonin reuptake inhibitor, SNRI: serotonin–norepinephrine reuptake inhibitor, CBT: cognitive behavioural therapy. Type* 1 = obsessions and checking, 2 = symmetry and ordering, 3 = cleanliness and washing, 4 = hoarding according to Leckman et al. 1997 [30].

4. Discussion

We reviewed here studies investigating the clinical effects of tDCS in patients with treatment-resistant OCD. Overall, our review included 12 studies, corresponding with a total sample of 77 patients with OCD. Results indicated that applying tDCS might show promising results to reduce OC symptoms. Little is known regarding the duration of this effect since it has not been systematically investigated. Two studies reported that the beneficial effects were still observed at a three-month [27] or seven-month follow-up [17]. In addition, it is interesting to note that some of the included studies also reported beneficial effects of tDCS on depression and anxiety that are common comorbid symptoms in patients with OCD. In line with this, a recent crossover study has investigated the effect of a single session of tDCS on obsession-induced anxiety after symptom provocation in patients with OCD. They reported a significant decrease in the severity of the obsession-induced anxiety following tDCS applied with the cathode over the medial PFC as compared with tDCS applied with the anode over the medial PFC and sham tDCS [16]. One may hypothesize that anxiety, depression, and OCD share abnormalities within brain networks that are targeted by cortical stimulation. However, the findings of beneficial effects of tDCS in OCD should be interpreted with caution and some methodological considerations should be noted.

First, none of the studies that are included in the present review was sham-controlled. One randomized study used a parallel arm design, but compared two active conditions [28]. To the best of our knowledge, only one randomized sham-controlled trial was conducted in OCD patients. This study included 20 patients with OCD and reported that active tDCS (2 mA, 20 min, 15 sessions) applied with the anode over the right DLPFC and the cathode over the left DLPFC improved decision-making abilities as compared to sham tDCS [14]. The authors thus showed that tDCS could have a pro-cognitive effect in patients with OCD, as reported in other psychiatric conditions [5]. However, this study did not provide direct clinical assessment of OC symptoms. Further studies are needed to determine the real effect of repeated sessions of active tDCS on OC symptoms, by comparing with sham. Indeed, previous sham-controlled studies have reported a large sham effect in patients with treatment-resistant OCD receiving repeated sessions of NIBS [11,31].

Second, most of the studies included in our review were case reports and only two studies included more than 10 patients [27,28]. Interpretation of results is thus limited by small sample size. Furthermore, tDCS parameters were highly heterogeneous across studies, in terms of electrode montage (see Figure 2), number of tDCS sessions, tDCS duration, and interval between sessions (from 2 h to 1 day). For instance, regarding electrode positioning, some studies targeted the DLPFC with the anode placed over the left DLPFC (F3) and the cathode over the right OFC [18], or the contralateral DLPFC [25]. Another study placed the cathode over the left DLPFC (F3) and the anode over the neck [20]. Other studies have proposed to target the left OFC (Fp1) or the right OFC (FP2) with the cathode combined with the anode over the right occipital cortex [19,22], the right cerebellum [26] or the temporo-parieto-occipital region [27]. These montages were based on neuroimaging studies showing hyperactivity within the left OFC and hypoactivity within the cerebellum in patients with OCD [9]. The pre-SMA was also commonly targeted in the reviewed studies either with the anode [17,21,23,28] or with the cathode [23,24,28]. In a randomized controlled trial comparing both montages (anode over the pre-SMA or cathode over the pre-SMA), D'Urso and colleagues suggested a better effect of the cathodal-tDCS montage on OC symptoms [28]. Nevertheless, based on these findings, it seems difficult to conclude regarding the optimal tDCS montage to adopt in order to alleviate symptoms in patients with OCD. However, in a computer head modelling study, Senço and colleagues reported interesting findings that may help us identifying the optimal electrode positioning [32]. More precisely, they found that the best theoretical montage to target the neurocircuitry involved in OCD would be with the cathode over the pre-SMA with an extra-cephalic anode, as done in D'Urso and colleagues' study [28].

Regarding the number and duration of tDCS sessions, the choice of delivering 10 to 20 sessions of 20 to 30 min has been mostly extrapolated from the data obtained in studies investigating the clinical effects of tDCS in patients with depression. However, it is not clearly established that increasing the duration and number of sessions leads to a better and longer clinical effect. The interval between consecutive tDCS sessions should also be considered. Indeed, some studies have shown that the inhibitory effects of a session of cathodal tDCS on motor corticospinal excitability were increased if a second tDCS session was performed during the after-effects of the first and were initially reduced and then re-established if the second tDCS session was performed 3 or 24 h after the first one [33]. Furthermore, it was reported in another study that the excitatory effects of anodal tDCS on motor corticospinal excitability were reduced, but prolonged when a second tDCS session was applied during the after-effects of the first (from 0 to 20 min after) but entirely abolished when the second tDCS session was applied 3 or 24 h after the first [34].

It is important to mention that most of the patients included in the reviewed studies were treated with different medication (in terms of duration and molecules) when they received tDCS. Most of the patients were treated with SSRIs, but in some studies, they were also treated with other medications, such as serotonin-norepinephrine reuptake inhibitors (SNRI), mood stabilizers or antipsychotics. The concomitant use of medication may influence the effects of tDCS [35]. For instance, studies investigating the effects of tDCS on motor corticospinal excitability have reported that both acute and chronic administration of the SSRI (citalopram) increased and prolonged the excitatory effects that are induced by anodal tDCS and reversed the inhibitory effects of cathodal tDCS into facilitation [36,37]. Furthermore, in a randomized-controlled trial in patients with major depressive disorder, Brunoni et al. have reported that combining tDCS with SSRI (sertraline hydrochloride) induced beneficial clinical improvements that were superior to each treatment taken separately (tDCS only or sertraline only) or sham [38]. Thus, future studies should take into account the concomitant use of medication when investigating the effects of tDCS on OC symptoms.

Clinical characteristics of patients should be taken into account when discussing the role of tDCS in the OCD treatment. For instance, the level of resistance was highly heterogeneous in the reviewed studies; some patients were resistant to several months of combination between SSRI and CBT (e.g., [18,22–26]), some others received ECT [17]. In addition, the subtypes of OCD (obsessions and checking; symmetry and ordering; cleanliness and washing; and, hoarding) [30] were also heterogeneous across studies and might be an important factor to report in future studies. These differences may also account to explain discrepancies observed between studies in term of symptoms improvement (from no effect on OC symptoms [20] to 80% decrease on YBOCS score [17]).

Another limitation is the brain state dependency that may have an impact on the tDCS clinical effect and should also be controlled in future studies. For instance, in the study reporting the largest beneficial effect of tDCS on OC symptoms, patients were not at rest during the stimulation session as in other studies but were required to listen to music and watch movies during the 30-min session duration [27]. In the same way, a single session of cathodal tDCS has been shown to have a beneficial effect when applied during exposure to anxiety [16]. Future studies should investigate the clinical effect of repeated sessions of tDCS when stimulation is applied during exposure to anxiety as compared to with being at rest.

Finally, up to now, no study has investigated the brain correlates of the symptom improvement following tDCS administration in OCD patients. Investigating biological effects of tDCS in patients with OCD will provide a better understanding of the pathophysiology of OCD (as done with other therapeutics, see [10,11]) and of tDCS' mechanisms of action. It could be speculated for example that hyperactive cortico-striatal pathways observed in patients with OCD may be down-regulated by either inhibitory stimulation of the OFC or SMA (with the cathode) or by excitatory stimulation (enhancement, with the anode) of the DLPFC. Neuroimaging or electrophysiological investigations are also needed to steer the parameter optimization. In this way, another transcranial electrical stimulation approach has been proposed recently by Klimke and colleagues [15]. In an open-label study including seven patients with OCD, the authors reported the clinical interest of transcranial alternating current stimulation (tACS) applied at gamma frequency (40 Hz). They observed that gamma-tACS applied in a bilateral fronto-temporal montage decreased OC symptoms by 52%, measured by the YBOCS. This novel protocol appears interesting and future studies are needed to further explore the effects of gamma-tACS in patients with OCD. Besides the optimization of stimulation parameters, further studies are also needed to determine the clinical and biological predictors of response, as done in studies on depression [39].

5. Conclusions

To conclude, only a few studies investigated the effects of tDCS in OCD, but they showed promising results, with some of them reporting a decrease >35% in YBOCS scores. This effect can be considered as clinically meaningful since the current definition of treatment response is at least a 35% reduction of Y-BOCS score [40]. However, these results are preliminary and further sham-controlled studies are needed to define the role of tDCS in the treatment of OCD and to determine the optimal stimulation parameters to deliver in this indication and subtypes of OCD. To date, regarding the high heterogeneity among studies in terms of the characteristics of patients (e.g., subtypes of OC symptoms, concomitant medication, age) and tDCS parameters (e.g., electrode montage, symptoms provocation paradigm during tDCS), it is difficult to draw a clear conclusion on the efficacy of tDCS in this indication and to propose guidelines for future investigations. Interestingly, based on these preliminary positive reports, randomized clinical trials have been initiated and are now recruiting participants around the world (as seen in clinical trials website: NCT 02407288, 02743715, 03304600). Results from these studies are expected before any conclusion on the relevance of tDCS in patients with OCD can be made.

Acknowledgments: The authors thank the "Conseil Scientific de la recherche du Centre Hospitalier le Vinatier" for financial support.

Author Contributions: J.B. and M.M. managed the literature search and assisted with the data collection. J.B., M.M. and R.B. wrote the first draft of manuscript. E.P. supervised searches. E.P., M.S. and U.P. critically revised the manuscript. All authors contributed to and have approved the final manuscript.

References

1. Ruscio, A.M.; Stein, D.J.; Chiu, W.T.; Kessler, R.C. The epidemiology of obsessive-compulsive disorder in the National Comorbidity Survey Replication. *Mol. Psychiatry* **2010**, *15*, 53–63. [CrossRef] [PubMed]
2. Fontenelle, I.S.; Fontenelle, L.F.; Borges, M.C.; Prazeres, A.M.; Rangé, B.P.; Mendlowicz, M.V.; Versiani, M. Quality of life and symptom dimensions of patients with obsessive-compulsive disorder. *Psychiatry Res.* **2010**, *179*, 198–203. [CrossRef] [PubMed]
3. Fineberg, N.A.; Reghunandanan, S.; Simpson, H.B.; Phillips, K.A.; Richter, M.A.; Matthews, K.; Stein, D.J.; Sareen, J.; Brown, A.; Sookman, D. Accreditation Task Force of The Canadian Institute for Obsessive Compulsive Disorders Obsessive-compulsive disorder (OCD): Practical strategies for pharmacological and somatic treatment in adults. *Psychiatry Res.* **2015**, *227*, 114–125. [CrossRef] [PubMed]
4. Pallanti, S.; Quercioli, L. Treatment-refractory obsessive-compulsive disorder: Methodological issues, operational definitions and therapeutic lines. *Prog. Neuropsychopharmacol. Biol. Psychiatry* **2006**, *30*, 400–412. [CrossRef] [PubMed]
5. Mondino, M.; Bennabi, D.; Poulet, E.; Galvao, F.; Brunelin, J.; Haffen, E. Can transcranial direct current stimulation (tDCS) alleviate symptoms and improve cognition in psychiatric disorders? *World J. Biol. Psychiatry* **2014**, *15*, 261–275. [CrossRef] [PubMed]
6. Lefaucheur, J.-P.; Antal, A.; Ayache, S.S.; Benninger, D.H.; Brunelin, J.; Cogiamanian, F.; Cotelli, M.; de Ridder, D.; Ferrucci, R.; Langguth, B.; et al. Evidence-based guidelines on the therapeutic use of transcranial direct current stimulation (tDCS). *Clin. Neurophysiol.* **2017**, *128*, 56–92. [CrossRef] [PubMed]
7. Nitsche, M.A.; Paulus, W. Excitability changes induced in the human motor cortex by weak transcranial direct current stimulation. *J. Physiol.* **2000**, *527*, 633–639. [CrossRef] [PubMed]
8. Keeser, D.; Meindl, T.; Bor, J.; Palm, U.; Pogarell, O.; Mulert, C.; Brunelin, J.; Moller, H.-J.; Reiser, M.; Padberg, F. Prefrontal Transcranial Direct Current Stimulation Changes Connectivity of Resting-State Networks during fMRI. *J. Neurosci.* **2011**, *31*, 15284–15293. [CrossRef] [PubMed]

9. Hou, J.; Wu, W.; Lin, Y.; Wang, J.; Zhou, D.; Guo, J.; Gu, S.; He, M.; Ahmed, S.; Hu, J.; et al. Localization of cerebral functional deficits in patients with obsessive-compulsive disorder: A resting-state fMRI study. *J. Affect. Disord.* **2012**, *138*, 313–321. [CrossRef] [PubMed]
10. Van der Straten, A.L.; Denys, D.; van Wingen, G. Impact of treatment on resting cerebral blood flow and metabolism in obsessive compulsive disorder: A meta-analysis. *Sci. Rep.* **2017**, *7*, 17464. [CrossRef] [PubMed]
11. Nauczyciel, C.; le Jeune, F.; Naudet, F.; Douabin, S.; Esquevin, A.; Vérin, M.; Dondaine, T.; Robert, G.; Drapier, D.; Millet, B. Repetitive transcranial magnetic stimulation over the orbitofrontal cortex for obsessive-compulsive disorder: A double-blind, crossover study. *Transl. Psychiatry* **2014**, *4*, e436. [CrossRef] [PubMed]
12. Rauch, S.L.; Jenike, M.A.; Alpert, N.M.; Baer, L.; Breiter, H.C.; Fischman, A.J. Regional cerebral blood flow measured during symptom provocation in obsessive-compulsive disorder using oxygen 15-labeled carbon dioxide and positron emission tomography. *Arch. Gen. Psychiatry* **1994**, *51*, 62–70. [CrossRef] [PubMed]
13. Milad, M.R.; Rauch, S.L. Obsessive-compulsive disorder: Beyond segregated cortico-striatal pathways. *Trends Cogn. Sci.* **2012**, *16*, 43–51. [CrossRef] [PubMed]
14. Yekta, M.; Rostami, R.; Fayyaz, E. Transcranial Direct Current Stimulation of Dorsolateral Prefrontal Cortex in Patients with Obsessive Compulsive Disorder to Improve Decision Making and Reduce Obsession Symptoms. *Pract. Clin. Psychol.* **2015**, *3*, 185–194.
15. Klimke, A.; Nitsche, M.A.; Maurer, K.; Voss, U. Case Report: Successful Treatment of Therapy-Resistant OCD with Application of Transcranial Alternating Current Stimulation (tACS). *Brain Stimul.* **2016**, *9*, 463–465. [CrossRef] [PubMed]
16. Todder, D.; Gershi, A.; Perry, Z.; Kaplan, Z.; Levine, J.; Avirame, K. Immediate Effects of Transcranial Direct Current Stimulation on Obsession-Induced Anxiety in Refractory Obsessive-Compulsive Disorder: A Pilot Study. *J. ECT* **2017**. [CrossRef] [PubMed]
17. Hazari, N.; Narayanaswamy, J.C.; Chhabra, H.; Bose, A.; Venkatasubramanian, G.; Reddy, Y.C.J. Response to Transcranial Direct Current Stimulation in a Case of Episodic Obsessive Compulsive Disorder. *J. ECT* **2016**, *32*, 144–146. [CrossRef] [PubMed]
18. Dinn, W.M.; Aycicegi-Dinn, A.; Göral, F.; Karamursel, S.; Yildirim, E.A.; Hacioglu-Yildirim, M.; Gansler, D.A.; Doruk, D.; Fregni, F. Treatment-resistant obsessive-compulsive disorder: Insights from an open trial of transcranial direct current stimulation (tDCS) to design a RCT. *Neurol. Psychiatry Brain Res.* **2016**, *22*, 146–154. [CrossRef]
19. Alizadeh Goradel, J.; Pouresmali, A.; Mowlaie, M.; Sadeghi Movahed, F. The Effects of Transcranial Direct Current Stimulation on Obsession-compulsion, Anxiety, and Depression of a Patient Suffering from Obsessive-compulsive Disorder. *Pract. Clin. Psychol.* **2016**, *4*, 75–80. [CrossRef]
20. Volpato, C.; Piccione, F.; Cavinato, M.; Duzzi, D.; Schiff, S.; Foscolo, L.; Venneri, A. Modulation of affective symptoms and resting state activity by brain stimulation in a treatment-resistant case of obsessive-compulsive disorder. *Neurocase* **2013**, *19*, 360–370. [CrossRef] [PubMed]
21. Narayanaswamy, J.C.; Jose, D.; Chhabra, H.; Agarwal, S.M.; Shrinivasa, B.; Hegde, A.; Bose, A.; Kalmady, S.V.; Venkatasubramanian, G.; Reddy, Y.C.J. Successful Application of Add-on Transcranial Direct Current Stimulation (tDCS) for Treatment of SSRI Resistant OCD. *Brain Stimul.* **2015**, *8*, 655–657. [CrossRef] [PubMed]
22. Mondino, M.; Haesebaert, F.; Poulet, E.; Saoud, M.; Brunelin, J. Efficacy of Cathodal Transcranial Direct Current Stimulation Over the Left Orbitofrontal Cortex in a Patient With Treatment-Resistant Obsessive-Compulsive Disorder. *J. ECT* **2015**, *31*, 271–272. [CrossRef] [PubMed]
23. D'Urso, G.; Brunoni, A.R.; Anastasia, A.; Micillo, M.; de Bartolomeis, A.; Mantovani, A. Polarity-dependent effects of transcranial direct current stimulation in obsessive-compulsive disorder. *Neurocase* **2016**, *22*, 60–64. [CrossRef] [PubMed]
24. Silva, R.M.; Brunoni, A.R.; Miguel, E.C.; Shavitt, R.G. Transcranial direct current stimulation for treatment-resistant obsessive-compulsive disorder: report on two cases and proposal for a randomized, sham-controlled trial. *Sao Paulo Med. J.* **2016**, *134*, 446–450. [CrossRef] [PubMed]
25. Palm, U.; Leitner, B.; Kirsch, B.; Behler, N.; Kumpf, U.; Wulf, L.; Padberg, F.; Hasan, A. Prefrontal tDCS and sertraline in obsessive compulsive disorder: A case report and review of the literature. *Neurocase* **2017**, *23*, 173–177. [CrossRef] [PubMed]

26. Bation, R.; Poulet, E.; Haesebaert, F.; Saoud, M.; Brunelin, J. Transcranial direct current stimulation in treatment-resistant obsessive-compulsive disorder: An open-label pilot study. *Prog. Neuropsychopharmacol. Biol. Psychiatry* **2016**, *65*, 153–157. [CrossRef] [PubMed]
27. Najafi, K.; Fakour, Y.; Zarrabi, H.; Heidarzadeh, A.; Khalkhali, M.; Yeganeh, T.; Farahi, H.; Rostamkhani, M.; Najafi, T.; Shabafroz, S.; et al. Efficacy of Transcranial Direct Current Stimulation in the Treatment: Resistant Patients who Suffer from Severe Obsessive-compulsive Disorder. *Indian J. Psychol. Med.* **2017**, *39*, 573–578. [CrossRef] [PubMed]
28. D'Urso, G.; Brunoni, A.R.; Mazzaferro, M.P.; Anastasia, A.; de Bartolomeis, A.; Mantovani, A. Transcranial direct current stimulation for obsessive-compulsive disorder: A randomized, controlled, partial crossover trial. *Depress. Anxiety* **2016**, *33*, 1132–1140. [CrossRef] [PubMed]
29. Goodman, W.K.; Price, L.H.; Rasmussen, S.A.; Mazure, C.; Delgado, P.; Heninger, G.R.; Charney, D.S. The Yale-Brown Obsessive Compulsive Scale. II. Validity. *Arch. Gen. Psychiatry* **1989**, *46*, 1012–1016. [CrossRef] [PubMed]
30. Leckman, J.F.; Grice, D.E.; Boardman, J.; Zhang, H.; Vitale, A.; Bondi, C.; Alsobrook, J.; Peterson, B.S.; Cohen, D.J.; Rasmussen, S.A.; et al. Symptoms of obsessive-compulsive disorder. *Am. J. Psychiatry* **1997**, *154*, 911–917. [PubMed]
31. Mansur, C.G.; Myczkowki, M.L.; de Barros Cabral, S.; Sartorelli, M.D.C.B.; Bellini, B.B.; Dias, A.M.; Bernik, M.A.; Marcolin, M.A. Placebo effect after prefrontal magnetic stimulation in the treatment of resistant obsessive-compulsive disorder: A randomized controlled trial. *Int. J. Neuropsychopharmacol.* **2011**, *14*, 1389–1397. [CrossRef] [PubMed]
32. Senço, N.M.; Huang, Y.; D'Urso, G.; Parra, L.C.; Bikson, M.; Mantovani, A.; Shavitt, R.G.; Hoexter, M.Q.; Miguel, E.C.; Brunoni, A.R. Transcranial direct current stimulation in obsessive-compulsive disorder: Emerging clinical evidence and considerations for optimal montage of electrodes. *Expert Rev. Med. Devices* **2015**, *12*, 381–391. [CrossRef] [PubMed]
33. Monte-Silva, K.; Kuo, M.F.; Liebetanz, D.; Paulus, W.; Nitsche, M.A. Shaping the Optimal Repetition Interval for Cathodal Transcranial Direct Current Stimulation (tDCS). *J. Neurophysiol.* **2010**, *103*, 1735–1740. [CrossRef] [PubMed]
34. Monte-Silva, K.; Kuo, M.-F.; Hessenthaler, S.; Fresnoza, S.; Liebetanz, D.; Paulus, W.; Nitsche, M.A. Induction of Late LTP-Like Plasticity in the Human Motor Cortex by Repeated Non-Invasive Brain Stimulation. *Brain Stimul.* **2013**, *6*, 424–432. [CrossRef] [PubMed]
35. McLaren, M.E.; Nissim, N.R.; Woods, A.J. The effects of medication use in transcranial direct current stimulation: A brief review. *Brain Stimul.* **2017**, *11*, 52–58. [CrossRef] [PubMed]
36. Nitsche, M.A.; Kuo, M.-F.; Karrasch, R.; Wächter, B.; Liebetanz, D.; Paulus, W. Serotonin Affects Transcranial Direct Current-Induced Neuroplasticity in Humans. *Biol. Psychiatry* **2009**, *66*, 503–508. [CrossRef] [PubMed]
37. Kuo, H.-I.; Paulus, W.; Batsikadze, G.; Jamil, A.; Kuo, M.-F.; Nitsche, M.A. Chronic Enhancement of Serotonin Facilitates Excitatory Transcranial Direct Current Stimulation-Induced Neuroplasticity. *Neuropsychopharmacology* **2016**, *41*, 1223–1230. [CrossRef] [PubMed]
38. Brunoni, A.R.; Valiengo, L.; Baccaro, A.; Zanão, T.A.; de Oliveira, J.F.; Goulart, A.; Boggio, P.S.; Lotufo, P.A.; Benseñor, I.M.; Fregni, F. The sertraline vs. electrical current therapy for treating depression clinical study: Results from a factorial, randomized, controlled trial. *JAMA Psychiatry* **2013**, *70*, 383–391. [CrossRef] [PubMed]
39. D'Urso, G.; Dell'Osso, B.; Rossi, R.; Brunoni, A.R.; Bortolomasi, M.; Ferrucci, R.; Priori, A.; de Bartolomeis, A.; Altamura, A.C. Clinical predictors of acute response to transcranial direct current stimulation (tDCS) in major depression. *J. Affect. Disord.* **2017**, *219*, 25–30. [CrossRef] [PubMed]
40. Lewin, A.B.; de Nadai, A.S.; Park, J.; Goodman, W.K.; Murphy, T.K.; Storch, E.A. Refining clinical judgment of treatment outcome in obsessive–compulsive disorder. *Psychiatry Res.* **2011**, *185*, 394–401. [CrossRef] [PubMed]

16

The Meaning in Life in Suicidal Patients: The Presence and the Search for Constructs

Alessandra Costanza [1,2,*], Massimo Prelati [2] and Maurizio Pompili [3]

1 Department of Psychiatry, Faculty of Medicine, University of Geneva (UNIGE), 1206 Geneva, Switzerland
2 Department of Psychiatry, ASO Santi Antonio e Biagio e Cesare Arrigo Hospital, 15121 Alessandria, Italy
3 Department of Neurosciences, Mental Health and Sensory Organs, Suicide Prevention Center, Sant'Andrea Hospital, Sapienza University of Rome, 00185 Rome, Italy
* Correspondence: alessandra.costanza@unige.ch

Abstract: *Background and Objectives:* Research on suicidal behavior (SB) has frequently focused more on risk factors than protective factors. Since the historic works of Viktor E. Frankl, who inquired how some Nazi concentration camps prisoners maintained their will to live though confronted with pervasive absurdity, Meaning in Life (MiL) has been interpreted as a potent resiliency factor. MiL then declined along a multitude of theoretical perspectives and was associated with various functioning domains of the individual. Surprising, few studies investigated the role of MiL on SB. We aimed to review and synthetize current literature on possible associations between MiL and SB, which included suicidal ideation (SI), suicidal attempts (SA), and completed suicide, focusing on two MiL constructs (the presence of MiL and search for MiL) from the Michael F. Steger's recent conceptualization. *Material and Methods:* A systematic strategy following PRISMA guidelines was used to search for relevant articles in Pubmed/MEDLINE, Scopus, PsycINFO, and ScienceDirect (January 1980–February 2019) and yielded 172 articles, 37 of which met our inclusion criteria. *Results:* MiL emerged as a protective factor against SI, SA, and completed suicides, directly or through mediation/moderation models with other SB-related variables. When distinguishing the presence of MiL and the search for MiL, a consensual protective impact was described for the former. Data for the latter were less consistent but rather oriented towards a non-protective impact *Conclusions:* These findings could have clinical repercussions for SB prevention, in both suicide risk assessment refinement and psychotherapeutic interventions. Further research is needed to examine the dynamic interplay of the two constructs.

Keywords: suicide; suicidal behavior; suicidal ideation; suicide attempt; meaning in life; suicide protective factors; suicide risk

---

1. Introduction

Research on suicidal behavior (SB) has frequently focused on suicide risk factors. In contrast, elements that can buffer stressors and protect an individual from SB have received less attention [1]. Historically, exploration into the adaptive and life-maintaining characteristics of non-suicidal people was originated by Viktor E. Frankl, who attempted to elucidate how some Nazi concentration camp prisoners were able to maintain the will to live and which subjective reasons protected them from a pervasive sense of absurdity [2]. He observed that individuals with a "will of meaning" (*Der Wille zum Sinn*) had the best chance of survival [2]. On this basis, Frankl elaborated the discovery path of Meaning in Life (MiL) against the "existential vacuum" as arising from three possible assumptions, uniquely concerning the human condition: (1) creativity (related to the sense of realization of an individual), (2) perception and a search for beauty (in relation to a sense of authenticity towards certain situations or encounters), and (3) the effort of an individual in trying to find a way to determine one's interior attitude, even when overwhelmed by miserable circumstances or unavoidable suffering [2].

Since Frankl's initial observations, Meaning in Life (MiL) has been described from a multitude of theoretical perspectives. One primary distinction has been made between a "global or existential" meaning and a "situational or specific" meaning, thereby discerning individuals' fundamental assumptions from meaning in the context of a particular environmental encounter [3–6]. In this latter area, the integrated model of "meaning-making", articulated by Crystal L. Park, is of particular interest [4]. In addition to the distinction between "global" and "situational" meaning, Park proposed the evaluation of "meaning-making efforts" and "meaning made", inscribing the possible effects of all these subconstructs in a meaning-making process aimed at adjusting one's experiences of events that are greatly discrepant with one's larger beliefs, plans, and desires [4].

In the recent psychological literature, Michael F. Steger has proposed that the greatest consensus in the conceptualization of MiL can be centered on two dimensions: "coherence", or a sense of the comprehensibility and self-concordant ability of making sense in one's life, and "purpose", or a sense of core goals, aims, and direction in life [7]. A third facet, "significance", which focuses on values, worth, and the importance of one's life, is receiving increasing attention [7]. "Coherence" refers to the cognitive component of MiL, focusing on the perception that stimuli are predictable and conform to recognizable personal patterns that transcend chaos. "Coherence" would be especially activated in situations where meaning is disrupted and the individual experiences distress and the related necessity to construct or reconstruct a framework to understand life [7]. While "purpose" is sometimes used synonymously with MiL, it should be explicitly considered separately from the general sense of MiL and understood as one of its components (the motivational one), based on one's goals and enthusiasm in life (e.g., spirituality and religiousness were shown to be correlated to MiL but not to "purpose", while optimism was correlated to "purpose" but not to MiL) [7]. "Significance" constitutes the evaluative component for MiL as it relates to how important, worthwhile, and inherently valuable one's life as a whole feels beyond trivial or momentary elements [7]. Both "purpose" and "significance" are value-laden concepts, but they differ in two essential aspects, based on their primary motivational versus evaluative nature. "Purpose" is about finding valuable goals future-oriented, while "significance" is about finding value in life, including the past, present, and future [7]. When all three components are taken together, a definition for MiL emerges from "the web of connections, interpretations, aspirations, and evaluations" that "(1) make our experiences comprehensible, (2) direct our efforts toward a desired future, and (3) provide a sense that our lives matter and are worthwhile" [7,8].

Steger's model divides MiL into two constructs: the presence of MiL and the search for MiL [9]. These two constructs were found not to be mutually exclusive [10]. The presence of MiL is uniformly thought to be beneficial for various functional aspects of life, including adaptive resources, overall psychological well-being, and positive affects [11]. By contrast, the search for MiL appears more controversial. Some researchers consider MiL the essence of human motivation [12,13], while others find it a dysfunctional sign that meaning has been frustrated or lost [14,15]. In a third perspective, the search for MiL can have either healthy or non-healthy connotations depending on the motivational [3] and personal characteristics of the individual [16]. Addressing this issue from a typological perspective, MiL profiles resulting from a combination of high scores in the presence of MiL and low scores in the search for MiL have been associated with better adjustment outcomes [17,18]. Both constructs are highly stable over time, suggesting that MiL more accurately reflects a trait aspect than a state aspect of individual functioning [18].

From a clinical viewpoint, exploring MiL in suicidal patients during psychiatric interviews would personalize and improve their SB risk assessments [19,20]. Interventions targeting MiL have also been found effective in reducing suicide risk [21] and represent a promising therapeutic opportunity [19,20,22].

Few studies have explored MiL in individuals presenting SB. With this review, we aimed to examine existing published data to investigate possible associations between MiL and suicidal ideation (SI), suicide attempts (SA), and completed suicide. Particular attention was given to studies that distinguished between the roles of the presence of MiL and the search for MiL. We hypothesized that MiL has a protective effect on SI, SA, and completed suicide. Specifically, for works that addressed the two constructs of MiL, we hypothesized that the presence of MiL would have a protective effect. The exiguity and contradictory nature of the data on the search for MiL did not allow us to formulate a specific hypothesis but only to perform exploratory analyses.

2. Methods

This review was conducted according to the Preferred Reporting Items for Systematic Reviews and Meta-Analyses (PRISMA) guidelines [23] and the Cochrane collaboration guidelines [24].

2.1. Information Sources and Search Strategy

We performed a systematic search in four major electronic databases comprising medical and social science research (PubMed/MEDLINE, Scopus, Science Direct, and PsychINFO) for relevant titles and abstracts published between January 1980 and February 2019. Additional articles were retrieved from the reference lists of relevant articles and from published reviews. The following combined search queries of free-text terms and exploded Medical Subject Headings (MeSH) terms were used for the Pubmed/MEDLINE database: "Meaning in Life" AND "Suicidal ideation" [MeSH] OR "Suicide, attempted" [MeSH] OR "Suicide" [MeSH] OR "Suicidal Behavior" OR "suicidality." This search strategy was adapted for use with the other databases.

2.2. Eligibility Criteria

Articles that explicitly mentioned a potential association between MiL and SB (OR suicidal ideation OR suicide attempts OR completed suicides) in non-clinical and clinical samples were included. When a title or abstract seemed to describe an eligible study, the full-text article was obtained and carefully examined to assess the study's relevance for our review. Our exclusion criteria were: (1) articles published before 1980, (2) articles with abstracts that did not directly mention an investigation into a potential association between MiL and SB, (3) articles not published in peer-reviewed journals, (4) articles not published in English, and (5) meta-analytic, systematic, or narrative reviews, or book chapters.

2.3. Study Selection and Data Collection

Studies were independently reviewed by two authors (A.C. and M.Pre.) using a two-step process. First, screening and selection were performed based on the article's title and abstract. Second, further screenings and selections were performed on retrieved full-text articles. A data extraction spreadsheet was developed [23]. The data were extracted by one author (A.C.) and supervised by another (M.Pre.). The data elements of interest were author(s), publication year, study design, sample characteristics (population type, sample size, and psychiatric diagnosis when appropriate), instrument(s) used to assess MiL, and the impact on SB-related variables (SI, SA, completed suicide, other SB-related variables, and/or main commentaries). At any stage of the article selection and data collection processes, disagreements were resolved through discussion with the senior reviewer (M.Pom.), who also independently read all the articles.

2.4. Summary Measures

As with previous studies [25,26], we assessed the selected studies for quality using the following criteria: (1) the representativeness of the sample for the general population, (2) the presence and representativeness of a control group, (3) the presence of longitudinal follow-up, (4) the evidence-based measures of MiL (e.g., a Meaning in Life Questionnaire, Purpose in Life Questionnaire, or other psychometric instruments), (5) the presence of raters who independently identified MiL, (6) the statistical evaluation of inter-rater reliability, and (7) evidence-based measures of SI or SA (e.g., a Suicidal Ideation Questionnaire, Suicide Risk Scale, Beck Hopelessness Scale, or other psychometric evaluation). A score of 0–2 points was attributed to each item, yielding a quality score ranging from 0 to 14. Studies were divided into 3 groups: (1) good quality (10–14 points), if most or all the criteria were fulfilled, or, where they were not met, the study conclusions were deemed very robust; (2) moderate quality (5–9 points), if some criteria were fulfilled or the study conclusions were deemed robust; or (3) low quality (0–4 points), if few criteria were fulfilled or the study conclusions were not deemed robust. Caution was adopted in interpreting the findings from the low-quality studies. Disagreements between reviewers were resolved by consensus.

3. Results

3.1. Included Studies

After removing 61 duplicates, a total of 172 potentially relevant articles were found. Figure 1 shows the flow through the identification, screening, and assessment of eligibility. Studies were excluded either because the exclusion criteria were met or because of low relevance compared to our primary theme. Finally, 37 studies met our inclusion criteria and were included in our qualitative synthesis for this review.

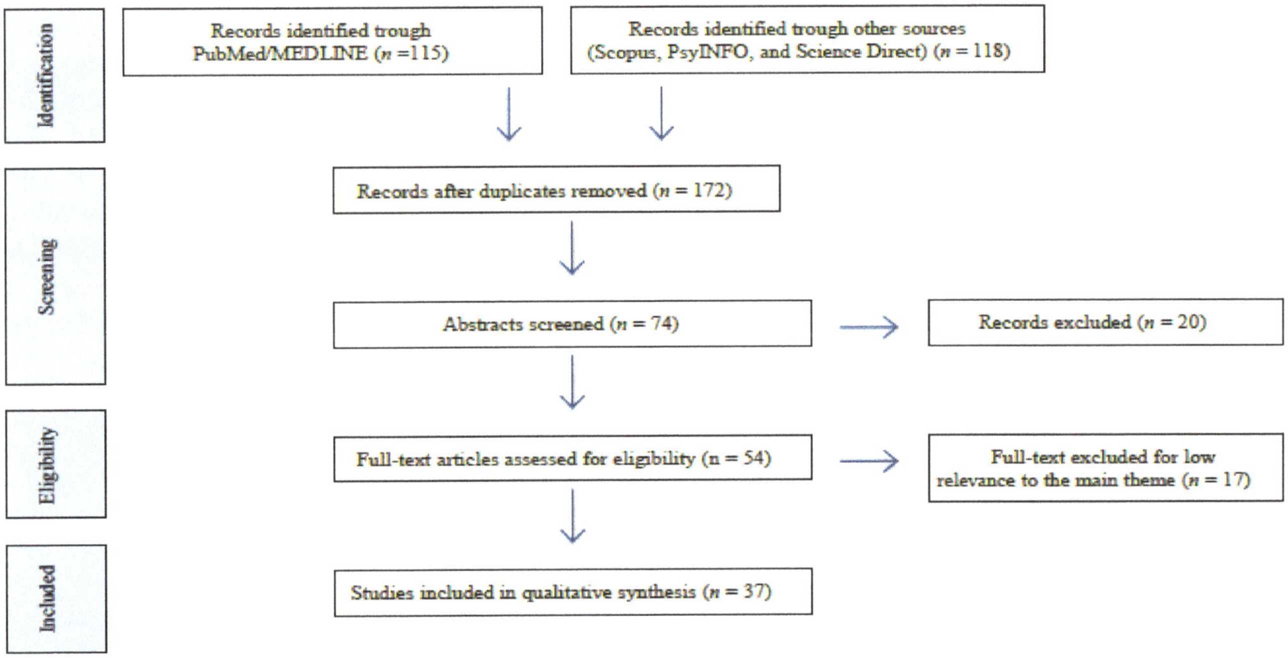

Figure 1. Flowchart for the search and selection process [23].

3.2. Characteristics of Included Studies (Study Designs and Samples)

The characteristics of the included studies are shown in Tables 1 and 2. In total, 24 studies were cross-sectional, nine were prospective and longitudinal, and five were qualitative (one was classified as both cross-sectional and longitudinal). Additionally, 20 were conducted using non-clinical populations (Tables 1 and 2), and 17 were conducted using psychiatric and non-psychiatric clinical populations (Tables 1 and 2). Among the non-clinical populations, undergraduate students and adolescents were the most frequently represented groups (n = 12) followed by elderly people (n = 7). Eight studies included individuals aged 12–70 years, one included only adults, and one included individuals aged at least 20 years and was based on the general population participating in the Nord-Trøndelag Health Study in Norway (the HUNT I cohort during 1984–1986 and the HUNT II cohort during 1995–1997). The specific studied populations were military personnel and veterans (n = 3), Chinese professional employees (n = 1), homeless people (n = 1), and disadvantaged African American female survivors of a recent SA (n = 1). Among studies performed using clinical populations, mood disorders were the most specifically addressed psychiatric diagnoses (n = 6), followed by borderline personality disorders (n = 3). Finally, five studies were performed based on various mental disorders (including mood and anxiety disorders, borderline and avoidant personality disorder, and post-traumatic stress disorder (PTSD), eating disorders, substance use disorder, and psychotic spectrum disorder), two were based on PTSD alone, and one was based on eating disorders. The only clinical non-psychiatric population studied was the population diagnosed as HIV-positive.

Of the studies that addressed the impact of the two MiL-distinct constructs (the presence of MiL and the search for MiL) (n = 5; Table 2), one was both cross-sectional and prospective, two were cross-sectional, and two were longitudinal and prospective. No qualitative studies were represented in this group. Three studies were conducted among non-clinical populations (two among undergraduate students and one among soldiers returning from deployment; Table 2), and two were conducted among clinical populations (one among patientss diagnosed with severe PTSD/depression and one among those diagnosed as HIV-positive; Table 2).

Interest in this research subject has increased over very recent years (32 of the included studies were published in 2013 or later). This was particularly evident among studies conducted using clinical populations (12 of these 17 studies were published in 2015 or later). Most of these (n = 7) were performed using Spanish clinical samples by Marco and colleagues. Of those performed using non-clinical samples of adolescents/undergraduate students, nearly half (5 of 12) were performed using Israeli samples, and four of these were performed by Wilchek-Aviad and colleagues. Notably, all the studies that focused on the impact of the two MiL-distinct constructs (presence of MiL and search for MiL) were published in 2013 or later, and all but one were published in 2016 or later. Notably, two of the three studies using samples of military personnel and veterans focused on these two constructs.

Table 1. Studies investigating associations between meaning in life (MiL) and suicidal behavior (SB)-related variables ($N = 32$).

Non-Clinical Populations ($n = 17$)								
Author(s)	Study Design	Sample		Instrument Assessing MiL	SB-Related Variables			
		Population	Size (N)		SI	SA	Completed Suicide	Other SB-Related Variables and/or Main Commentaries
Edwards and Holden, 2001 [27]	Cross-sectional	Undergraduate students	298	PIL, Sense of Coherence Scale	↓	↓	–	↓ Self-reported likelihood of future SB
Orbach et al., 2003 (study 2) [28]	Cross-sectional	Undergraduate students	98	LRI	–	–	–	MiL inversely related to mental pain
Wang et al., 2007 [1]	Cross-sectional	Undergraduate students	416	PIL	↓	↓	–	Mediation model: MiL mediated relationships between stress, coping, SI, and SA indirectly via an inverse effect on depression
Heisel and Flett, 2008 [29]	Cross-sectional	Elderly	107	GSIS Perceived MiL subscale	↓	–	–	–
Bjerkeset et al., 2010 [30]	Longitudinal prospective	Individuals aged 20+ yr, based on the Norwegian HUNT general population cohort	141,117	Self-reported measure of sense of MiL (n.sp.)	n.sp.	n.sp.	↓	A lower sense of MiL associated with increased suicide risk after controlling for common mental disorders that emerged during the survey
Kleiman et al., 2013 [31]	Longitudinal prospective	Undergraduate students	209	MLQ	↓	–	–	Mediated moderation model: gratitude and grit work synergistically to enhance MiL and confer resiliency to suicide by increasing MiL
Henry et al., 2014 [32]	Cross-sectional	Undergraduate students	2936	3-item MLQ	↓	–	–	Mediation model (female population): MiL could explain how bullying victimization leads to SI; moderation model (male population): effect of victimization on SI was attenuated as MiL increased
Wilchek-Aviad, 2015 [33]	Cross-sectional	Adolescents (Ethiopian immigrant and native-born Israeli)	277	PIL	–	–	–	↓ Suicidal tendencies (measured while accounting for depression and anxiety/emotional state) beyond one's immigrant and native-born status
Denneson et al., 2015 [22]	Qualitative	Veterans	34	Semi-structured interviews	↓	–	–	
Heisel and Flett, 2016 [34]	Longitudinal prospective	Elderly	126	EMIL, PIL	↓	–	–	–

Table 1. *Cont.*

Non-Clinical Populations (n = 17)								
Author(s)	**Study Design**	**Sample**		**Instrument Assessing MiL**	**SB-Related Variables**			
		Population	**Size (N)**		**SI**	**SA**	**Completed Suicide**	**Other SB-Related Variables and/or Main Commentaries**
Heisel et al., 2016 [35]	Longitudinal prospective	Elderly	109	EMIL	↓	–	–	Mediation model: MiL mediated associations between "Reasons for Living" and SI; it also explained the significant unique variance in SI
Wilchek-Aviad and Malka, 2016 [36]	Cross-sectional	Adolescents (Jewish religious and secular)	450	PIL	–	–	–	↓ Suicidal tendency (see above) beyond religiosity
Wilchek-Aviad et al., 2017 [37]	Cross-sectional	Adolescents (having different types of leisure time activities)	450	PIL	↓	–	–	MiL was greatest among adolescents involved in social endeavors, lower among those involved in solitary activities, and lowest among those not involved in any leisure activity
Wilchek-Aviad and Ne'eman-Haviv, 2018 [38]	Cross-sectional	Adolescent girls (disadvantaged at different stages of rehabilitation and normative)	209	PIL	–	–	–	↓ Suicidal potential (equivalent to the suicidal tendency, see above) among normative and disadvantaged adolescent girls residing in boarding schools
Schnell et al., 2018 [39]	Cross-sectional	Undergraduate students	300	Crisis of Meaning Scale	↓	↓	–	Crisis of meaning was distinguished from depression and predicted suicidality in youth independent of depression
Liu et al., 2018 [40]	Cross-sectional	Chinese professional employees	687	MLM	↓	–	–	Mediation model: MiL mediated relationships between psychological strain and SI
Testoni et al., 2018 [41]	Qualitative	Homeless people	55	Thematic and interpretative phenomenological analysis	↓	–	–	MiL was the most important reason for living; when it was considered unworkable, addiction/alcoholism represented a strategy to endure life in the street. Neither religiosity nor meaning of death were protective factors for addiction/alcoholism or SI

(A)

Table 1. *Cont.*

Clinical Populations (n = 15)									
Author(s)	Study Design	Sample			Instrument Assessing MiL	SB-Related Variables			
		Population	Size (N)	Psychiatric Diagnosis		SI	SA	Completed Suicide	Other SB-Related Variables and Main Commentaries
Moore, 1997 [42]	Qualitative	Elderly	11	Depression	Hermeneutic analysis	↓	–	–	MiL descriptions were always tied to relational contexts: meaninglessness relative to missing (or perceived to be missing) connectedness
Heisel and Flett, 2004 [43]	Cross-sectional	Adults	49	Various	PIL	↓	–	–	MiL accounted for significant variance in SI—also, a mediation model between satisfaction in life and SI and a moderation model between depression and SI
van Orden et al., 2012 [44]	Longitudinal prospective	Elderly	65	Depression, anxiety	GSIS Perceived MiL subscale	–	–	–	"Perceived burdensomeness" might contribute to suicide morbidity and mortality by eroding MiL
Holm et al., 2014 [45]	Qualitative	Elderly	9	Mood disorder	Hermeneutic analysis	↓	–	–	MiL in the experience of SI was associated with existential aloneness: "Being alone without MiL"
García-Alandete et al., 2014 [46]	Cross-sectional	16–60 yr old	80	Borderline personality disorder	PIL-10	–	–	–	↓ Suicide risk (measured accounting for general suicide risk factors), ↓ depression,↓ hopelessness
van Orden et al., 2015 [47]	Qualitative	Elderly	101	Various	Semi-structured interviews	–		–	"Thwarted belongingness" was associated with more lethal methods and increased re-attempts
Braden et al., 2015 [48]	Cross-sectional	Veterans	110	Depressive disorder	LRI Framework subscale	↓	–	–	The relationship between MiL and SI remained significant after accounting for depressive symptoms, past SA, prior inpatient psychiatric hospitalization, and poor physical health
Marco et al., 2016 [19]	Cross-sectional	13–68 yr old	224	Various	PIL-10	–	–	–	Moderation model: MiL buffered associations between suicide risk factors and hopelessness
Marco et al., 2017a (study 2) [20]	Cross-sectional	13–70 yr old	80	Borderline personality disorder	PIL-10	–	↓	–	MiL was also negatively correlated with other behavioral symptoms of borderline personality disorders, including suicidal threats, high-risk behaviors, drug overdoses, and aggressive behavior

Table 1. *Cont.*

Clinical Populations (*n* = 15)									
Author(s)	**Study Design**	**Sample**			**Instrument Assessing MiL**	**SB-Related Variables**			
		Population	**Size (*N*)**	**Psychiatric Diagnosis**		**SI**	**SA**	**Completed Suicide**	**Other SB-Related Variables and Main Commentaries**
Marco et al., 2017b [49]	Cross-sectional	13–56 yr old	124	Borderline personality disorder	PIL-10	–		–	Moderation model: MiL buffered associations between suicide risk factors and hopelessness
Marco et al., 2017c [50]	Cross-sectional case-control	12–60 yr old	474	Eating disorder	PIL	↓	–	–	Patients with eating disorders had lower MiLs and greater SI than the controls; MiL predicts greater levels of both eating disorder psychopathologies and SI
Pérez Rodriguez et al., 2017a [51]	Cross-sectional	18–60 yr old	150	Various	PIL-10	–	NS	–	Hopelessness (specifically its affective component) differentiated between patients with non-suicidal self-injuries and those with SA but not MiL, which underlies the continuum of self-harm
Pérez Rodriguez et al., 2017b [52]	Cross-sectional	12–60 yr old	348	Various (mainly eating disorder)	PIL-10	–	↓	–	Lower levels of MiL and higher levels of hopelessness, borderline symptoms, and non-suicidal self-injuries were associated with SA in the previous year
Lamis et al., 2018 [53]	Cross-sectional	19–65 yr old	112	Bipolar disorder	SWBS (EWB + RWB)	↓	–	–	Existential MiL but not religious well-being acted as a protective factor against SI among bipolar disorder patients and those who experienced childhood sexual abuse
Florez et al., 2018 [54]	Longitudinal prospective	Disadvantaged African American female survivors of a recent SA	113	PTSD	SWBS (EWB + RWB)	↓	–	–	Mediation model: existential MiL, but not religious well-being, mediated the relationship between PTSD severity and both hopelessness and SI level

(B)

Note: MiL = Meaning in Life; SB = suicidal behavior; SI = suicidal ideation; SA = suicide attempt; PIL = Purpose in Life test; LRI = Life Regard Index; GSIS = Geriatric Suicide Ideation Scale; n.sp. = not specified; MLQ = Meaning in Life Questionnaire; 3-item MLQ = 3-item shortened version of the MLQ; EMIL = Experienced Meaning in Life instrument; PIL-10 = 10-item shortened version of the PIL; MLM = Meaningful Life Measure; yr = years; NS = not significant; SWBS = Spiritual Well-Being Scale; EWB = Existential Well-Being subscale; RWB = Religious Well-Being subscale.

Table 2. Studies investigating the associations between the the presence of MiL and the search for MiL and SB-related variables ($N = 5$).

Non-Clinical Populations ($n = 3$)								
Author(s)	**Study Design**	**Sample**		**Instrument Assessing MiL**	**SB-Related Variable**			
		Population	**Size (*N*)**		**SI**	**SA**	**Completed Suicide**	**Other SB-Related Variables and/or Main Commentaries**
Kleiman and Beaver, 2013 [55]	Cross-sectional and longitudinal prospective	Undergraduate students	670 (cross-sectional analysis); 585 (prospective analysis)	MLQ	↓ SI over time for both presence of MiL and search for MiL (greater effect for presence of MiL; minor effect for search for MiL)	↓ lifetime SA odds for presence of MiL	–	Additional findings: The presence of MiL, but not the search for MiL, mediated the relationship between MiL and the burdensomeness or thwarted belongingness and SI
Kim et al., 2017 [56]	Longitudinal prospective	Soldiers returning from deployment	970	MLQ	↓ for presence of MiL(miao)and ↑ for search for MiL	↓ for presence of MiL and(miao)↑ for search for MiL	–	Suicide risk (including four dimensions of SI and SB): ↑ for the search for MiL; (miao)↓ for the presence of MiL (the latter was described by the authors as consistent but not significant)
Collins et al., 2018 [57]	Cross-sectional	Undergraduate students	93	MLQ (the presence of MiL subscal only)	–	–	–	An experimentally-enhanced presence conferred resilience to the interpersonal adversity ("perceived burdensomeness" or "thwarted belongingness") implicated in suicide risk

(A)

Clinical Populations ($n = 2$)									
Author(s)	**Study Design**	**Sample**			**Instrument Assessing MiL**	**SB-Related Variables**			
		Population	**Size (*N*)**	**Psychiatric Diagnosis**		**SI**	**SA**	**Completed Suicide**	**Other SB-Related Variables and/or Main Commentaries**
Sinclair et al., 2016 [58]	Cross-sectional	Military personnel and veterans	393	Elevated PTSD and depression	MLQ	–	–	–	Mediation model: The presence of MiL, but not search for MiL negatively mediated the relationship between PTSD or depression and the trajectory from SI to SA
Lu et al., 2018 [59]	Longitudinal prospective	HIV-positive patients	113	–	MLQ	↓ for presence of MiL, NS search for MiL	NS for presence of MiL; NS for search for MiL	–	Moderation model: The presence of MiL buffered the relationship between depressive symptoms and SI (no moderating effect between depressive symptoms and SA)

(B)

Note: MiL = Meaning in life; SB = suicidal behavior; SI = suicidal ideation; SA = suicide attempt; MLQ = Meaning in Life Questionnaire; PTSD = post-traumatic stress disorder; NS = not significant.

3.3. *Quality Assessments*

Based on our quality scoring system, the mean score of the included studies was 7.2. Most ($n = 16$) were of moderate quality, followed by those of low quality ($n = 14$) and those of good quality ($n = 7$).

3.4. *Primary Findings*

3.4.1. Studies of Associations between MiL and SB-Related Variables

The primary findings of the included studies that aimed to elucidate associations between MiL and SB-related variables are shown in Table 1. In these studies, MiL was assessed using either the Purpose in Life test [60] or its 10-item shortened version [61], the Geriatric Suicide Ideation Scale, the Perceived MiL subscale [62], the Experienced Meaning in Life instrument [63], the Life Regard Index [64,65], the Sense of Coherence Scale [66], the Crisis of Meaning Scale [67], the Meaningful Life Measure [68], the Spiritual Well-Being Scale (including the Existential Well-Being subscale and the Religious Well-Being subscale [69]), and qualitative analysis. Steger's Meaning in Life Questionnaire (MLQ) and its three-item shortened version [70] were also utilized, but without separate measures for the presence of, and search for, constructs.

Most studies investigated the impact of MiL on SI, and an inverse association was reported as direct [22,27,29,34,36,39,41–43,45,48,50,53] and/or through mediation and moderation models. MiL was found to mediate the relationships between SI and a variety of factors: stress/coping (via an inverse effect on depression) [1], "Reason for Living" [35], psychological strain [40], and satisfaction in life [43]. It was also found to mediate the relationship of both SI and hopelessness with PTSD severity [54]. Additionally, MiL was found to moderate associations between SI and depression [43] and between risk factors for suicide and hopelessness [19,49]. Both the mediation and moderation effects of MiL was found for gratitude and grit, which were shown to work synergistically to enhance MiL and confer resiliency to suicide by increasing MiL [31]. In bullying, a mediation model was reported in the female population, in which MiL explained how victimization can lead to SI, while a moderation model was reported in the male population, in which MiL attenuated the victimization effect on SI [32].

An inverse association between MiL and SA has been found in many studies [20,27,39,52]. Similar to the findings with SI, MiL was found to mediate the relationship between SA and stress/coping (via an inverse effect on depression) [1]. However, a moderation model was not described.

Only 1 study showed an inverse association between MiL and completed suicides. This result was based on two large cohorts of the general population [30]. The association remained significant after controlling for a common mental disorder that emerged during the survey. Unfortunately, only a published abstract was available for this study.

Inverse associations were also reported between MiL and suicidal tendency or suicidal potential (a measure accounting for depression, anxiety, and emotional state) [33,36,38] and between MiL and suicide risk (taking into account general suicide risk factors) [46].

Mental pain was inversely related to MiL [28] (study 2). Two variables of the Interpersonal-Psychology Theory of Suicide (IPTS) [71,72] were explored in relation to MiL. "Perceived burdensomeness" could contribute to suicide morbidity and mortality by eroding MiL [44], and "thwarted belongingness" was associated with more lethal methods for SA and increased SA [47]. Although not formally related to the IPTS, two additional context-relational variables were tied to meaninglessness in the SI experience: aloneness [45] and missing (or perceived missing) connectedness [42]. MiL, but neither religiosity [41] nor religious well-being [53,54], acted as protective factors against SI [41,53] and mediated the relationship between PTSD severity and both hopelessness and SI [54].

3.4.2. Studies of Associations between the Presence of MiL and the Search for MiL and SB-Related Variables

The primary findings of the included studies that aimed to elucidate associations between the presence of MiL and the search for MiL and SB-related variables are shown in Table 2. These two constructs of MiL were assessed using Steger's MLQ, which consists of a self-reported 10-item inventory measuring the extent to which individuals feel their lives are meaningful (the presence of MiL, five items) and the extent to which they are actively seeking meaning (the search for MiL, five items) [70].

Presence of MiL

The presence of MiL predicted decreased SI over time and lowered the lifetime odds of SA among undergraduate students in the longitudinal prospective analyses (with an average follow-up of 2 months) and cross-sectional analyses, respectively, from the same study [55]. These findings remained significant above and beyond the effects of low levels of psychopathology (depression and anxiety symptoms) and high levels of protective factors (gratitude and social support) [55]. In a study examining the factors related to changes in suicide risk among soldiers returning from deployment in Iraq and Afghanistan, surveyed 6 and 12 months following their return, the negative association between the presence of MiL and suicide risk became greater, but this finding was not statistically significant [56]. In this study, suicide risk was assessed using the Suicide Behavior Questionnaire-Revised, which includes four dimensions of SI and SB (lifetime SI and/or SA, frequency of SI over the past 12 months, the threat of SA, and self-reported likelihood of SB in the future) [73]. Among military personnel and veterans with severe PTSD and depression, the presence of MiL negatively mediated the relationship between PTSD or depression and the trajectory leading from the emergence of SI to SA [58]. The presence of MiL was found to moderate the association between depressive symptoms and SI but not the association between depressive symptoms and SA in HIV-positive patients 6 to 12 months following diagnosis [59]. Data for completed suicides were not available.

The presence of MiL mediated the relationships between MiL and the IPTS variables of "perceived burdensomeness" and "thwarted belongingness" and SI [55]. Additionally, the experimentally enhanced presence of MiL conferred resilience to perceived "burdensomeness and "thwarted belongingness" [57]. Both studies were performed using undergraduate students [55,57].

Search for MiL

The search for MiL predicted a decreased SI over time, but with a lower threshold for statistical significance than the presence of MiL, and it did not predict the lifetime odds of SA among undergraduate students [55]. In particular, the search for MiL was shown to predict post-deployment suicide risk, which increased among soldiers returning from deployment in Iraq and Afghanistan based on surveys administered 6 and 12 months following their return [56]. The strength of the association between initial depressive symptoms and becoming a high post-deployment suicide risk was diminished after accounting for the search for MiL. The search for MiL did not negatively mediate the relationship between PTSD or depression and the trajectory from SI to SA among military personnel and veterans [58]. Data for completed suicides were not available.

The search for MiL did not mediate the relationships between MiL and "perceived burdensomeness" or "thwarted belongingness" and SI [55], and it was not investigated in experimentally-enhanced conditions of interpersonal adversity [57] among undergraduate students [55,57].

4. Discussions

With this review, we have aimed to investigate the associations between MiL and SB, including SI, SA, and completed suicide. These associations have been examined in studies that considered MiL and those that distinguished the two MiL constructs (the presence of MiL and the search for MiL), according to Steger's model. We placed a particular focus on the latter.

The included studies consensually showed the protective impact of MiL on SI, SA, and completed suicide, whether conducted using clinical or non-clinical populations. In studies distinguishing the two MiL constructs (the presence of MiL and the search for MiL), a unanimous protective impact on SB-related variables was described only for the former. Correlations between the latter and SB-related variables were less consistent but were globally oriented towards a non-protective impact.

However, comparisons within the first group of studies are limited by an important heterogeneity in the neuropsychological assessment of MiL (Purpose in Life test, Geriatric Suicide Ideation Scale, Perceived MiL subscale, Experienced Meaning in Life instrument, Life Regard Index, Sense of Coherence Scale, Crisis of Meaning Scale, Meaningful Life Measure, Spiritual Well-Being Scale, and MLQ), presupposing different MiL conceptualizations that can overlap but cannot be considered synonymous [3,5,6]. By contrast, only one instrument, the MLQ [70], was utilized in the second group of studies, implying a more uniform MiL conceptualization upstream that includes the distinction between the presence of MiL and search for MiL.

Non-unanimous findings of the role of the search for MiL in SB reflect the debate surrounding the role of search for MiL in other functional aspects of individuals. In their longitudinal analysis of undergraduate students, Kleiman and Beaver [55] found that both the presence of MiL and the search for MiL predicted decreased SI over time, even if the statistical effect of the search for MiL was more marginal. Their cross-sectional analysis at baseline revealed, instead, that only the presence of MiL was associated with lower lifetime odds of SA. They argued that the search for MiL can only act as a protective factor against less severe manifestations of suicidality, which they supposed to be SI compared to SA. Their findings were especially interesting because the presence of MiL was shown to confer suicide resiliency independent of low levels of risk factors, such as psychopathology (depression and anxiety symptoms), and protective factors (gratitude and social support). However, they recognized a number of study limitations, which included the use of a non-clinical population, a large majority of female representatives in their sample, self-reporting of anxiety and depression symptoms, and a relatively small number of participants with a SA history, leading to an underpowered analysis based on SA [55].

The two studies performed using military personnel and veterans concluded only partially concordant findings on the beneficial versus deleterious impacts of the presence of MiL and search for MiL. Kim and colleagues [56] surveyed the suicide risk among soldiers returning from Iraq and Afghanistan twice during their first year post-deployment, observing that suicide risk increased significantly between the 6th and 12th months. Greater levels of search for MiL and perceived stress were associated with becoming a high suicide risk. The strength of the association between initial depressive symptoms and suicide risk was attenuated after accounting for these measures. On the other hand, they found a consistent negative association between the presence of MiL and becoming a high suicide risk post-deployment, but this relationship was not statistically significant [56]. The primary finding made by Sinclair and colleagues [58] in a study of military personnel and veterans with elevated levels of PTSD and depression was that the presence of MiL negatively mediated the relationship between PTSD or depression and the trajectory from SI to SA, particularly during acute experiences of mood disturbances. They estimated that this mediation was crucial for explaining why some military personnel and veterans do not become suicidal despite the correlation between their clinical conditions (PTSD/depression) and suicide risk. Contrary to their expectations, they found that search for MiL did not show the same mediation effect, suggesting that the active pursuit of MiL is not central to the trajectory from SI to SA [58].

In a clinical non-psychiatric cohort of HIV-positive patients surveyed 6 and 12 months after diagnosis (a population at high risk for both SI and SA), Lu and colleagues [59] reported that depressive symptoms were the primary predictors of changes in both SI and SA. Among the examined psychosocial factors, they found that only the presence of MiL buffered the relationship between depressive symptoms and SI. Neither the presence of MiL nor search for MiL showed a similar moderating effect on the relationship between depressive symptoms and SA [59].

Finally, Kleiman and Beaver [55] and Collins and colleagues [57] described the protective effect of the presence of MiL (but not the search for MiL) deployed on SI through two IPTS variables ("perceived burdensomeness" and "thwarted belongingness") described by Joiner and colleagues [71,72], in two cohorts of undergraduate students. According to IPTS, "perceived burdensomeness" and "thwarted belongingness" combine to produce SI [71,72]. The findings in the student samples mentioned above [55,57] were valorized because they potentially offered an additional way to explain and weaken the SI risk conferred by interpersonal adversities. However, both constructs were assessed in the former study [55], but only the presence of MiL was investigated (and manipulated in experimental conditions) in the latter study [57]. Inspired by IPTS, which marked a crucial turning point in suicide theories by distinguishing the emergence of SI from the progression from SI to SA (mediated in this case by the coexistence of a third variable, the "acquired suicidal capability"), another "Ideation-to Action" framework was proposed by Klonsky and May: the Three-Step Theory of Suicide (3ST) [74]. This framework posits that SI first results from the combination of pain (usually psychological pain) and hopelessness. Second, among those experiencing both these conditions, connectedness is a key protective factor against SI escalation. Third, the progression from SI to SA is facilitated by dispositional, acquired, and practical contributors to the capacity to make SA [74]. In the theories of Joiners and colleagues and Klonsky and May, connectedness represents an essential resource and a fundamental step in the passage from suicidal ideation to suicidal action. As previously noted [20], connectedness can be considered similar to MiL in its reference to one's attachment to a work, to a role, or to shared projects and interests that keep one invested in living. Thus, their negative predictions for the role of SI could also be conceptually linked.

Taken together, these findings show that exploring the presence of MiL and the search for MiL contribute to refining the SB risk assessment. By widening the boundaries of diagnostic interviews to these two constructs, new entry points to SI could possibly be determined in both clinical and non-clinical populations [55], but particularly in populations that (1) can have silent/occult SI and (2) can abruptly experience out-of-the-ordinary experiences (e.g., veterans) [22].

Moreover, the presence of MiL and the search for MiL could constitute a useful target for psychotherapeutic interventions designed to decrease SB risk. These two constructs can be dealt with from different perspectives. Therapeutic modalities were initially systematized according to the classical assumptions of the existential–humanistic Logotherapy of Viktor E. Frankl [75]. Subsequently, Meaning-Centered Counseling, consisting of a cognitive-behavioral reformulation of Logotherapy [76], and Meaning-Centered Counseling and Therapy, consisting of an eclectic model that integrates different theories with MiL as its central and unifying theme [77], were proposed. Finally, a program aimed at achieving meaningful personal goals has been described [21], which, in patients with a borderline personality disorder, could be articulated with Dialectical Behavioral Therapy [20,49]. Although not specifically, the first three models [75–77] address both constructs, while the last model [20,21,49] is more focused on the presence of the Mil construct. Considering all these previous, precious, contributions (and after we have acquired more knowledge on the dynamic interplay of the two constructs), a specific approach for both the presence of Mil and the search for MiL could provide a promising psychotherapeutic area of study.

5. Limitations

This review has several limitations. First, it is based on studies of various natures. In qualitative and retrospective studies, clinical variables are not always readily available. Second, the studies investigated very heterogeneous populations. Some were conducted using non-clinical individuals of various ages and socio-professional conditions, while others used clinical populations with various psychiatric diagnoses, who were either outpatients or inpatients. Some studies also considered mixed samples of patients belonging to different age groups with various psychiatric diagnoses and in various stages of a given disorder. Third, these studies used varied instruments to examine the possible links between SB and the constructs in question. Furthermore, the SB risk was sometimes evaluated using differing methods. Given these factors, the data were often difficult to make generalizable.

We did not carry out a meta-analysis because the data from most of these studies did not permit such an approach. The studies used different measures and had differing outcomes, assessed patients at differing time points, and had several methodological problems, which often made the results difficult to interpret. Moreover, most of the studies considered nonhomogeneous samples, analyzed only a few variables, and did not include a control group. Finally, there are a limited number of articles in the literature concerning the topic of this review, particularly when distinguishing between the presence of MiL and the search for MiL.

6. Conclusions

In conclusion, considering the important limitations stated, MiL nonetheless emerges as a protective factor against suicidality. This has been demonstrated particularly for the MiL construct presence of MiL on SI and its inclusion among non-clinical psychiatric populations. These findings have clinical repercussions on SB prevention in both SB assessment and psychotherapeutic interventions. However, further research is needed to confirm the role of the presence of MiL and to clarify its interplay with the search for MiL, particularly in (1) clinical psychiatric populations (to possibly quantify their impacts on SB risk despite clinical conditions), (2) longitudinally designed cohorts, and (3) studies addressing SAs.

Author Contributions: A.C. drafted the primary manuscript, contributed to the conceptualization of the study, and participated to study selection/data collection; M.P. (Massimo Prelati) corrected/reviewed the manuscript, contributed to the conceptualization of the study, and participated to study selection/data collection; M.P. (Maurizio Pompili) corrected/reviewed the manuscript, conceptualized the study, supervised the work, and provided the intellectual impetus. All authors approved the final manuscript.

Acknowledgments: The authors are grateful to A. Canuto, M. Baertschi, and K. Weber.

References

1. Wang, M.C.; Richard Lightsey, O.; Pietruszka, T.; Uruk, A.C.; Wells, A.G. Purpose in life and reasons for living as mediators of the relationship between stress, coping, and suicidal behavior. *J. Posit. Psychol.* **2007**, *2*, 195–204. [CrossRef]
2. Frankl, V.E. *Man's Search for Meaning. From Death Camp to Existentialism*, 1st ed.; Beacon Press: New York, NY, USA, 1959.
3. Reker, G.T. Theoretical perspective, dimensions, and measurement of existential meaning. In *Exploring Existential Meaning: Optimizing Human Development Across the Life Span*; Recker, G.T., Chamberlain, K., Eds.; SAGE Publications Inc.: New York, NY, USA, 2000; pp. 39–55.
4. Park, C.L. Making sense of the meaning literature: An integrative review of meaning making and its effects on adjustment to stressful life events. *Psychol. Bull.* **2010**, *136*, 257–301. [CrossRef] [PubMed]
5. Wong, P.T.P. Introduction: A roadmap for meaning research and applications. In *The Human Quest for Meaning: Theories, Research, and Applications*; Wong, P., Ed.; Routledge, Taylor Francis Group: New York, NY, USA, London, UK 2012; pp. xxvii–xliv.
6. Glaw, X.; Kable, A.; Hazelton, M.; Inder, K. Meaning in life and meaning of life in mental health care: An integrative literature review. *Issues Ment. Health Nurs.* **2017**, *38*, 243–252. [CrossRef] [PubMed]
7. Martela, F.; Steger, M.F. The three meanings of meaning in life: Distinguishing coherence, purpose, and significance. *J. Posit. Psychol.* **2016**, *11*, 531–545. [CrossRef]
8. Steger, M.F. Experiencing meaning in life: Optimal functioning at the nexus of well-being, psychopathology, and spirituality. In *The Human Quest for Meaning: Theories, Research, and Applications*; Wong, P.T.P., Ed.; Routledge, Taylor Francis Group: New York, NY, USA; London, UK, 2012; pp. 165–184.

9. Steger, M. Meaning in life. In *The Oxford Handbook of Positive Psychology*; Lopez, S., Snyder, C., Eds.; Oxford University Press: Oxford, UK, 2009; pp. 679–688.
10. Steger, M.F.; Oishi, S.; Kesebir, S. Is a life without meaning satisfying? The moderating role of the search for meaning in satisfaction with life judgments. *J. Posit. Psychol.* **2011**, *6*, 173–180. [CrossRef]
11. Steger, M.; Kashdan, T. Search for meaning in life. In *Encyclopedia of Social Psychology*; Baumeister, R., Vohs, K., Eds.; Sage Publications: Thousand Oaks, CA, USA, 2007; pp. 783–785.
12. Frankl, V.E.; Crumbaugh, J.C.; Gerz, H.O.; Maholick, L.T. *Psychotherapy and Existentialism: Selected Papers on Logotherapy*; Simon and Schuster: New York, NY, USA, 1967; pp. 71–75.
13. Maddi, S.R. The search for meaning. In *Nebraska Symposium on Motivation*; Page, M., Ed.; University of Nebraska Press: Lincoln, NE, USA, 1970; pp. 137–186.
14. Baumeister, R.F. *Meanings of Life*; Guilford Press: New York, NY, USA, 1991.
15. Klinger, E. The search for meaning in evolutionary perspective and its clinical implications. In *The Human Quest for Meaning: A Handbook of Psychological Research and Clinical Application*; Wong, P.T.P., Fry, P.S., Eds.; Lawrence Erlbaum Associates: Mahwah, NJ, USA, 1998; pp. 25–70.
16. Steger, M.F.; Kashdan, T.B.; Sullivan, B.A.; Lorentz, D. Understanding the search for meaning in life: Personality, cognitive style, and the dynamic between seeking and experiencing meaning. *J. Pers.* **2008**, *76*, 199–228. [CrossRef]
17. Dezutter, J.; Casalin, S.; Wachholtz, A.; Luyckx, K.; Hekking, J.; Vandewiele, W. Meaning in life: An important factor for the psychological well-being of chronically ill patients? *Rehabil. Psychol.* **2013**, *58*, 334–341. [CrossRef]
18. Dezutter, J.; Luyckx, K.; Wachholtz, A. Meaning in life in chronic pain patients over time: Associations with pain experience and psychological well-being. *J. Behav. Med.* **2015**, *38*, 384–396. [CrossRef]
19. Marco, J.H.; Pérez, S.; García-Alandete, J. Meaning in life buffers the association between risk factors for suicide and hopelessness in participants with mental disorders. *J. Clin. Psychol.* **2016**, *72*, 689–700. [CrossRef]
20. Marco, J.H.; Pérez, S.; García-Alandete, J.; Moliner, R. Meaning in life in people with borderline personality disorder. *Clin. Psychol. Psychother.* **2017**, *24*, 162–170. [CrossRef]
21. Lapierre, S.; Dubé, M.; Bouffard, L.; Alain, M. Addressing suicidal ideations through the realization of meaningful personal goals. *Crisis* **2007**, *28*, 16–25. [CrossRef] [PubMed]
22. Denneson, L.M.; Teo, A.R.; Ganzini, L.; Helmer, D.A.; Bair, M.J.; Dobscha, S.K. Military veterans' experiences with suicidal ideation: Implications for intervention and prevention. *Suicide Life Threat. Behav.* **2015**, *45*, 399–414. [CrossRef] [PubMed]
23. Moher, D.; Liberati, A.; Tetzlaff, J.; Altman, D.G. Preferred Reporting Items for Systematic Reviews and Meta-Analyses: The PRISMA statement. *BMJ* **2009**, *339*, b2535. [CrossRef] [PubMed]
24. Higgins, J.P.T.; Green, S. *Cochrane Handbook for Systematic Reviews of Interventions Version 5.1.0 [Updated March 2011]*; The Cochrane Collaboration: London, UK, 2014.
25. Serafini, G.; Muzio, C.; Piccinini, G.; Flouri, E.; Ferrigno, G.; Pompili, M.; Girardi, P.; Amore, M. Life adversities and suicidal behavior in young individuals: A systematic review. *Eur. Child Adolesc. Psychiatry* **2015**, *24*, 1423–1446. [CrossRef] [PubMed]
26. Serafini, G.; Calcagno, P.; Lester, D.; Girardi, P.; Amore, M.; Pompili, M. Suicide risk in Alzheimer's disease: A systematic review. *Curr. Alzheimer Res.* **2016**, *13*, 1083–1099. [CrossRef]
27. Edwards, M.J.; Holden, R.R. Coping, meaning in life, and suicidal manifestations: Examining gender differences. *J. Clin. Psychol.* **2001**, *57*, 1517–1534. [CrossRef] [PubMed]
28. Orbach, I.; Mikulincer, M.; Gilboa-Schechtman, E.; Sirota, P. Mental pain and its relationship to suicidality and life meaning. *Suicide Life Threat. Behav.* **2003**, *33*, 231–241. [CrossRef]
29. Heisel, M.J.; Flett, G.L. Psychological resilience to suicide ideation among older adults. *Clin. Gerontol.* **2008**, *31*, 51–70. [CrossRef]
30. Bjerkeset, O.; Nordahl, H.M.; Romundstad, P.R.; Gunnell, D. PW01-253-personality traits, self-esteem and sense of meaning in life as predictors for suicide: The Norwegian HUNT cohort. *Eur. Psychiatry* **2010**, *25*, 1681. [CrossRef]
31. Kleiman, E.M.; Adams, L.M.; Kashdan, T.B.; Riskind, J.H. Gratitude and grit indirectly reduce risk of suicidal ideations by enhancing meaning in life: Evidence for a mediated moderation model. *J. Res. Personal.* **2013**, *47*, 539–546. [CrossRef]

32. Henry, K.L.; Lovegrove, P.J.; Steger, M.F.; Chen, P.Y.; Cigularov, K.P.; Tomazic, R.G. The potential role of meaning in life in the relationship between bullying victimization and suicidal ideation. *J. Youth Adolesc.* **2014**, *43*, 221–232. [CrossRef] [PubMed]
33. Wilchek-Aviad, Y. Meaning in life and suicidal tendency among immigrant (Ethiopian) youth and native-born Israeli youth. *J. Immigr. Minor. Health* **2015**, *17*, 1041–1048. [CrossRef] [PubMed]
34. Heisel, M.J.; Flett, G.L. Does recognition of meaning in life confer resiliency to suicide ideation among community-residing older adults? A longitudinal investigation. *Am. J. Geriatr. Psychiatry* **2016**, *24*, 455–466. [CrossRef] [PubMed]
35. Heisel, M.J.; Neufeld, E.; Flett, G.L. Reasons for living, meaning in life, and suicide ideation: Investigating the roles of key positive psychological factors in reducing suicide risk in community-residing older adults. *Aging Ment. Health* **2016**, *20*, 195–207. [CrossRef] [PubMed]
36. Wilchek-Aviad, Y.; Malka, M. Religiosity, meaning in life and suicidal tendency among Jews. *J. Relig. Health* **2016**, *55*, 480–494. [CrossRef] [PubMed]
37. Wilchek-Aviad, Y.; Ne'eman-Haviv, V.; Malka, M. Connection between suicidal ideation, life meaning, and leisure time activities. *Deviant Behav.* **2017**, *38*, 621–632. [CrossRef]
38. Wilchek-Aviad, Y.; Ne'eman-Haviv, V. The relation between a sense of meaning in life and suicide potential among disadvantaged adolescent girls. *Int. J. Offender Ther. Comp. Criminol.* **2018**, *62*, 1474–1487. [CrossRef] [PubMed]
39. Schnell, T.; Gerstner, R.; Krampe, H. Crisis of meaning predicts suicidality in youth independently of depression. *Crisis* **2018**, *39*, 294–303. [CrossRef] [PubMed]
40. Liu, Y.; Usman, M.; Zhang, J.; Gul, H. Making sense of Chinese employees' suicidal ideation: A psychological strain—Life Meaning Model. *Psychol. Rep.* **2018**. [CrossRef]
41. Testoni, I.; Russotto, S.; Zamperini, A.; De Leo, D. Addiction and religiosity in facing suicide: A qualitative study on meaning of life and death among homeless people. *Ment. Illn.* **2018**, *10*, 16–24. [CrossRef] [PubMed]
42. Moore, S.L. A phenomenological study of meaning in life in suicidal older adults. *Arch. Psychiatr. Nurs.* **1997**, *11*, 29–36. [CrossRef]
43. Heisel, M.J.; Flett, G.L. Purpose in life, satisfaction with life, and suicide ideation in a clinical sample. *J. Psychopathol. Behav. Assess.* **2004**, *26*, 127–135. [CrossRef]
44. Van Orden, K.A.; Bamonti, P.M.; King, D.A.; Duberstein, P.R. Does perceived burdensomeness erode meaning in life among older adults? *Aging Ment. Health* **2012**, *16*, 855–860. [CrossRef] [PubMed]
45. Holm, A.L.; Lyberg, A.; Berggren, I.; Åström, S.; Severinsson, E. Going around in a circle: A Norwegian study of suicidal experiences in old age. *Nurs. Res. Pract.* **2014**, *2014*, 734635. [CrossRef] [PubMed]
46. García-Alandete, J.; Salvador, M.; José, H.; Pérez Rodríguez, S. Predicting role of the meaning in life on depression, hopelessness, and suicide risk among borderline personality disorder patients. *Univ. Psychol.* **2014**, *13*, 1545–1555. [CrossRef]
47. Van Orden, K.A.; Wiktorsson, S.; Duberstein, P.; Berg, A.I.; Fässberg, M.M.; Waern, M. Reasons for attempted suicide in later life. *Am. J. Geriatr. Psychiatry* **2015**, *23*, 536–544. [CrossRef]
48. Braden, A.; Overholser, J.; Fisher, L.; Ridley, J. Life meaning is associated with suicidal ideation among depressed veterans. *Death Stud.* **2015**, *39*, 24–29. [CrossRef]
49. Marco, J.H.; Guillén, V.; Botella, C. The buffer role of meaning in life in hopelessness in women with borderline personality disorders. *Psychiatry Res.* **2017**, *247*, 120–124. [CrossRef]
50. Marco, J.H.; Cañabate, M.; Pérez, S.; Llorca, G. Associations among meaning in life, body image, psychopathology, and suicide ideation in Spanish participants with eating disorders. *J. Clin. Psychol.* **2017**, *73*, 1768–1781. [CrossRef]
51. Perez Rodriguez, S.; Marco Salvador, J.H.; García-Alandete, J. The role of hopelessness and meaning in life in a clinical sample with non-suicidal self-injury and suicide attempts. *Psicothema* **2017**, *29*, 323–328.
52. Pérez, S.; Marco, J.H.; García-Alandete, J. Psychopathological differences between suicide ideators and suicide attempters in patients with mental disorders. *Clin. Psychol. Psychother.* **2017**, *24*, 1002–1013. [CrossRef]
53. Lamis, D.A.; Kapoor, S.; Evans, A.P. Childhood sexual abuse and suicidal ideation among bipolar patients: Existential but not religious well-being as a protective factor. *Suicide Life Threat. Behav.* **2018**, *49*, 401–412. [CrossRef]
54. Florez, I.A.; Allbaugh, L.J.; Harris, C.E.; Schwartz, A.C,; Kaslow, N.J. Suicidal ideation and hopelessness in PTSD: Spiritual well-being mediates outcomes over time. *Anxiety Stress Coping* **2018**, *31*, 46–58. [CrossRef]

55. Kleiman, E.M.; Beaver, J.K. A meaningful life is worth living: Meaning in life as a suicide resiliency factor. *Psychiatry Res.* **2013**, *210*, 934–939. [CrossRef]
56. Kim, H.M.; Levine, D.S.; Pfeiffer, P.N.; Blow, A.J.; Marchiondo, C.; Walters, H.; Valenstein, M. Postdeployment suicide risk increases over a 6-month period: Predictors of increased risk among Midwestern Army National Guard soldiers. *Suicide Life Threat. Behav.* **2017**, *47*, 421–435. [CrossRef]
57. Collins, K.R.; Legendre, M.N.; Stritzke, W.G.; Page, A.C. Experimentally-enhanced perceptions of meaning confer resilience to the interpersonal adversity implicated in suicide risk. *J. Behav. Ther. Exp. Psychiatry* **2018**, *61*, 142–149. [CrossRef]
58. Sinclair, S.; Bryan, C.J.; Bryan, A.O. Meaning in life as a protective factor for the emergence of suicide ideation that leads to suicide attempts among military personnel and veterans with elevated PTSD and depression. *Int. J. Cogn. Ther.* **2016**, *9*, 87–98. [CrossRef]
59. Lu, H.F.; Sheng, W.H.; Liao, S.C.; Chang, N.T.; Wu, P.Y.; Yang, Y.L.; Hsiao, F.H. The changes and the predictors of suicide ideation and suicide attempt among HIV-positive patients at 6–12 months post diagnosis: A longitudinal study. *J. Adv. Nurs.* **2018**, *75*, 573–584. [CrossRef]
60. Crumbaugh, J.C.; Maholick, L.T. *Manual of Instructions for the Purpose-in-Life Test*; Viktor Frankl Institute of Logotherapy: Saratoga, CA, USA, 1969.
61. García-Alandete, J.; Martínez, E.R.; Nohales, P.S. Estructura Factorial y Consistencia Interna de una Versión Española del Purpose-In-Life Test [Factorial Structure and Internal Consistency of a Spanish Version of the Purpose in Life Test]. *Univ. Psychol.* **2013**, *12*, 517–530. [CrossRef]
62. Heisel, M.J.; Flett, G.L. The development and initial validation of the Geriatric Suicide Ideation Scale. *Am. J. Geriatr. Psychiatry* **2006**, *14*, 742–751. [CrossRef]
63. Heisel, M.J. Assessing experienced meaning in life among older adults: The development and initial validation of the EMIL. *Int. Psychogeriatr.* **2009**, *21*, S172–S173.
64. Batista, J.; Almond, R. The development of meaning in life. *Psychiatry* **1973**, *36*, 409–427. [CrossRef]
65. Debats, D.L. Measurement of Personal Meaning: The Psychometric Properties of the Life Regard Index. In *The Human Quest for Meaning: A Handbook of Psychological Research and Clinical Applications*; Wong, P.T.P., Fry, P.S., Eds.; Lawrence Erlbaum Associates Publishers: Mahwah, NJ, USA, 1998; pp. 237–259.
66. Antonovsky, A. The structure and properties of the sense of coherence scale. *Soc. Sci. Med.* **1993**, *36*, 725–733. [CrossRef]
67. Schnell, T. The Sources of Meaning and Meaning in Life Questionnaire (SoMe): Relations to demographics and well-being. *J. Posit. Psychol.* **2009**, *4*, 483–499. [CrossRef]
68. Morgan, J.; Farsides, T. Measuring meaning in life. *J. Happiness Stud.* **2009**, *10*, 197–214. [CrossRef]
69. Ellison, C.W. Spiritual well-being: Conceptualization and measurement. *J. Psychol. Theol.* **1983**, *11*, 330–338. [CrossRef]
70. Steger, M.F.; Frazier, P.; Oishi, S.; Kaler, M. The meaning in life questionnaire: Assessing the presence of and search for meaning in life. *J. Couns. Psychol.* **2006**, *53*, 80–93. [CrossRef]
71. Joiner, T.E. *Why People Die by Suicide*; Harvard University Press: Cambridge, MA, USA, 2005.
72. Van Orden, K.A.; Witte, T.K.; Cukrowicz, K.C.; Braithwaite, S.R.; Selby, E.A.; Joiner, T.E., Jr. The interpersonal theory of suicide. *Psychol. Rev.* **2010**, *117*, 575–600. [CrossRef]
73. Osman, A.; Bagge, C.L.; Gutierrez, P.M.; Konick, L.C.; Kopper, B.A.; Barrios, F.X. The Suicidal Behaviors Questionnaire-Revised (SBQ-R): Validation with clinical and nonclinical samples. *Assessment* **2001**, *8*, 443–454. [CrossRef]
74. Klonsky, D.E.; May, A.M. The Three-Step Theory (3ST): A New Theory of Suicide Rooted in the "Ideation-to-Action" Framework. *Int. J. Cogn. Ther.* **2015**, *8*, 114–129. [CrossRef]
75. Frankl, V.E. *The Will to Meaning: Foundations and Applications of Logotherapy*; New American Library: New York, NY, USA, 1988.
76. Wong, P.T.P. Meaning-centered counseling: A cognitive-behavioral approach to Logotherapy. *Int. Forum Logother.* **1997**, *20*, 85–94.
77. Wong, P.T.P. Towards an integrative model of meaning-centered counseling and therapy. *Int. Forum Logother.* **1998**, *22*, 47–55.

Permissions

All chapters in this book were first published by MDPI; hereby published with permission under the Creative Commons Attribution License or equivalent. Every chapter published in this book has been scrutinized by our experts. Their significance has been extensively debated. The topics covered herein carry significant findings which will fuel the growth of the discipline. They may even be implemented as practical applications or may be referred to as a beginning point for another development.

The contributors of this book come from diverse backgrounds, making this book a truly international effort. This book will bring forth new frontiers with its revolutionizing research information and detailed analysis of the nascent developments around the world.

We would like to thank all the contributing authors for lending their expertise to make the book truly unique. They have played a crucial role in the development of this book. Without their invaluable contributions this book wouldn't have been possible. They have made vital efforts to compile up to date information on the varied aspects of this subject to make this book a valuable addition to the collection of many professionals and students.

This book was conceptualized with the vision of imparting up-to-date information and advanced data in this field. To ensure the same, a matchless editorial board was set up. Every individual on the board went through rigorous rounds of assessment to prove their worth. After which they invested a large part of their time researching and compiling the most relevant data for our readers.

The editorial board has been involved in producing this book since its inception. They have spent rigorous hours researching and exploring the diverse topics which have resulted in the successful publishing of this book. They have passed on their knowledge of decades through this book. To expedite this challenging task, the publisher supported the team at every step. A small team of assistant editors was also appointed to further simplify the editing procedure and attain best results for the readers.

Apart from the editorial board, the designing team has also invested a significant amount of their time in understanding the subject and creating the most relevant covers. They scrutinized every image to scout for the most suitable representation of the subject and create an appropriate cover for the book.

The publishing team has been an ardent support to the editorial, designing and production team. Their endless efforts to recruit the best for this project, has resulted in the accomplishment of this book. They are a veteran in the field of academics and their pool of knowledge is as vast as their experience in printing. Their expertise and guidance has proved useful at every step. Their uncompromising quality standards have made this book an exceptional effort. Their encouragement from time to time has been an inspiration for everyone.

The publisher and the editorial board hope that this book will prove to be a valuable piece of knowledge for researchers, students, practitioners and scholars across the globe.

List of Contributors

Carla Gramaglia and Patrizia Zeppegno
Institute of Psychiatry, Università degli Studi del Piemonte Orientale, 28100 Novara, Italy
S.C. Psichiatria, Azienda Ospedaliero Universitaria Maggiore della Carità, 28100 Novara, Italy

Raffaella Calati
Department of Psychology, University of Milano-Bicocca, 20126 Milan, Italy
Nîmes University Hospital, 30029 Nîmes, France

Anita Ribeiro Blanchard
Faculty of Psychology, University of Barcelona, 08035 Barcelona, Spain

William Edgar Comfort
Social and Cognitive Science Laboratory, Centre for Health and Biological Sciences, Mackenzie Presbyterian University, São Paulo 01241, Brazil

Leo Sher and René S. Kahn
James J. Peters Veterans' Administration Medical Center, Bronx, New York, NY 10468, USA
Icahn School of Medicine at Mount Sinai, New York, NY 10029, USA

Mark Schechter
North Shore Medical Center, 81 Highland Avenue, Salem, MA 01970, USA

Elsa Ronningstam, Benjamin Herbstman and Mark J. Goldblatt
Harvard Medical School, 25 Shattuck Street, Boston, MA 02115, USA
McLean Hospital, 115 Mill Street, Belmont, MA 02478, USA

Sabine B.-E. Baumgart
Faculty of Medicine, Institute for Health and Nursing Sciences, Martin Luther University Halle-Wittenberg, 06108 Halle, Germany

Anja Baumbach-Kraft
M.Sc. Public Health, 24105 Kiel, Germany

Juergen Lorenz
Department of Biomedical Engineering, Faculty of Life Science, University of Applied Sciences, 21033 Hamburg, Germany

Marion Rochet and Boriana Atanasova
UMR 1253, iBrain, Université de Tours, Inserm, 37200 Tours, France

Wissam El-Hage
UMR 1253, iBrain, Université de Tours, Inserm, 37200 Tours, France
CHRU de Tours, Clinique Psychiatrique Universitaire, 37044 Tours, France

Sami Richa
Department of Psychiatry, Faculty of Medicine, Saint-Joseph University, 11-5076 Beirut, Lebanon

François Kazour
UMR 1253, iBrain, Université de Tours, Inserm, 37200 Tours, France
Psychiatric Hospital of the Cross, 60096 Jal Eddib, Lebanon

Luca Bonanni, Flavia Gualtieri, Giulia Falcone and Adele Nardella
Psychiatry Residency Training Program, Faculty of Medicine and Psychology, Sapienza University of Rome, 00189 Rome, Italy

David Lester
Psychology Program, Stockton University, Galloway, NJ 08205, USA

Andrea Fiorillo
Department of Psychiatry, University of Campania Luigi Vanvitelli, 80138 Naples, Italy
Department of Psychiatry, University of Campania "L. Vanvitelli", Largo Madonna Delle Grazie, 80139 Naples, Italy

Maurizio Pompili
Department of Neurosciences, Mental Health and Sensory Organs, Suicide Prevention Center, Sant'Andrea Hospital, Sapienza University of Rome, 00189 Rome, Italy

Djamila Bennabi and Emmanuel Haffen
Department of Clinical Psychiatry, CIC-1431 INSERM, CHU de Besançon, EA Neurosciences, University Bourgogne Franche-Comte, FondaMental Foundation, 94000 Creteil, France

Rebecca Boehme
Center for Social and Affective Neuroscience, Linköping University, 58185 Linköping, Sweden
Center for Medical Image Science and Visualization (CMIV), 58185 Linköping, Sweden

Xenia Gonda
Department of Psychiatry and Psychotherapy, Semmelweis University, Faculty of Medicine, 1125 Budapest, Hungary
National Institute of Psychiatry and Addictions, Laboratory for Suicide Research and Prevention, 1135 Budapest, Hungary
MTA-SE Neuropsychopharmacology, Neurochemistry Research Group, Hungarian Academy of Sciences, 1089 Budapest, Hungary
NAP-2-SE New Antidepressant Target Research Group, Hungarian Brain Research Program, Semmelweis University, 1089 Budapest, Hungary

Peter Dome and Zoltan Rihmer
Department of Psychiatry and Psychotherapy, Semmelweis University, Faculty of Medicine, 1125 Budapest, Hungary
National Institute of Psychiatry and Addictions, Laboratory for Suicide Research and Prevention, 1135 Budapest, Hungary

Helene van Ettinger-Veenstra and Björn Gerdle
Center for Medical Image Science and Visualization (CMIV), 58185 Linköping, Sweden
Pain and Rehabilitation Centre, and Department of Health, Medicine and Caring Sciences, Linköping University, 58185 Linköping, Sweden

Håkan Olausson
Center for Social and Affective Neuroscience, Linköping University, 58185 Linköping, Sweden
Center for Medical Image Science and Visualization (CMIV), 58185 Linköping, Sweden
Department of Clinical Neurophysiology, Linköping University, 58185 Linköping, Sweden

Saad S. Nagi
Center for Social and Affective Neuroscience, Linköping University, 58185 Linköping, Sweden
Department of Clinical Neurophysiology, Linköping University, 58185 Linköping, Sweden

Isabella Berardelli and Denise Erbuto
Department of Neurosciences, Mental Health and Sensory Organs, Suicide Prevention Center, Sant'Andrea Hospital, Sapienza University of Rome, 00185 Rome, Italy

Bruno Müller-Oerlinghausen
Charité, Universitätsmedizin Berlin, 10117 Berlin, Germany

Gabriele Cocco
Faculty of Medicine and Psychology, Sapienza University of Rome, 00185 Rome, Italy

Salvatore Sarubbi and Elena Rogante
Department of Psychology, Sapienza University of Rome, 00185 Rome, Italy

Michael Hawkins
Department of Psychiatry, University of Toronto, Toronto, ON M4B 1B4, Canada
Department of Psychiatry, University of Toronto, Toronto, ON M5S, Canada

Norbert Hemrich
Berufsfachschule für Massage am Universitätsklinikum Würzburg, 97080 Würzburg, Germany

Michaela Maria Arnold
Medizinische Fakultät, Julius-Maximilians-Universität Würzburg, 97070 Würzburg, Germany
Berufsfachschule für Massage am Universitätsklinikum Würzburg, 97080 Würzburg, Germany

Dominikus Bönsch
Medizinische Fakultät, Julius-Maximilians-Universität Würzburg, 97070 Würzburg, Germany
Bezirkskrankenhaus für Psychiatrie, Psychotherapie und Psychosomatische Medizin, 97816 Lohr am Main, Germany

Giovanna Fico, Vito Caivano, Francesca Zinno, Marco Carfagno, Gaia Sampogna and Mario Luciano
Department of Psychiatry, University of Campania "L. Vanvitelli", Largo Madonna Delle Grazie, 80139 Naples, Italy

Luca Steardo Jr.
Department of Health Sciences, Psychiatric Unit, University Magna Graecia of Catanzaro, Viale Europa, 88100 Catanzaro CZ, Italy

Joel Paris
Institute of Community and Family Psychiatry, McGill University, 4333 chemin de la cote ste. Catherine, Montreal, QC H3T1E4, Canada

Jérôme Brunelin and Marine Mondino
INSERM, U1028, Lyon Neuroscience Research Center, PSY-R2 team, F-69000 Lyon, France
CNRS, UMR5292, Lyon Neuroscience Research Center, PSY-R2 Team, F-69000 Lyon, France
University Lyon, F-69000 Lyon, France
Centre Hospitalier le Vinatier, F-69678 Bron, France

Ulrich Palm
Department of Psychiatry and Psychotherapy, Klinikum der Universität München, D-80336 Munich, Germany

Rémy Bation and Mohamed Saoud
INSERM, U1028, Lyon Neuroscience Research Center, PSY-R2 team, F-69000 Lyon, France
CNRS, UMR5292, Lyon Neuroscience Research Center, PSY-R2 Team, F-69000 Lyon, France
University Lyon, F-69000 Lyon, France
Centre Hospitalier le Vinatier, F-69678 Bron, France
Psychiatry Unit, Wertheimer Hospital, CHU Lyon, F-69500 Bron, France

Emmanuel Poulet
INSERM, U1028, Lyon Neuroscience Research Center, PSY-R2 team, F-69000 Lyon, France
CNRS, UMR5292, Lyon Neuroscience Research Center, PSY-R2 Team, F-69000 Lyon, France
University Lyon, F-69000 Lyon, France
Centre Hospitalier le Vinatier, F-69678 Bron, France
Psychiatry Emergency Unit, Edouard Herriot Hospital, CHU, F-69000 Lyon, France

Alessandra Costanza
Department of Psychiatry, Faculty of Medicine, University of Geneva (UNIGE), 1206 Geneva, Switzerland

Massimo Prelati
Department of Psychiatry, ASO Santi Antonio e Biagio e Cesare Arrigo Hospital, 15121 Alessandria, Italy

Index

www.ingramcontent.com/pod-product-compliance
Lightning Source LLC
LaVergne TN
LVHW082158200926
848484LV00008B/2180